IMAGING OF ATHLETIC INJURIES

IMAGING OF ATHLETIC INJURIES

A Multimodality Approach

JOSEPH R. MARTIRE, M.D.

*Attending Radiologist, The Union Memorial Hospital
and Sports Medicine Center
Attending Radiologist, The Children's Hospital
and Bennett Institute for Sports Medicine
Consulting Radiologist, The Johns Hopkins University
Division of Sports Medicine and Intercollegiate Athletic Teams
Baltimore, Maryland*

E. MARK LEVINSOHN, M.D., F.A.C.R.

*Professor and Director of Musculoskeletal Radiology
Department of Radiology, SUNY Health Science Center
Attending Radiologist, The Crouse-Irving Memorial Hospital
Syracuse, New York*

McGRAW-HILL, INC.
Health Professions Division

New York   St. Louis   San Francisco   Auckland   Bogotá   Caracas   Lisbon   London   Madrid
Mexico   Milan   Montreal   New Delhi   Paris   San Juan   Singapore   Sydney   Tokyo   Toronto

IMAGING OF ATHLETIC INJURIES

1234567890   HALHAL   987654321

ISBN 0-07-040728-2

This book was set in Times Roman by Ruttle, Shaw & Wetherill, Inc.
The editors were Edward M. Bolger and Muza Navrozov;
the production supervisor was Richard Ruzycka;
the book design and page layout were done by José Fonfrias;
the index was prepared by Tony Greenberg, M.D.
Arcata Graphics/Halliday was printer and binder.

LIBRARY OF CONGRESS CATALOGING-IN-PUBLICATION DATA

Martire, Joseph R.
    Imaging of athletic injuries : a multimodality approach / Joseph R. Martire, E. Mark Levinsohn.
        p.   cm.
    Includes bibliographical references and index.
    ISBN 0-07-040728-2 :
    1. Sports—Accidents and injuries—Imaging.   I. Levinsohn, E. Mark.   II. Title.
    [DNLM: 1. Athletic Injuries—diagnosis.   2. Diagnostic Imaging.
QT 260 M386i]
RD97.M37   1992
617.1'027—dc20
DNLM/DLC
for Library of Congress   91-25470
                                                                    CIP

This book is dedicated to our families:

To our wives—Jeannette Levinsohn and Carol Martire

*To our children—Mary, Robert, Daniel, and Susan Levinsohn
and Andrew Martire*

*Without their constant support and encouragement,
this book could not have been written.
Their understanding and patience
during the many nights and weekends we spent writing this book
are lovingly appreciated.*

CONTENTS

FOREWORD

INTEREST IN PHYSICAL FITNESS through exercise and sports continues to grow not only in the United States but throughout the world, ushering in an unprecedented expansion in the field of sports medicine. For decades, radiography, fluoroscopy, and tomography were the only tools for imaging sites of injury. Then, in the 1970s, computed tomography (CT) and skeletal radionuclide imaging with ^{99m}Tc diphosphonates and the scintillation camera appeared, followed a decade later by magnetic resonance imaging (MRI). All these modalities have markedly altered the investigation of athletic injuries. While this work focuses on the optimal application of the newer imaging modalities, the importance of radiography, including special projection films, is not neglected.

Computed tomography often defines anatomic detail, fracture extent, and other bony abnormalities better than radiographs. MRI best defines lesions in the marrow and surrounding soft tissues, including ligaments, fibrocartilage, menisci, muscles, intervertebral disks, spinal cord, and nerves. The importance of T_1- and T_2-weighted sequences, proton density sequences, and gradient-recalled echo (GRE) sequences is emphasized, particularly for spinal lesions.

The authors stress the importance of three-phase bone scintigraphy with ^{99m}Tc methylene diphosphonate and the scintillation camera—i.e., *phase one,* rapid sequential 1- to 2-second images immediately after injection during the ''first transit'' of radioactivity through the region of interest, to assess relative differences in perfusion between ipsilateral and contralateral limbs or between adjacent vertebra; *phase two,* early images within the first few minutes to assess increases or decreases in ''blood pool,'' and *phase three,* detailed images after 3 to 5 hours, to detect local differences in skeletal concentration. This imaging modality covers large

areas of the body easily, an advantage when multiple injuries are suspected. Imaging of injuries is technically more demanding than is required for certain other lesions. For example, multiple metastases often need not be localized with such anatomic precision as traumatic lesions. Hence, the latter usually require imaging with high-resolution parallel collimators or sometimes pinhole collimation with long exposure times. Radionuclide imaging tends to be more helpful in occult or stress fractures or in assisting localization of acute or chronic pain, when images with other modalities are negative or nearly normal. In addition, negative radionuclide images of known chronic lesions may help to indicate that they are quiescent or healed. In acute fractures, radionuclide images always become positive beyond 48 hours after the injury. The time interval for images to revert to normal with healing fractures varies, but 90 percent do so by 2 years.

About half of all athletic injuries involve the distal extremities, about equally divided between upper and lower extremities. The authors have clearly shown that the relative value of each imaging modality varies in the different regions of the body. In knee injuries, for example, CT is important for demonstrating bony abnormalities and MRI for the many types of soft tissue injury, with the role of radionuclide imaging being relatively minor. On the other hand, for the leg and thigh regions, three-phase skeletal imaging becomes more important for demonstrating occult and stress fractures, shin splints, rhabdomyolysis, and reflex sympathetic dystrophy. Moreover, ultrasound is useful for demonstrating cysts and masses, and duplex Doppler sonography for detecting deep venous thrombosis. For lesions of the foot and ankle, high-resolution thin section CT and MRI are frequently helpful additions to radiography. Radionuclide imaging often reveals focal lesions such as stress fractures of the metatarsals, but more diffusely increased activity is extremely common in asymptomatic active athletes.

In the upper extremities, the authors have found MRI studies important for soft tissue injuries of the shoulder such as rotator cuff tear. Single- or double-contrast arthrography, including CT arthrography, is sometimes required. Radionuclide imaging may best demonstrate arthritis or synovitis. For wrist lesions, MRI again demonstrates ligamentous injuries, and high-resolution CT is often indicated for such lesions as occult carpal fractures. Triple-injection arthrograms may be needed. Radionuclide triple-phase bone imaging may indicate reflex sympathetic dystrophy. As a general principle, a concept expressed in the discussion of wrist injury applies to all regions—i.e., to call an injury a ''sprain'' is no longer an adequate diagnosis. One must seek to define the soft tissue anatomic structure involved and the nature of its injury.

In spinal injuries, CT localization of skeletal lesions and CT myelography as well as MRI are important for demonstrating lesions of the spinal cord, nerve roots, ligaments, disks, and marrow. For lesions of the spine, pelvis, and hips, SPECT has become a valuable adjunct to planar radionuclide imaging for occult hip or pelvic fractures as well as microfractures of the spine and diskitis and osteomyelitis. These lesions are now often detected by SPECT even when planar images are negative or nearly normal. Stress-related increased uptake of the posterior elements of the lower lumbar vertebrae with localized pain and tenderness is frequently found only on SPECT imaging.

Although I have had an interest in skeletal imaging for over two decades, I learned a great deal from reading this book. It is just the right length. It perks your interest, enticing you to delve for more details in the authors' abundant references.

JOHN G. MCAFEE, M.D.
Professor of Radiology
Department of Radiology
Division of Nuclear Medicine
The George Washington University
  Medical Center
Washington, D.C.

PREFACE

THE NEED FOR A BOOK of this type reflects two major developments: the dramatic growth in participation in athletic activities by men and women of all ages since the 1970s and a revolution in imaging capability. The specialty of sports medicine grew out of the need to address the unique problems of the competitive athlete, which include prevention, diagnosis, and treatment of injury. Drawn into this field, along with other medical specialists, were radiologists seeking to combine their expertise in musculoskeletal imaging with their personal interest in sports medicine. Armed with the tools of three-dimensional and magnetic resonance imaging (MRI), computed tomography (CT), and radionuclide triple-phase bone scanning (TPBS), radiologists are able now more than ever before to provide accurate diagnoses even in those frustrating circumstances in which conventional tests are unable to establish a diagnosis.

The highly competitive athlete, reluctant to tolerate inactivity or delay in diagnosis when injured, puts great pressure on the team physician and trainer to expedite diagnosis and treatment. Since the risk of serious reinjury, which may be career- if not life-threatening, exists if athletes inappropriately return to activity, radiologists are in a position to play an increasingly important role in securing the correct diagnosis. Similarly, the appropriate application of advanced imaging techniques to the diagnosis of injuries sustained by the recreational athlete is emphasized.

Advances in sports medicine, including the application of modern tools to the assessment of sports injury, have benefited the entire medical community. A vast number of injured athletes with both common and complex problems provide us with what amounts to a field laboratory for diagnosis and treatment. Our modern understanding of overuse and stress injuries comes from our experience in analyzing these problems in athletes over the last 25 years. The major advances in reconstructive orthopedic bone and joint injury, including tendon and ligament transplant attempts, have grown out of the need to develop newer and better surgical techniques in an effort to return injured athletes to peak performance.

This book, which is organized along anatomic divisions, represents our attempt to demonstrate the usefulness of TPBS, CT, and MRI in helping to diagnose athletic injuries. TPBS has been widely used in assessing orthopedic diseases since the early 1970s. Better than any other imaging modality, it provides a metabolically oriented image depicting dynamic soft tissue and bony events. By assessing the degree and timing of nuclide activity as determined by triple-phase techniques (blood flow, blood pool, and delayed images), this examination becomes a "physiologic scan" which can detect the chronicity and activity of bony abnormalities. A development of the mid- to late 1970s, CT superbly demonstrates bony structure and, to a lesser extent, the intramedullary space and the soft tissues. Some hint of vascularity can be determined from contrast administration with dynamic CT scanning, but the metabolic activity and age of abnormality cannot be determined with the degree of certainty that the TPBS provides for us.

MR imaging blossomed in the middle to late 1980s. More than any other modality, MR provides superb soft tissue contrast allowing the diagnosis of muscular, cartilaginous, ligamentous, and tendinous injuries. Additionally, MR expands our ability to assess the intramedullary space so that such entities as bone contusion and acute avascular necrosis can now be recognized.

In preparing this book, both of us have relied on our extensive experience in utilizing these advanced imaging modalities to diagnose athletic injuries. Each of us has worked closely for nearly two decades with orthopedists and team physicians in the Syracuse and Baltimore areas, and we have drawn from this experience illustrative material which forms the basis of this book.

Each chapter begins with an orthopedic overview written by a prominent orthopedist, who provides a personal approach to the use of modern imaging in securing the diagnosis. An introductory section follows, which discusses the relative strengths and weaknesses of each modality in the area being imaged and summarizes injuries peculiar to the area. Each chapter then deals first with acute and then with chronic problems. Where appropriate, these are supplemented with illustrations and tables. Chapters close with sections on diagnostic problems covering those nonathletic entities which may mimic athletic injuries. These create possible pitfalls if the attending physician is not sensitive to such entities.

This book is not simply an interesting collection of sports medicine cases. It is a combined text and atlas of athletic injuries, emphasizing the appropriate use of the most advanced imaging modalities in demonstrating the appearance of athletic injuries. Both common and unusual clinical entities are presented, including their appearance as demonstrated by TPBS, MRI, and CT. Occasionally, other modalities such as arthrography, sonography, and three-dimensional reconstruction techniques are demonstrated where indicated. The text is abundantly referenced for those readers who wish to explore the topics in greater depth. It is our hope that the organization and presentation of this material will demonstrate for the reader the appropriate use of these advanced imaging techniques in providing greater accuracy in the diagnosis of athletic injuries.

JOSEPH R. MARTIRE, M.D.
E. MARK LEVINSOHN, M.D.

ACKNOWLEDGMENTS

A PROJECT OF THIS SIZE could only be successful with the support of our private practice groups and hospital facilities. In Syracuse, we thank the SUNY Health Science Center and Harrison Center Radiology (affiliated with University Radiology Associates). In Baltimore, we thank The Union Memorial Hospital and the Children's Hospital and Center for Reconstructive Surgery (and their respective sports medicine centers) as well as Drs. Schultze, Snider & Associates, P.A. (with a special thank-you to Robin Tolkoff Levy, group administrator).

We have had the opportunity in both Baltimore and Syracuse to work with many outstanding specialists at the above-named hospitals. We are especially indebted to the seven orthopedic surgeons—Dr. Bruce Baker, Dr. Andy Palmer, and Dr. Hansen Yuan in Syracuse and Dr. Kenneth Gertsen, Dr. John O'Donnell, Dr. Michael Scheerer, and Dr. Charles Silberstein in Baltimore—who greatly added to this book by writing orthopedic overviews for all chapters. Their personal perspective is testimony to the fact that radiologists and sports medicine physicians must communicate and work closely so that diagnostic imaging becomes a successful tool to accurately diagnose difficult athletic injuries.

Special thanks are extended to Dr. Edwin D. Cacayorin (Professor of Radiology and Neurosurgery, Division of Neuroradiology), Dr. Leo Hochhauser (Assistant Professor of Radiology, Division of Neuroradiology), Dr. John J. Wasenko (Assistant Professor of Radiology, Division of Neuroradiology), and Dr. Jeffrey Winfield (Associate Professor of Neurosurgery) of the SUNY Health Science Center at Syracuse for their efforts as contributing authors in Chapter 7 ("The Spine"). While we gladly accepted the challenge of writing the book ourselves, we wisely asked for their expertise in neuroradiology and neurosurgery in order to assist us in completing this final chapter. Additionally, Dr. Lawrence E. Holder, Dr. Stuart Rabinowitz, and Dr. Andrew Yang in Baltimore and Dr. Zachary Grossman and Dr. F. Deaver Thomas in Syracuse were also kind in lending us several cases from their teaching files to be used in this book. Finally, Dr. John G. McAfee honored us by agreeing to write the Foreword.

The tremendous task of photographing and duplicating over 300 cases was performed by Mr. John G. Hodgson (SUNY Health Science Center). In Baltimore, Mr. Dan Beisel provided all the original medical drawings displayed throughout the book.

In the area of research, administrative and secretarial assistance, and manuscript transcription, we want to thank many individuals. The large task of transcribing the manuscript was performed in Syracuse by Maria Pembrook and Marci Guyer and in Baltimore by Kim Koehrer and Nancy Hawkins. Additional secretarial assistance and researching case files were given in Baltimore by Kate Smith, Christy Holthaus, Dolores Fosque, Aaron Flaks, and Randy Nolan. Finally, Pat Spilman deserves special recognition for her tireless efforts in the areas of case and photographic coordination, library research, and computerization of the bibliography.

The high level of diagnostic imaging displayed in this text is a result of the dedication and efforts of technologists in both Syracuse and Baltimore. At the sake of omitting some names, we feel obligated to mention the special efforts of the Licensed Registered Technologists (LRT) in Syracuse, Gail L. Bailey, Diane L. Cole, Catherine S. Collins, Kevin L. Draht, Michael Formikell, Amber J. Keeler, Melinda J. Lockwood, Mary Martin, Anne M. Perkins, Tina M. Saya, and Lynn Seabridge and in Baltimore, the senior Certified

Nuclear Medicine Technologists (CNMT) Lisa Cole, Melanie Cook, Aaron Flaks, Debbie Hollidge, Nellie Kelty, Georgeanne Kroen, Jane Machin, Patti Sheehan, and Pat Webb.

Finally, a special thank-you to Mariapaz Ramos Englis, Muza Navrozov, Roger Kasunic, José Fonfrias, Jack Farrell, and the entire staff of the Health Professions Division of McGraw-Hill.

JOSEPH R. MARTIRE
E. MARK LEVINSOHN

IMAGING OF ATHLETIC INJURIES

Orthopedic overview

With the recent increase in recreational and competitive athletic interests by the general population, injuries to the knee associated with these activities have become a common cause of disability in a broad range of age groups. These injuries include disruption of the menisci, ligamentous tears, fractures, chondral defects with loose bodies, dislocation of the patella, and overuse syndromes, such as patellar tendinitis, stress fracture and patellofemoral pain syndrome.

The initial evaluation of a patient with complaints related to the knee includes the history. If the mechanism of injury is known, this becomes significant in determining the type of structure injured. For example, a direct lateral blow to the knee in a contact sport with abduction and external rotation is likely to produce injury to the medial collateral ligament, possibly the medial meniscus and the anterior cruciate ligament. A fall on the tibial tubercle on a firm surface may produce disruption of the posterior cruciate ligament with an isolated instability. The presence of an effusion shortly after the injury indicates a significant intracapsular injury, and statistically there is a high incidence of ligament disruption and meniscal tear associated with this finding.

Physical examination with evidence of laxity of the knee may help to explain the specific structure injured. If no laxity exists, but there is an effusion, there still is significant potential for disruption of ligament and/or meniscal structures in addition to other problems, such as chondral fractures. Routine radiographs, including anteroposterior, lateral, oblique, tunnel, and merchant views are helpful in identifying such injuries as avulsion fractures of the tibial spine, which may indicate an anterior cruciate ligament injury in an immature individual. An avulsion from the lateral tibial plateau (Segond fracture) may indicate an anterior cruciate ligament insufficiency secondary to a recent injury. Merchant views can be helpful in determining whether there is a predisposition for a subluxation or dislocation of the patella. A tunnel view allows visualization of the areas near the intercondylar notch, which are most commonly the site of an osteochondritis dissecans defect. Stress views, helpful in determining the extent of ligamentous laxity secondary to an injury, are most important when there is consideration for an epiphyseal fracture of the distal femur associated with a valgus stress. A determination of the type of injury is important when considering treatment in the skeletally immature individual.

Many times, the patient will not allow enough relaxation to occur to adequately examine the knee. Examination under anesthesia and arthroscopy are means by which specific information can be obtained about the integrity of the knee, both by stressing the knee while under anesthesia and also by directly visualizing the structures in the intracapsular region. Prior to examination under anesthesia and arthroscopy, MRI is an extremely useful diagnostic tool. There is no other study that allows the visualization of the soft tissues, including the ligaments and tendons about the knee, as well as the integrity of the menisci. When concern exists specifically about the ligaments or the menisci, MRI is the diagnostic procedure of choice.

CHAPTER 1

KNEE

This is frequently followed by examination under anesthesia with arthroscopy for diagnosis and, in many cases, treatment.

When significant trauma has occurred and consideration is made for the possibility of fracture about the knee, in addition to plain films, CT scanning is helpful in determining whether an injury such as a depressed plateau fracture may have occurred. This can be done in addition to bone scanning for clarification of the anatomy and determination of the extent of injury.

With overuse syndromes and chronic changes, the use of bone scanning is significantly helpful in terms of specifically isolating the area of injury, thereby allowing physicians to make recommendations to patients about their activity patterns. For example, the runner who has chronic pain about the knee may be dealing with a stress fracture. If the bone scan is positive, then appropriate treatment, to include limitation of activity, is indicated. If the bone scan is negative and no other structural changes are evident, then consideration can be made for modification of the activity pattern without total limitation. This can be extremely important for the competitive athlete in particular.

The treatment of the injured knee in the competitive and recreational athlete is a constant challenge for the physician. The appropriate use of adjunctive clinical imaging techniques, such as MRI, CT scanning, and bone scanning, provides a more accurate and definitive means of diagnosing the problems, thereby allowing the physician to prescribe the appropriate treatment for the patient.

BRUCE E. BAKER, M.D.
Syracuse University Athletic Department
Syracuse, New York

AS THE LARGEST and perhaps the most complex joint, the knee is particularly vulnerable to athletic injury. In addition to flexion and extension, there is rotatory motion of the femoral condyles as they slide over the menisci. The intra- and extraarticular structures stabilize the tibiofemoral articulation. The menisci provide an adaptive surface, which allows stable articulation of the femur and tibia over a wide range of motion. Stress and shearing forces caused by this motion subject the menisci and cruciate ligaments to potential injury. In order to better visualize injury about the knee, a number of diagnostic imaging tools have been developed.

Arthrography was first introduced in 1905 but did not become a widely accepted procedure until the 1940s. Considerable experience was gained with single- and double-contrast arthrography, and in the 1960s through 1980s a number of studies were done that showed the arthrogram to be a highly accurate and dependable examination. The development of arthroscopy paralleled the development of arthrography, and each examination had both proponents and critics. Although both examinations are invasive, arthroscopy provides a tool to correct the visualized abnormality not possible with arthrography.

With the advent of computed tomography (CT) and magnetic resonance imaging (MRI), it became possible to noninvasively visualize intraarticular structures of the knee.[1–8] The accuracy of each of these modalities when done by experienced radiologists is somewhat comparable (Table 1-1). The invasive nature of arthrography, the technical skill demanded of the radiologist to perform a high-quality examination, and the high degree of accuracy of MRI have led to a virtual replacement of knee arthrography by magnetic resonance scanning.[9–11] CT scanning of intraarticular structures, although shown to be an accurate diagnostic tool,[12] has not become a popular modality. Similarly, sonography of the menisci has not proved useful.[13]

In the knee, triple-phase bone scanning (TPBS) cannot compete with magnetic resonance imaging of either the menisci or ligaments. Some attempts to identify meniscal pathology with TPBS have not obtained popular support be-

TABLE 1-1

Comparative accuracy of diagnosis of meniscal tears, percent

	Arthrography	Arthroscopy	CT	MR
Medial meniscus	82–97[22,24,26,27]	70–95[22,24,27]	89.2–91.5[6,23]	95[10,35]
Lateral meniscus	69–93[22,24,26,27]	76–95[22,24,27]	91.6–96.1[4,23]	95[10,35]
Anterior cruciate ligament	50–95[20,22,24,27]	97–100[22,27]	NR	90–95[1,10,37]
Posterior cruciate ligament	NR	NR	NR	95–100[10]
Chondromalacia	55[27]	100[27]	97.1[75]	NR

NR = not reported.

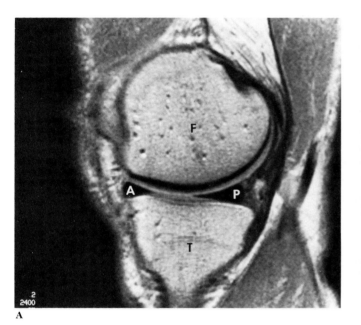

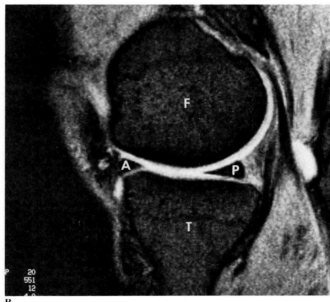

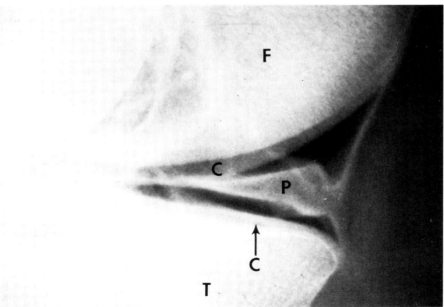

Figure 1-1 Normal Medial Meniscus. **A.** *Sagittal image at T1-weighted sequence.* **B.** *Sagittal image at short TR gradient echo (FISP 20°) sequence.* **C.** *Arthrogram of the posterior horn. The medial meniscus normally is a triangular-shaped structure with low-signal intensity on T1- and T2-weighted sequences. The sagittal scans demonstrate the normally smaller anterior and larger posterior horns of the meniscus. The articular cartilage, adjacent bones, and periarticular soft tissue structures are demonstrated. The arthrogram nicely shows the articular surface of the meniscus. Without a surface tear, contrast does not enter the substance of the meniscus. F = femur; T = tibia; A = anterior horn; P = posterior horn; C = articular cartilage.*

cause of the insufficient anatomic detail provided by this modality.[14] TPBS is valuable, however, in diagnosing some causes of chronic knee pain including fractures (occult or stress) that have negative or equivocal radiographs. The development of single photon emission computed tomography (SPECT) imaging has increased the sensitivity of nuclide scanning, providing useful diagnostic information even when planar imaging is equivocal.[15]

Although MRI is a new diagnostic tool, it has enjoyed enormous interest as applied to diagnosis of intra- and periarticular problems about the knee. Not only does it have the

potential to superbly demonstrate abnormalities of the menisci, cruciate ligaments, extensor mechanism, collateral ligaments, and periarticular soft tissues, it additionally displays the cortical, trabecular, and marrow features of stress fracture, osteonecrosis, and infiltrating marrow disorders.[10,16] As with other areas in the musculoskeletal system, plain radiographs should be taken prior to MRI in order to exclude bony abnormalities, which may not be visible on magnetic resonance scanning. The normal anatomic features of TPBS and MRI of the menisci are shown in Figs. 1-1 to 1-5.

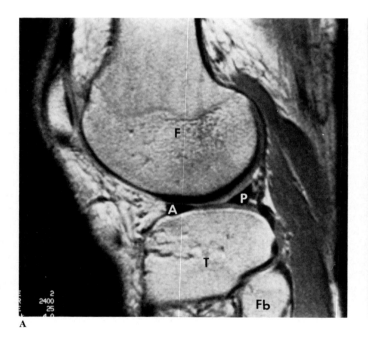

A

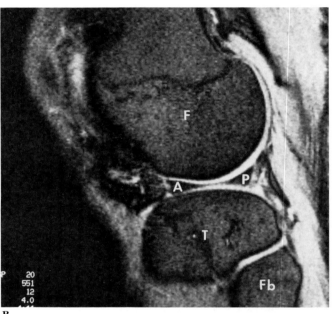

B

Figure 1-2　Normal Lateral Meniscus. **A.** *Sagittal image at T1-weighted sequence.* **B.** *Short TR gradient echo sequence (FISP 20°).* **C.** *Sagittal T1-weighted image. The lateral meniscus demonstrates low-signal intensity causing it to appear dark. It has a C-shaped appearance unlike the comma-shaped appearance of the medial meniscus. Part C demonstrates the normal transverse meniscal ligament which runs from the anterior aspect of the lateral meniscus transversely across the knee to the anterior aspect of the medial meniscus. F = femur; T = tibia; A = anterior horn; P = posterior horn; C = articular cartilage; Fb = fibula; TL = transverse ligament.*

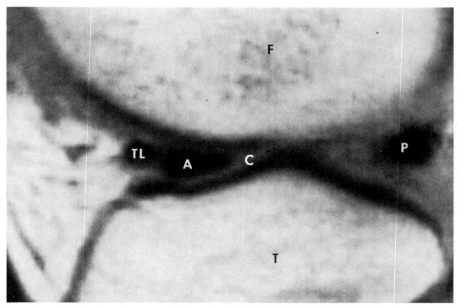

C

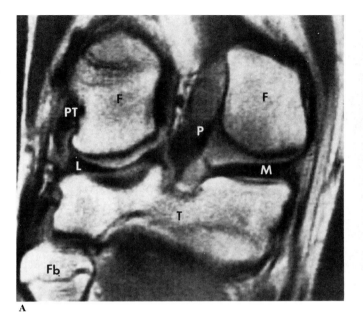
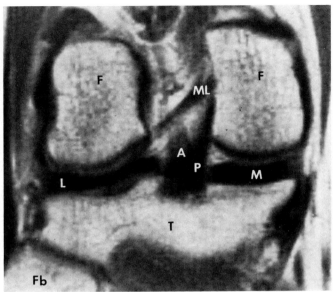
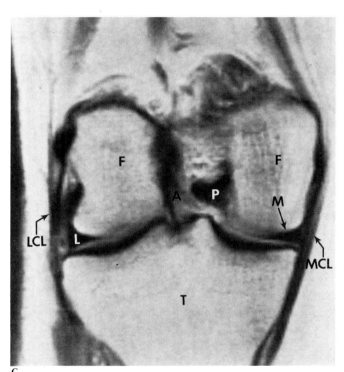
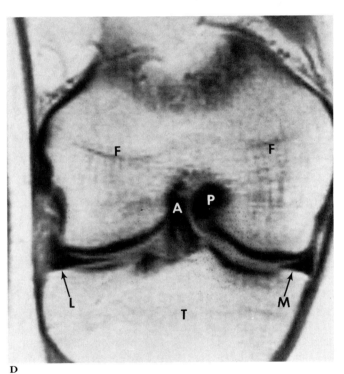

Figure 1-3 Normal Coronal Anatomy. **A.** *Coronal image at T1-weighted sequence through the posterior aspect of the knee demonstrates the central attachments of the medial and lateral menisci to the tibia. The posterior cruciate ligament, lateral collateral ligament, and popliteus tendon are seen.* **B.** *Coronal image at T1-weighted sequence through the midposterior aspect of the knee show the anterior and posterior cruciate ligaments overlapping normally and the*

meniscofemoral fibers. **C.** *Coronal midanterior image at T1-weighted sequence shows the attachment of the anterior and posterior cruciate ligaments within the intercondylar notch. The popliteus tendon, lateral collateral ligament, menisci, and medial collateral ligament are seen.* **D.** *Coronal image anteriorly through the joint at T1-weighted sequence shows the attachments of the anterior and posterior cruciate ligaments, the medial collateral ligament, and the*

menisci. F = femur; Fb = fibula; T = tibia; M = medial meniscus; L = lateral meniscus; A = anterior cruciate ligament; P = posterior cruciate ligament; ML = meniscofemoral ligament; PT = popliteus tendon; MCL = medial collateral ligament; LCL = lateral collateral ligament.

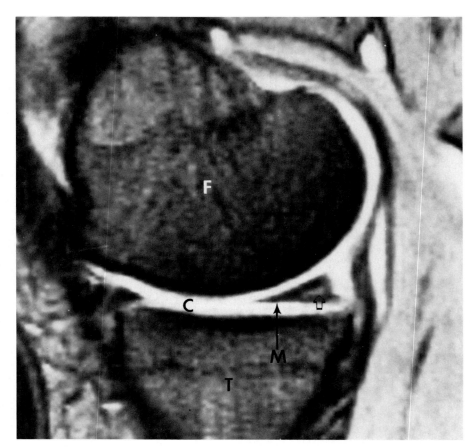

Figure 1-4 Normal Intrameniscal Signal. *Sagittal scan at short TR gradient echo sequence through the medial meniscus demonstrates grade 2 increased signal within the posterior horn. Increased signal which does not extend to the articulating margin is a normal finding not representing meniscal tear. M = medial meniscus; open arrow = region of increased signal; C = articular cartilage; F = femur; T = tibia.*

ACUTE PROBLEMS

Probably the most productive imaging examination to be performed on the athlete presenting with an acute intraarticular knee injury is the magnetic resonance scan. The accuracy of magnetic resonance imaging in the detection of abnormalities of the menisci is approximately 95 percent and equals or surpasses that of the arthrogram and arthroscopic examination.[17–27] In addition to the usual normal features demonstrated in Figs. 1-1 to 1-4, several anatomic variations occur which may mimic meniscal tears. The approximation of the meniscofemoral ligament to the posterior horn of the lateral meniscus (Fig. 1-3) and of the transverse meniscal ligament to the anterior horns of the medial and lateral menisci (Fig. 1-2) may be mistaken for meniscal tears if not recognized.[28,29]

Meniscal tears (Figs. 1-6 to 1-11)

The normal meniscus is a triangular structure with a smooth articular surface. The medial meniscus is teardrop-shaped with a large posterior horn and a smaller anterior horn. The C-shaped lateral meniscus is uniform in size from anterior to posterior. Normally each meniscus is composed of uniform fibrocartilagenous tissue, which demonstrates homogeneously low signal on all imaging sequences. Not infrequently, some increased signal may be present within the meniscus[30,31] (Fig. 1-4). The increased signal is graded 0–3[32,33] (Table 1-2). Menisci demonstrating no signal (grade 0) histologically are found to be normal. In those menisci with punctate areas of increased signal or linear areas of increased signal (grades 1 and 2) focal regions of mucoid degeneration are found. It is likely that some patients with grade 2 increased signal have symptoms associated with mucoid degeneration. Arthroscopic examination of those knees is usually normal. Patients with increased signal extending out to the articular surface (grade 3A) or with loss of the usual contour of the menisci (grade 3B) histologically demonstrate meniscal tears (Figs. 1-6 to 1-11).

Cruciate ligament tears (Figs. 1-12 to 1-16)

The magnetic resonance examination is clearly superior to the arthrogram in the evaluation of the cruciate ligaments. The identification of anterior cruciate ligament tears is greater than 90 percent with magnetic resonance scanning and approaches 100 percent for assessment of the posterior cruciate ligament.

TABLE 1-2

Pathologic significance of meniscal signal

Meniscal signal grade	MR appearance	Pathologic significance	Symptoms
0	Uniformly dark	Normal	No
1	Tiny foci of increased signal	Normal	No
2	Intrameniscal linear band of increased signal	Mucoid degeneration	Possibly
3a	Linear band of increased signal extending to the articular surface	Meniscal tear	Yes
3b	Fragmentation of meniscus with loss of normal shape	Meniscal tear	Yes

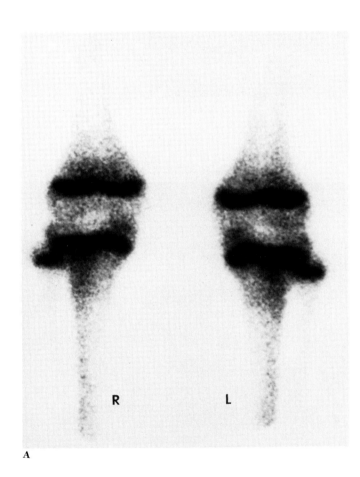

Figure 1-5   Delayed Images of Normal Knee (TPBS). **A.** *Anteroposterior view.* **B.** *Medial-lateral view. These delayed images of a TPBS demonstrate increased activity in the growth plates of the long bones about the knee seen in adolescent athletes before growth plate fusion. Uptake in the patella in a normal patient is equal to or less than the adjacent long bones.*

A

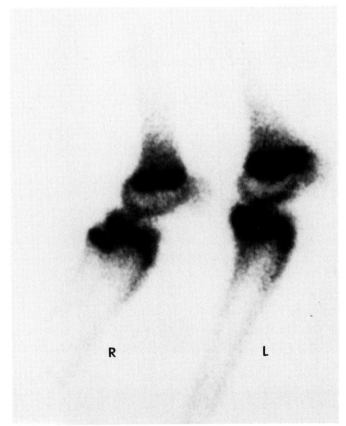

B

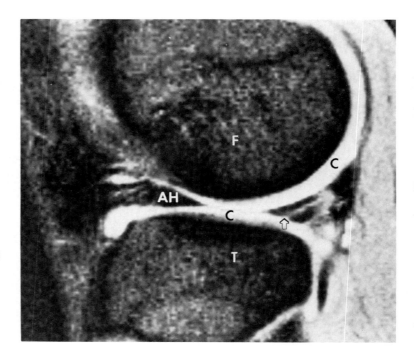

Figure 1-6 Medial Meniscus Tear. *Sagittal image at short TR gradient echo sequence demonstrates an oblique tear of the posterior horn of the medial meniscus. The area of increased signal extends to involve the articulating surface of the meniscus. Open arrow = tear; AH = anterior horn; C = articular cartilage; F = femur; T = tibia.*

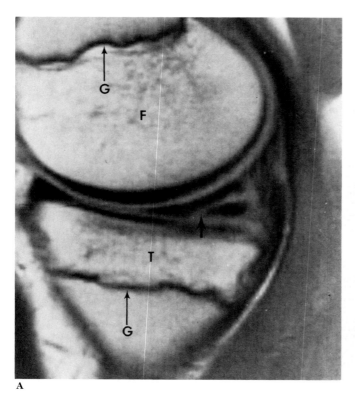

A

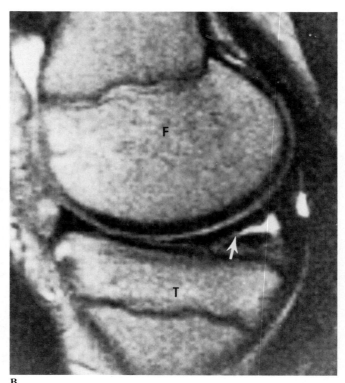

B

Figure 1-7 Medial Meniscus Tear. **A.** *Sagittal image at T1-weighted sequence shows increased signal in the posterior horn of the medial menis-* *cus.* **B.** *A similar image at T2-weighted sequence shows joint fluid with high-signal intensity filling the tear. This "arthrogram effect" clearly outlines the ex-* *tent of tear. Arrow = meniscal tear; F = femur; T = tibia; G = growth plate.*

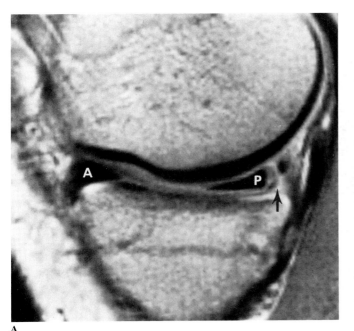

A

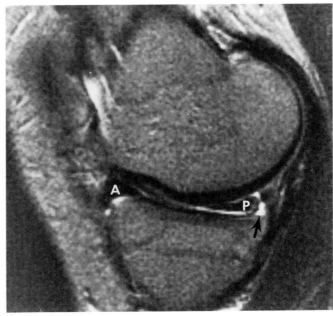

B

Figure 1-8 Medial Meniscus Tear (Peripheral). **A.** *Sagittal image at T1-weighted sequence shows area of increased signal at the periphery of the* *posterior horn of the medial meniscus.* **B.** *Sagittal image at T2-weighted sequence shows high signal corresponding to joint fluid filling the meniscal tear* *and creating an arthrogram effect. A = anterior horn; P = posterior horn; arrow = tear.*

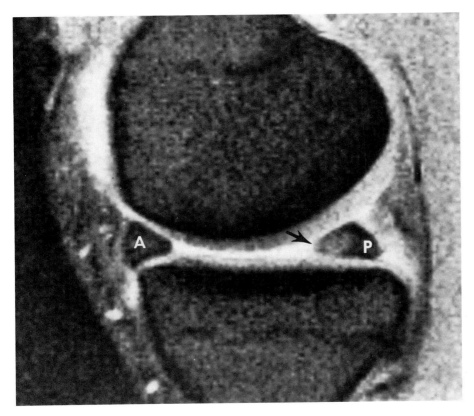

Figure 1-9 Medial Meniscus Tear. *Sagittal image at short TR gradient echo sequence shows increased signal within the central edge of the posterior horn of the medial meniscus. Additionally, there is blunting of the meniscus noted. Since the increased signal extends out to the articular surface, a meniscal tear is present. A = anterior horn; P = posterior horn; arrow = abnormal central edge of medial meniscus.*

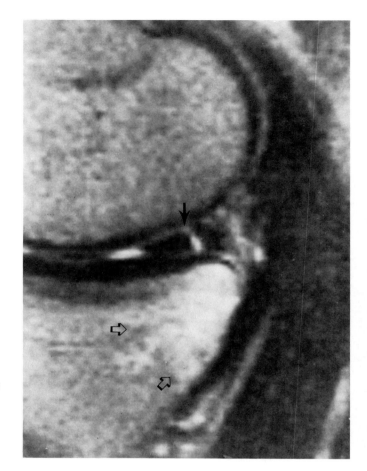

Figure 1-10 Vertical Tear Medial Meniscus with Adjacent Bone Bruise. *Sagittal image at T2-weighted sequence demonstrates fluid creating high signal filling a vertical tear of the posterior horn of the medial meniscus. There is a diffuse area of high signal within the adjacent tibia representing a focus of bone bruise. The overlying tibial cortex is intact. Arrow = meniscal tear; open arrows = bone bruise.*

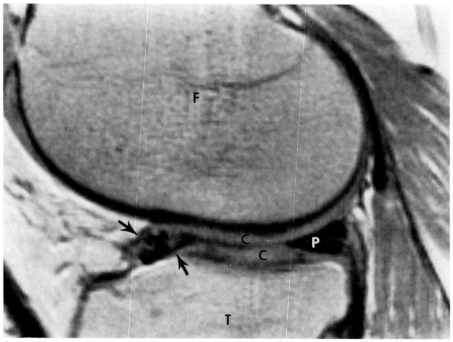

Figure 1-11 Lateral Meniscal Tear. **A.** *Sagittal image at T1-weighted sequence demonstrates fragmentation of the anterior horn of the meniscus.* (Fig. 1-11B and C continues on the opposite page.)

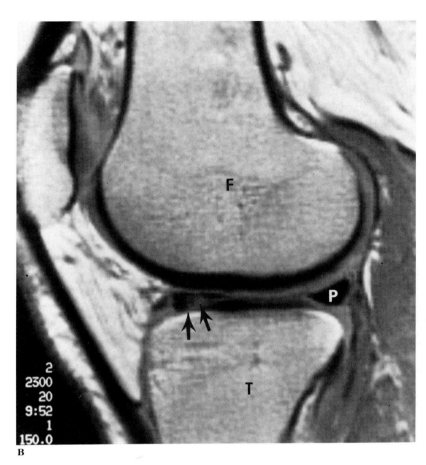

B

Figure 1-11 Lateral Meniscal Tear (Continued). **B.** *Sagittal image at proton density sequence demonstrates tear of the anterior horn of the lateral meniscus causing loss of the usual triangular shape. A tear involves the central edge and inferior aspect of the meniscus.* **C.** *Coronal image at proton density sequence shows loss of the triangular shape of the middle sector of the lateral meniscus representing a lateral meniscal tear. Arrows = fragmented and torn anterior horn; P = posterior horn; F = femur; T = tibia; C = articular cartilage.*

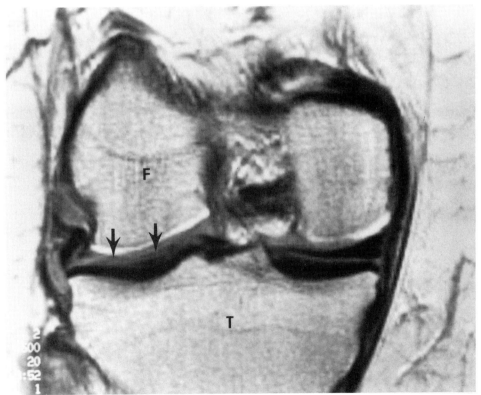

C

The normal posterior cruciate ligament is a hockey stick–shaped structure extending posteriorly from the intercondylar eminence of the tibia to the medial aspect of the intercondylar notch (Fig. 1-12). It demonstrates homogeneously low-signal intensity and when normal is visualized in the sagittal plane in virtually all patients.[34] In 30 to 58 percent of patients, meniscofemoral fibers extending medially off the central edge of the posterior horn of the lateral meniscus are noted along the anterior surface and less often along the posterior surface of the posterior cruciate ligament.[35] Tears of the posterior cruciate ligament cause increased signal and deformity of that structure[36] (Figs. 1-13 and 1-14). Avulsion of the bony attachment of the posterior cruciate ligament causes a similar appearance on the magnetic resonance scan (Fig. 1-15). The bony fragment may not be seen without radiographs.

The anterior cruciate ligament (ACL) extends at a 10 to 20° oblique angle from the anterior aspect of the tibial plateau posterolaterally to insert on the intercondylar notch (Fig. 1-12). Its signal characteristics differ substantially from the posterior cruciate ligament. The anterior cruciate ligament is composed of parallel bands of low-signal fibers separated by intermediate signal tissue. Tears of the ACL demonstrate increased signal and loss of fiber continuity[37] (Fig. 1-16).

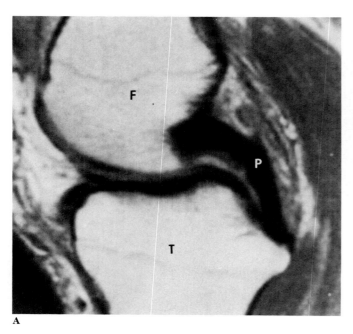

A

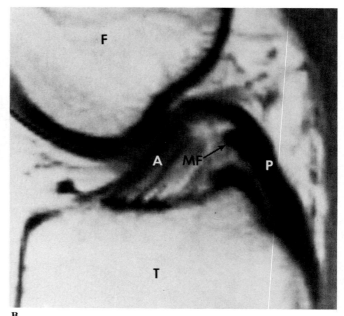

B

Figure 1-12   Anterior and Posterior Cruciate Ligaments. **A.** *Sagittal image at T1-weighted sequence through the knee just medial to midline shows the normal "hockey stick" appearance of the posterior cruciate ligament.* **B.** *Sagittal image at T1-weighted sequence through the midportion of the knee shows a portion of the posterior cruciate ligament overlapping a portion of the anterior cruciate ligament. The posterior cruciate ligament shows uniformly low signal throughout its course. A structure adjacent to the anterior surface of the posterior cruciate ligament represents the normal anterior meniscofemoral fibers seen in 30 percent of examinations. The anterior cruciate ligament demonstrates alternating bands of low and intermediate signal intensity.* **C.** *Sagittal image at T1-weighted sequence through the knee just lateral to the midline shows the substance of the anterior cruciate ligament. (Fig. 1-12D continues on the opposite page.)*

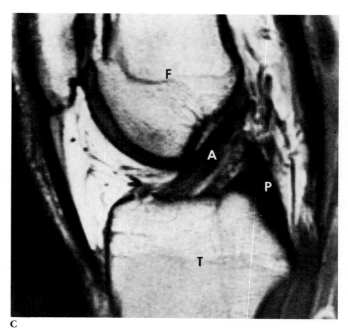

C

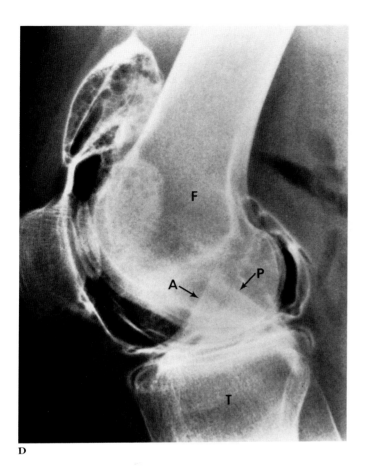

D

Figure 1-12   Anterior and Posterior Cruciate Ligaments (Continued).   **D.** *Lateral radiograph from an arthrogram shows the anterior and posterior cruciate ligaments. P = posterior cruciate ligament; A = anterior cruciate ligament; MF = anterior meniscofemoral ligament; F = femur, T = tibia.*

Figure 1-13   Posterior Cruciate Ligament Tear. *Sagittal image at T1-weighted sequence shows increased signal within the substance of the posterior cruciate ligament indicating tear of that structure. The anterior cruciate ligament appears to be normal. A = anterior cruciate ligament; arrows = torn posterior cruciate ligament; F = femur; T = tibia.*

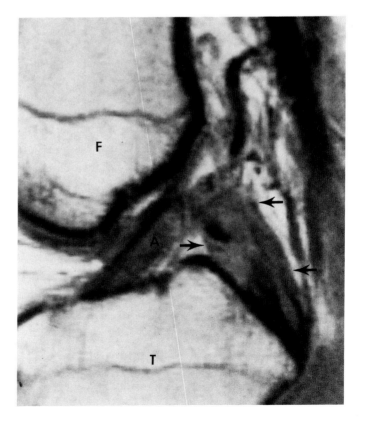

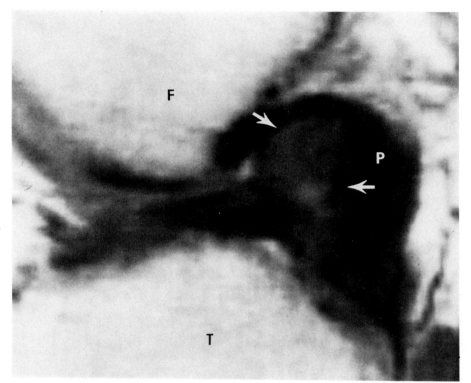

Figure 1-14   Incomplete Posterior Cruciate Ligament Tear. *Sagittal image at T1-weighted sequence shows deformity of the posterior cruciate ligament with an expansile region of intermediate signal anteriorly. This indicates partial tear with hematoma involving the posterior cruciate ligament. P = posterior cruciate ligament; arrows = hematoma; F = femur; T = tibia.*

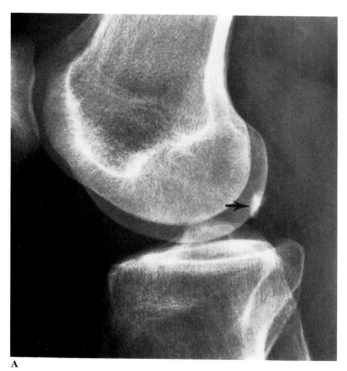

A

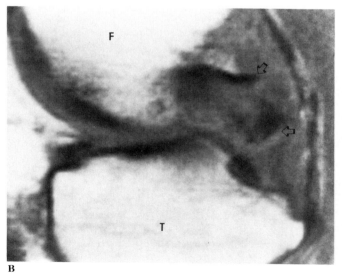

B

Figure 1-15   Torn Posterior Cruciate Ligament with Bony Avulsion. **A.** *Lateral radiograph demonstrates bony fragment superimposed over usual projection of posterior cruciate ligament.* **B.** *Sagittal image at T1-weighted sequence shows disruption of posterior cruciate ligament. Arrow = bony fragment; open arrows = torn posterior cruciate ligament; F = femur; T = tibia.*

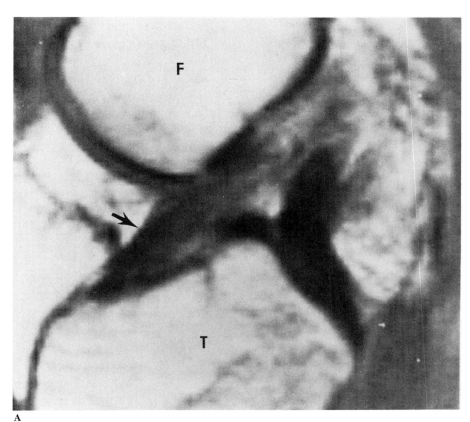

A

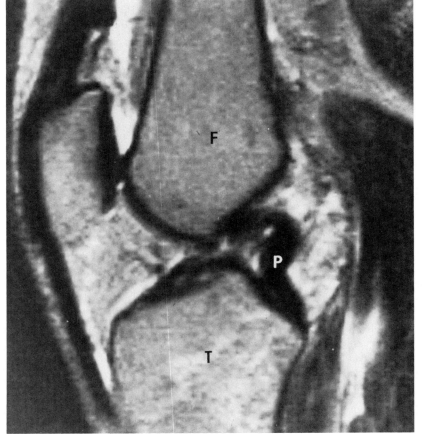

B

Figure 1-16   Anterior Cruciate Ligament Tear. **A.** *Sagittal image at T1-weighted sequence shows an inhomogeneous appearance to the anterior cruciate ligament with lack of normal structure. This indicates tear of the anterior cruciate ligament.* **B.** *Sagittal image at T2-weighted sequence shows a buckled appearance of the posterior cruciate ligament. This deformity results from underlying tear of the anterior cruciate ligament. Arrow = torn anterior cruciate ligament; P = buckled posterior cruciate ligament; F = femur; T = tibia.*

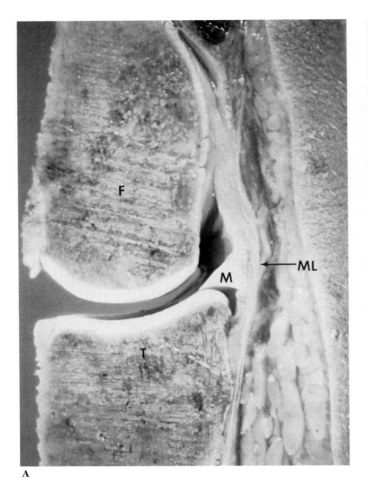

A

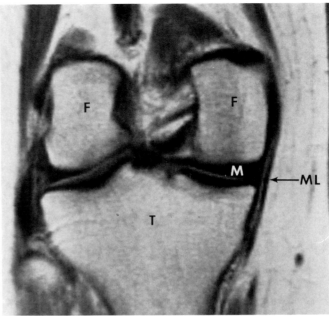

B

Figure 1-17   Normal Medial Collateral Ligament.
A. *Coronal section through the knee shows the medial meniscus, loose fibrofatty connective tissue, and medial collateral ligament.* **B.** *Coronal MR image at T1-weighted sequence demonstrates normal medial collateral ligament, normal medial meniscus, and fibrofatty zone between those structures. M = medial meniscus; ML = medial collateral ligament (superficial layer); F = femur; T = tibia.*

Figure 1-18   Medial Collateral Ligament Tear. **A.** *Anteroposterior radiograph from an arthrogram shows leakage of contrast into the medial soft tissues. This is diagnostic of medial collateral ligament tear.* (Fig. 1-18B and C continues on the opposite page.)

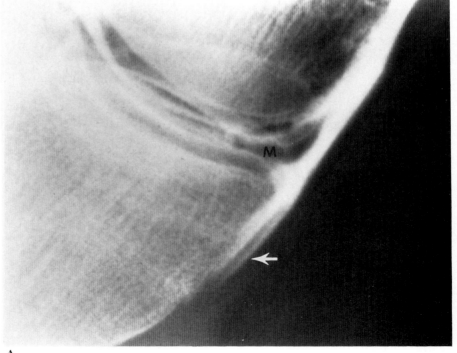

A

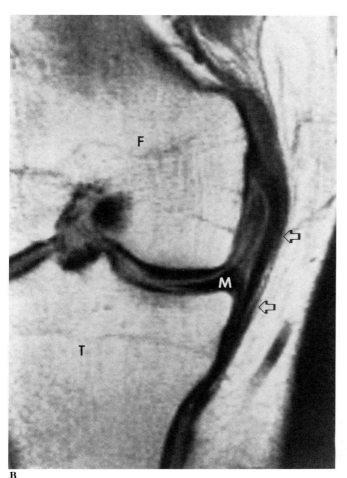

B

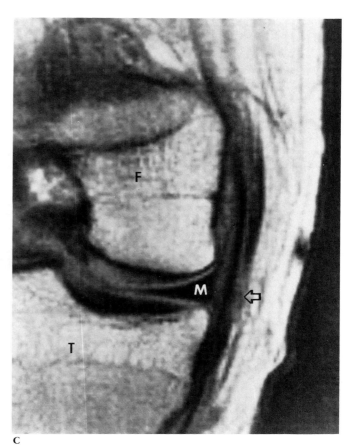

C

Figure 1-18 Medial Collateral Ligament Tear (Continued).
B. *Coronal MR image at T1-weighted sequence shows thickening of the medial collateral ligament indicating grade 2 partial tear.* **C.** *Coronal MR image at T1-weighted sequence shows thickening of the medial collateral ligament and associated soft tissues indicating grade 2 tear. Arrow = leakage of contrast into medial soft tissues; open arrow = thickening and abnormality of medial collateral ligament; M = medial meniscus; F = femur; T = tibia.*

Collateral ligament injury (Figs. 1-17 and 1-18)

The medial collateral ligament (MCL) is the most frequently injured of the collateral ligaments of the knee and is nicely evaluated on magnetic resonance scans (Fig. 1-17). Injuries to the MCL (Fig. 1-18) are classified as grades 1–3. Grade 1 injuries are those in which the ligament appears normal but in which there is a soft tissue swelling in the subcutaneous tissues adjacent to the MCL. Grade 3 injury indicates complete disruption of the MCL with associated soft tissue swelling and hemorrhage. Grade 2 injury is intermediate. Injury to the lateral collateral ligament is less frequent but is characterized by discontinuity, widening, distortion, and in-

creased signal within that ligament with edema and hemorrhage present in the adjacent soft tissues.

Extensor mechanism injury (Figs. 1-19 and 1-20)

Disruptions of the extensor mechanism from either a quadriceps tendon tear (Fig. 1-19) or a patellar ligament injury (Fig. 1-20) are optimally visualized on magnetic resonance scans.[38,39] Although ultrasound and CT may be positive for quadriceps tendon or patellar ligament abnormality, the magnetic resonance scan is superior.

Figure 1-19   Quadriceps Tendon Rupture. *Sagittal MR scan* ▶
at T2-weighted sequence demonstrates disruption of the
quadriceps tendon at its attachment to the patella. Secondary
wrinkling of the patellar tendon has resulted. Arrows =
quadriceps tendon tear; open arrows = wrinkled patellar
tendon; F = femur; T = tibia; P = patella.

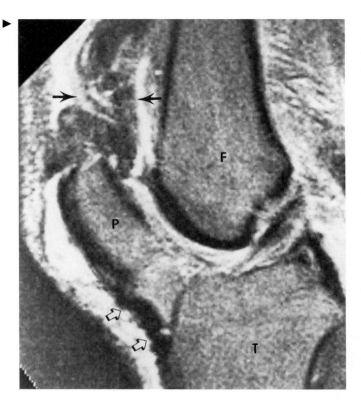

Figure 1-20   Abnormalities of the Patellar
Tendon. **A.** *Sagittal MR image at proton density*
sequence demonstrates thickening of the patellar
tendon just distal to its attachment to the patella
with increased signal within that portion of tendon.
This represents early degenerative change of the
tendon. **B.** *Sagittal MR image at T1-weighted*
sequence demonstrates two ossicles to be present
within the patellar tendon. This anatomic variation
lacks pathologic significance. **C.** *Ossicle at the*
attachment site of patellar tendon to tibia. (Fig.
1-20D and E continues on the opposite page.)
▼

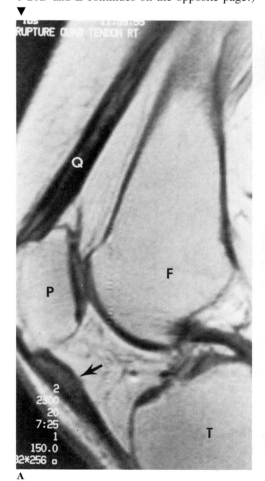

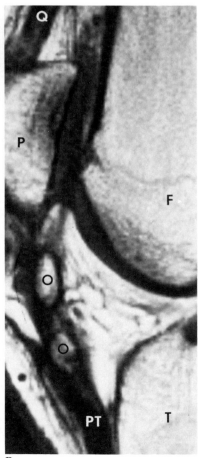

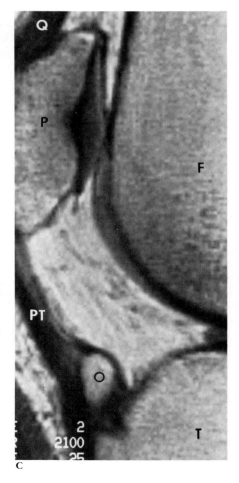

A

B

C

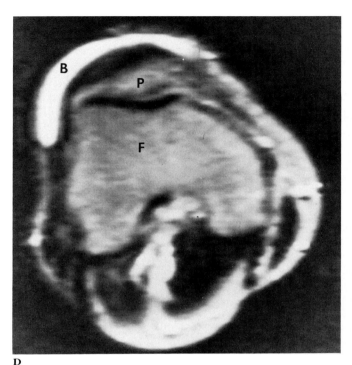

D

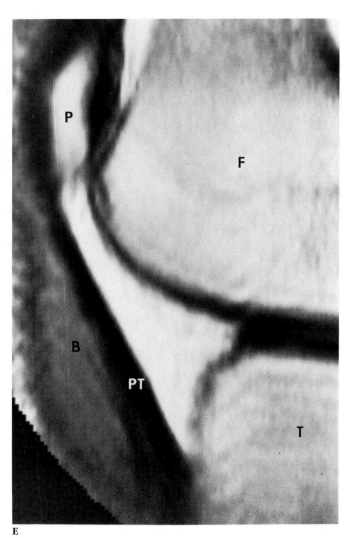

E

Figure 1-20 Abnormalities of the Patellar Tendon (Continued). **D.** *Axial image at T2-weighted sequence demonstrates fluid within the prepatellar bursa indicating prepatellar bursitis.* **E.** *Same case as above. Sagittal image at T1-weighted sequence demonstrates diffuse intermediate signal anterior to the patellar tendon indicating prepatellar bursitis. The patellar tendon is normal. Q = quadriceps tendon; PT = patellar tendon; O = ossicles; B = fluid in prepatellar bursa; F = femur; T = tibia; P = patella; arrow = abnormal patellar tendon.*

Bone contusion (Fig. 1-21)

Athletes with acute knee trauma and/or sudden onset of pain are usually referred for initial radiographs if bony pathology is suspected. If radiographs are either negative or equivocal, then TPBS is the test of choice.[40–42] TPBS can be used not only to detect occult fracture but also to evaluate intermediate and long-term healing.[41,43] MRI is also being used to evaluate acute bony abnormalities and is more sensitive than plain radiographs in detecting clinically significant traumatic bone injuries.[44] Three different types of image findings are recognized on magnetic resonance scan[45,46] (Table 1-3). A type 1 finding (Fig. 1-21) demonstrates diffuse, reticulated signal intensity in the metaphyseal and epiphyseal regions of bone. This signal pattern indicates a bony contusion (and/or microfracture) often associated with ligamentous injury that occurred at the time of injury. Type 1 injury indicates regions of bone that may be at increased risk for developing insuf-

ficiency fracture. A type 2 (Fig. 1-21) abnormality is associated with interruption in the smooth low-signal cortical line and associated loss of signal of the adjacent trabecular bone. These injuries are rarely visualized on plain radiographs. They are commonly associated with tears of the anterior cruciate ligament and of the collateral ligaments. A type 3 injury demonstrates intact cortical bone with subcortical signal loss. This appearance may be indistinguishable from degenerative bony change. Osteochondral fracture, stress fracture, and fracture of the tibial plateau (Figs. 1-22 and 1-23) and supracondylar region of the femur may also be identified both on MRI and on TPBS. Despite normal radiographs, when physical findings and the injury mechanism raise a high index of suspicion for bone pathology, TPBS and MRI can be used to identify otherwise nonvisible fractures even within the first 24 h following injury.[40,41,47]

TABLE 1-3

Magnetic resonance appearance of posttraumatic bony changes

Type of signal pattern	Signal appearance		Pathologic significance	Associated ligamentous injury
	T1	T2		
I	Homogenous intermediate-to-low signal in metaphyseal and epiphyseal bone	Homogeneous high signal	Microfracture (bone bruise/contusion)	Likely
II	Homogenous low signal in metaphyseal and epiphyseal bone with loss of cortical continuity	Homogenous high signal in metaphyseal and epiphyseal bone with loss of cortical continuity	Completed fracture with trabecular microfracture	Likely
III	Intact cortical bone with subcortical signal loss	Homogenous low signal involving cortical and subcortical bone	Healed compression injury	Not likely

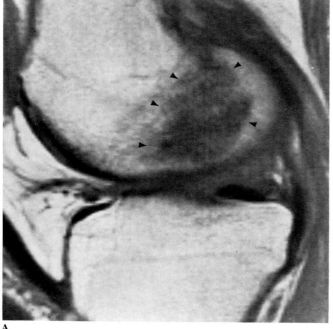

A

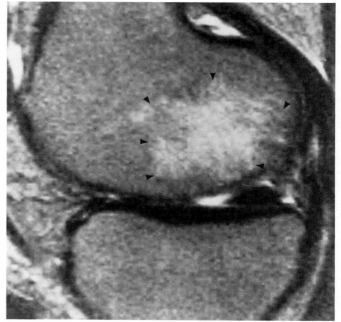

B

Figure 1-21 Bone Bruise. **A.** *Sagittal MR image at T1-weighted sequence shows diffuse low signal within the distal condyle of the femur.* **B.** *Same patient with sagittal MR image at T2-weighted sequence demonstrates high signal intensity within that area. These combined findings indicate edematous change of the distal femoral condyle consistent with type I bone bruise. The femoral cortex remains intact.* (Fig. 1-21C continues on the opposite page.)

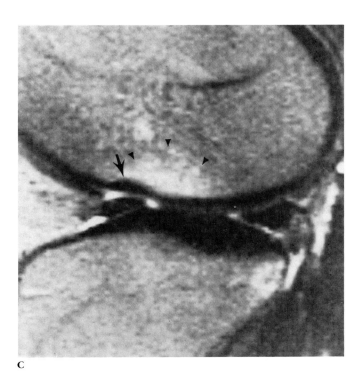

C

Figure 1-21   Bone Bruise (Continued). **C.** *Sagittal MR image at T2-weighted sequence shows high signal adjacent to the distal articulating surface of femur. The femoral cortex is irregular. These features indicate type 2 bone bruise with cortical disruption. Arrowheads = trabecular abnormality; arrow = cortical abnormality.*

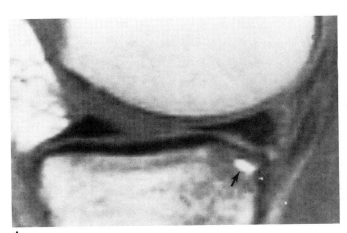

A

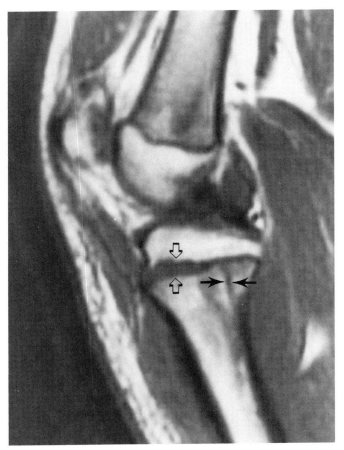

B

Figure 1-22   Focal Tibial Plateau Fracture. **A.** *Sagittal MR image at T1-weighted sequence shows a focus of high-signal intensity beneath the posterior aspect of the medial tibial plateau representing hemorrhage from a focal plateau fracture. The adjacent posterior horn of the medial meniscus is irregular on its inferior surface representing a tear. Arrow = subcortical hemorrhage at fracture site. [From Levinsohn EM: MR imaging of extremities excels in knee evaluation,* Diagnostic Imaging *11(5):102, 1989. Reproduced with permission.]* **B.** *Sagittal MR image at T1-weighted sequence shows widening of the proximal tibial growth plate with fracture line extending through the proximal metaphysis of the tibia. This represents a Salter 2 fracture of the tibia. Open arrows = widened growth plate; arrows = fracture line.*

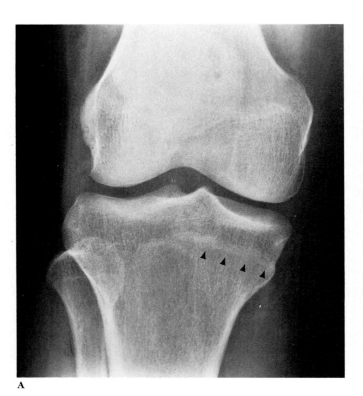

A

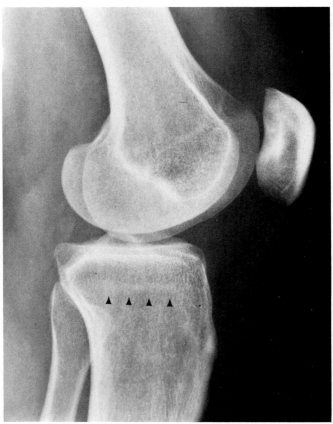

B

Figure 1-23   Tibial Plateau Fracture. **A.** *Anteroposterior radiograph of right knee.* **B.** *Lateral radiograph of right knee. Multiple arrowheads demonstrate faint line of increased bony density thought to be suspicious finding for nondepressed tibial plateau fracture. TPBS performed to determine if this represented an acute finding.* **C.** *Medial-lateral blood pool images of both knees. Increased activity in anterior right tibial plateau (arrow). Faint increased activity in the anterior aspect of the patella (arrowhead).* (Fig. 1-23D continues on the opposite page.)

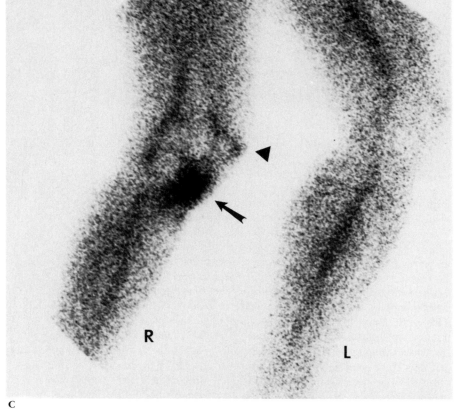

C

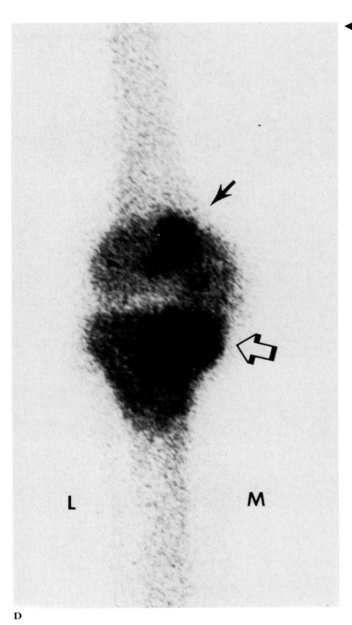

D

◀ **Figure 1-23** Tibial Plateau Fracture (Continued). **D.** *Delayed anterior view of right knee. Open arrow identifies focal intense nuclide activity in medial aspect of right tibial plateau. Black arrow demonstrates minimal to mildly increased activity in patella (consistent with bone bruise; not intense enough to represent fracture). Notice generalized increased activity on both sides of the joint associated with this acute traumatic event representing generalized hyperemia in the juxtaarticular portion of the right knee. M = medial; L = lateral.*

Tibial plateau fracture (Figs. 1-22 and 1-23)

Failure to diagnose this fracture may result in a depressed fragment requiring surgery and internal fixation. In an acutely injured patient, it is not uncommon to overlook associated occult tibial plateau fracture while focusing on acute ligamentous or meniscal damage (Fig. 1-22). TPBS is a very reliable test to answer the question of acute bony fracture associated with joint injury[54–56] (Fig. 1-23). Routine thin section tomography and/or CT scanning with sagittal and coronal reformatting are useful tools in assessing the location and degree of plateau depression following a tibial plateau fracture. MR has been shown to be sensitive in helping to detect small avulsion fractures at tendon attachment sites.[57]

Patellar fracture (Fig. 1-24)

As with fractures elsewhere, magnetic resonance imaging is sensitive in demonstrating edema and hemorrhage adjacent to and within the fracture area. TPBS should be positive on all phases, with acute patellar fracture demonstrating diffuse intense activity of the entire patella. Occasionally the patella sustains a less severe injury with only minimal or focal nuclide activity that is not the typical fracture pattern. This has been termed a *bone bruise* (Fig. 1-23).[48–50] An occult patellar fracture may be identified on TPBS despite normal radiographs. Stress fractures will essentially have the same TPBS appearance as acute fracture, with the distinction being made clinically as to whether the injury was due to a single traumatic event or overuse.[51–53]

Spontaneous osteonecrosis (Fig. 1-25)

Middle-aged athletes have their own unique spectrum of injuries.[58] Spontaneous or idiopathic osteonecrosis of the femoral condyle should always be considered in evaluating acute knee pain in a middle-aged or elderly patient with normal radiographs. There are multiple theories to explain this problem.[59,60] TPBS is very sensitive in helping to detect this entity. Nuclide activity accumulates in that area of bone believed to represent the revascularizing or healing phase.[61,62] Magnetic resonance imaging is sensitive and specific for this entity.[63,64] Additionally, MR affords an opportunity to evaluate the overlying hyaline cartilage and to assess early secondary osteoarthritis. Radiographs may never become positive if the condition is detected early enough and successfully treated with nonweight bearing.[65]

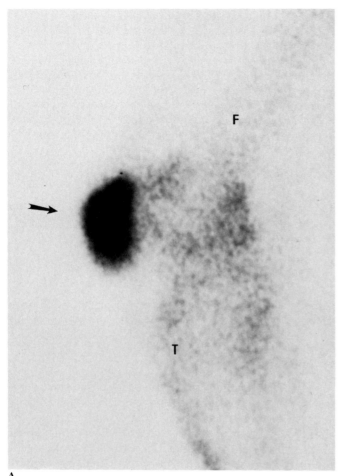

A

Figure 1-24 Acute Patellar Fracture (with Normal Radiographs, not shown). **A.** *Lateral view.* **B.** *Antero-posterior view. High-resolution delayed images of TPBS demonstrate intense nuclide activity in the entire patella (arrow). With acute injury, all three phases should be positive. F = femur; T = tibia.*

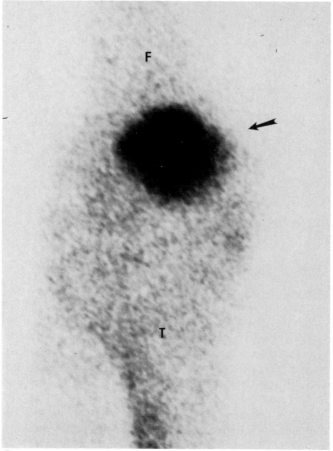

B

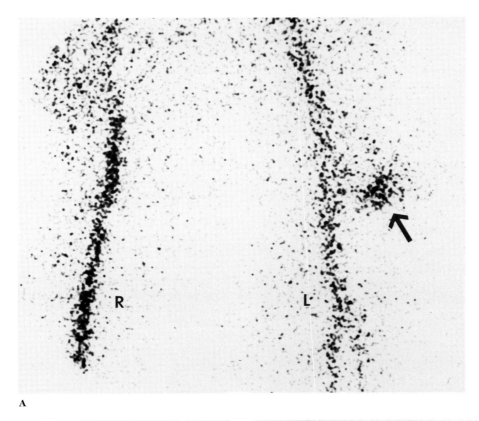

A

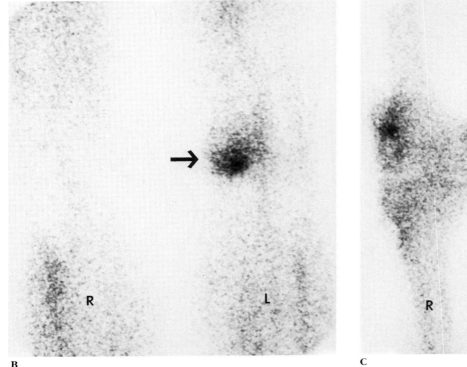

B
C

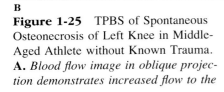

Figure 1-25 TPBS of Spontaneous Osteonecrosis of Left Knee in Middle-Aged Athlete without Known Trauma. **A.** *Blood flow image in oblique projection demonstrates increased flow to the* *left knee (arrow).* **B.** *Immediate blood pool image shows increased activity in medial aspect of left knee (arrow).* **C.** *High-resolution delayed images in anterior projection show large focal area* *of increased activity in the left medial femoral condyle apparently extending to the articular surface (arrow).*

CHRONIC PROBLEMS (Drawing I)

The sports medicine physician faces a daily dilemma in sorting the multiple causes of chronic knee pain: tendinitis, arthritis, chondromalacia, stress fracture, muscle injury, ligament damage, calcium deposition, meniscal or synovial cyst, plica syndrome, etc. If the radiograph is negative, consider TPBS and MRI. Even with a positive radiograph, TPBS may indicate the activity of the lesion, helping to explain pain (Table 1-4). MRI may demonstrate an anatomic abnormality not positive on TPBS.

Patellofemoral syndrome (Fig. 1-26)

Extensive research has been devoted to the patellofemoral joint in an attempt to identify the biomechanical problem causing pain and to classify the pathology.[66-68] *Patellofemoral arthralgia,* or *patellalgia,* are newer terms that describe the symptom complex.[69] The degree of nuclide activity noted on TPBS in the patellofemoral joint has been correlated to the severity of observed clinical symptoms.[70] Chondromalacia probably accounts for a small portion, less than

20 percent, of patellofemoral syndrome.[69,71] When present, moderate and severe chondromalacia are demonstrable on magnetic resonance imaging.[72] Combined CT arthrography has been shown to be a very sensitive way to assess patellar chondromalacia.[73-77]

TABLE 1-4

Disorders causing chronic knee pain optimally evaluated by TPBS

Patellofemoral syndrome
Tricompartment arthritis
Jumper's knee (infrapatellar tendinitis)
Osteochondritis dissecans
Pellegrini-Stieda disease
Painful bipartite patella
Osgood-Schlatter disease
Patellar stress fracture
Reflex sympathetic dystrophy
Tibial plateau stress fracture

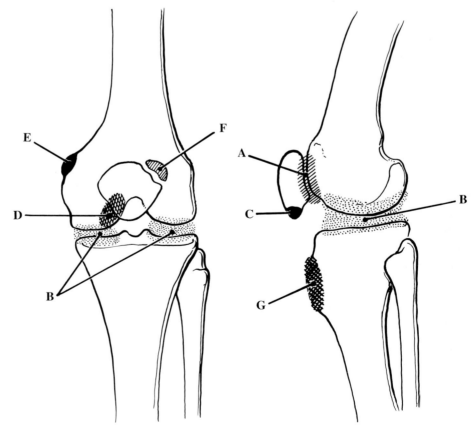

Drawing I   *Anterior and lateral views of the knee demonstrate the common causes and the anatomic locations of chronic knee pain in athletes.* **A.** *Patellofemoral syndrome.* **B.** *Arthritis.* **C.** *Infrapatellar tendinitis (jumper's knee).* **D.** *Osteochondritis dissecans.* **E.** *Pellegrini-Stieda disease.* **F.** *Painful bipartite patella.* **G.** *Osgood-Schlatter syndrome.*

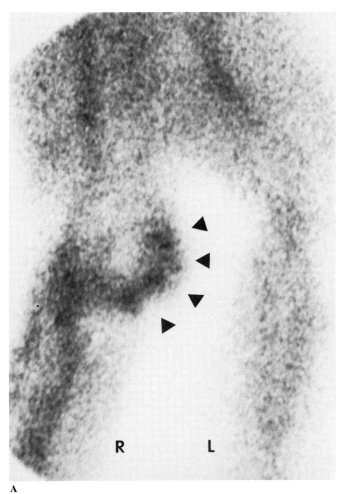

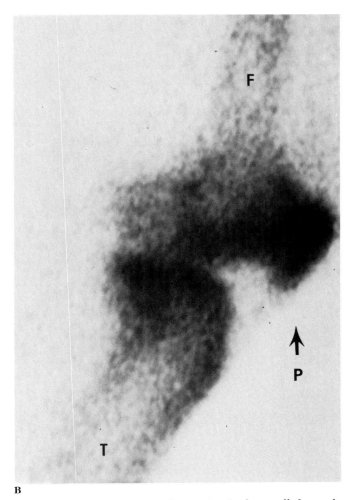

A

B

Figure 1-26 Patellofemoral Syndrome. **A.** *Medial-lateral blood pool views of both knees demonstrates increased activity in the right femoropatellar region (arrowheads).* **B.** *High resolution delayed lateral image of right* knee shows increased activity in the right patella and anterior aspect of the right distal femur with obliteration of the patellofemoral space. P = patella; F = femur; T = tibia. This abnormal nonspecific finding is consistent with hyperemia/inflammation in the patellofemoral space. Activity is increased above the normal appearance and is greater than the opposite knee.

Tricompartment arthritis (Fig. 1-27)

In middle-aged and older athletes, arthritis involving all three compartments of the knee is not infrequent. TPBS and magnetic resonance scanning are both useful in evaluating the extent and severity of degenerative cartilage loss, associated bony reactive change, and inflammatory reaction. The appearance on blood flow and blood pool images helps to determine if an inflammatory component is present. Gadolinium-enhanced MR imaging has also been shown to help separate inflammatory from noninflammatory arthritis.[78]

Osteochondritis dissecans (Figs. 1-28 and 1-29)

Osteochondritis dissecans is a familiar problem with a predilection for the lateral aspect of the medial femoral condyle

accounting for 75 percent of the cases involving the knee. The articular surfaces of the condyles account for 20 percent of cases, and the patella the remaining 5 percent of cases.[79–81] The etiology is thought to be due to repeated microtrauma associated with focal avascular necrosis.[82,83] CT scanning following contrast injection into the joint and magnetic resonance both allow determination of whether the overlying articular cartilage is intact and whether the bony fragment is loose.[84,85] In those circumstances, where there is a tear of the overlying articular cartilage with synovial fluid interposed between the bony fragment and adjacent native bone, the osteochondritis dissecans fragment will not heal without surgical intervention. TPBS can measure the degree of healing or of progression of osteochondritis dissecans better than they can be determined from the radiographs[86,87] (Drawing II).

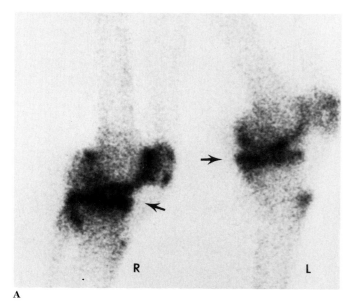

A

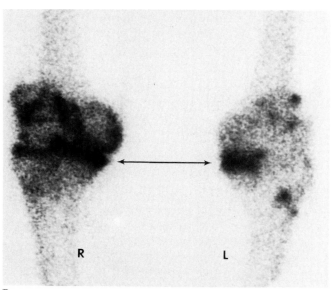

B

Figure 1-27 Bilateral Knee Arthritis in Middle-Aged Patient. **A.** *Medial-lateral views of both knees.* **B.** *Anterior images of both knees. Arrows indicate areas of increased uptake in the juxtaarticular portions of the long bones (femur and tibia) causing obliteration of the joint space. Note that, on the right, there is increased activity in the patella, especially in the patellofemoral space. On the right, the increased activity in the medial, lateral, and patellofemoral region is compatible with tricompartment arthritis. This TPBS allows the clinician to be comfortable in the diagnosis of arthritis rather than occult fracture, spontaneous osteonecrosis, stress fracture, or other more serious knee problem.* (Fig. 1-27C and D continues on the opposite page.)

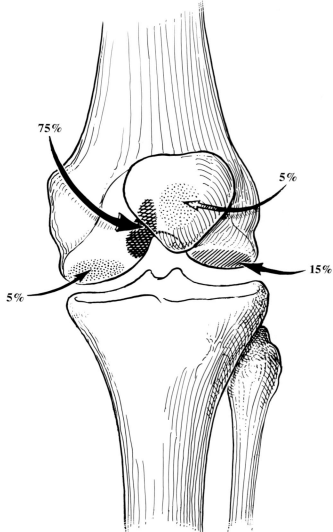

Drawing II *Anterior view of the knee demonstrates the distribution of osteochondritis dissecans: lateral aspect of medial femoral condyle (75 percent), articular surfaces of condyles (20 percent), patella (5 percent).*

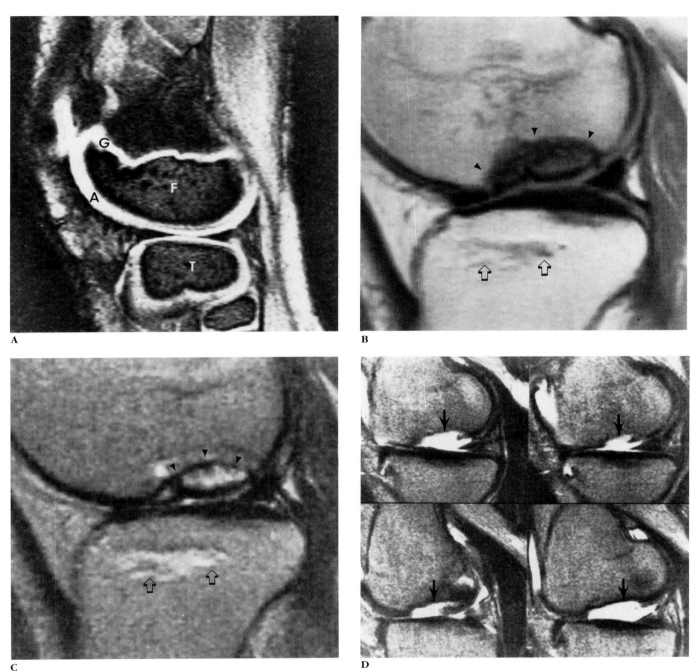

Figure 1-28 Osteochondritis Dissecans. **A.** *Sagittal image at short TR gradient echo sequence shows the normal
cartilaginous structures demonstrating
high-signal intensity. The trabecular
bone and cartilage both appear normal.
G = growth cartilage; A = articular
cartilage; F = distal femoral epiphysis;
T = proximal tibial epiphysis.* **B.** *Healed
osteochondritis dissecans with intact
overlying cartilage. Sagittal image at
T1-weighted sequence shows focal abnormality of the distal articulating surface of the medial femoral condyle representing healed osteochondritis
dissecans. A linear region of intermediate signal intensity within the proximal
portion of tibia represents stress fracture. Arrowheads = healed osteochondritis dissecans fragment; open arrow =
stress fracture.* **C.** *Sagittal image at T2-
weighted sequence through this same
area again shows the healed osteochondritis dissecans with intact overlying cartilage. A linear focus of increased signal
intensity within the proximal portion of
tibia represents a stress fracture. Arrowheads = healed osteochondritis dissecans fragment; open arrow = stress
fracture.* **D.** *Sagittal images at T2-
weighted sequences show a defect in the
distal articulating surface of medial femoral condyle from a displaced fragment
of underlying osteochondritis dissecans.
Arrows = bony defect.*

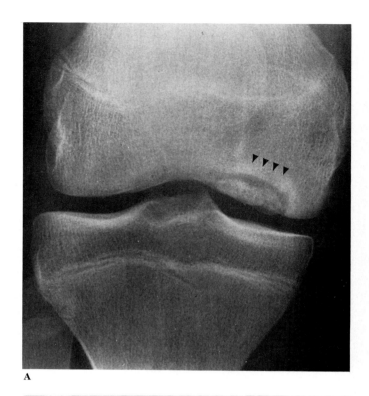

Figure 1-29   Osteochondritis Dissecans of the Right Knee in Adolescent Male Patient.   **A.** *Anteroposterior radiograph of the right knee demonstrates typical appearance of osteochondritis dissecans on the articular surface of the right medial femoral condyle (arrowheads).* **B.** *Delayed high-resolution anterior image of right knee. Arrow shows increased activity in medial aspect of femoral condyle. M = medial; L = lateral.* **C.** *High-resolution delayed lateral image of right knee. Arrow shows increased activity in articular portion of medial femoral condyle anteriorly (corresponding to findings on anterior view). Arrowhead shows mildly increased uptake in the anterior tibial tubercle consistent with the anterior tibial tubercle apophysitis (Osgood-Schlatter disease) probably in a healing phase since it was not identified on blood flow or blood pool images.*

A

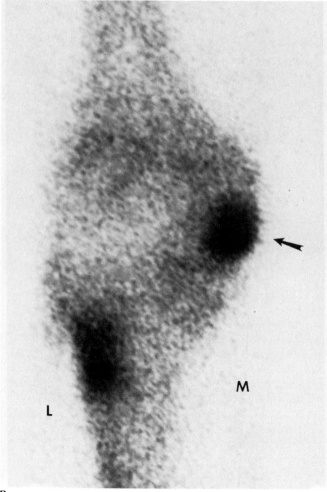

B

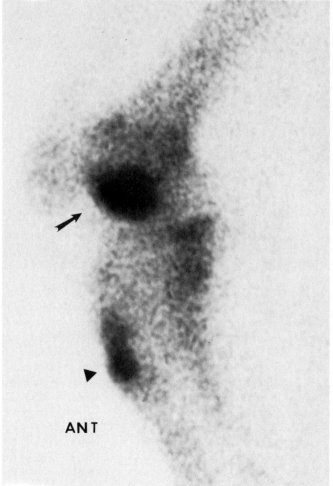

C

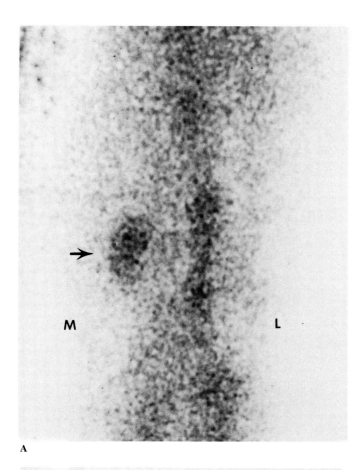

A

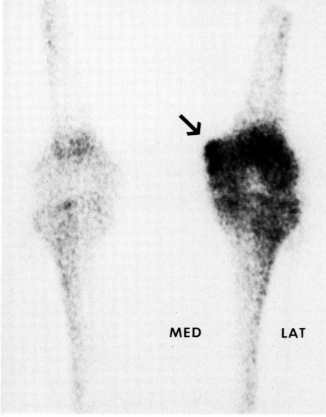

MED   LAT

B

Figure 1-30   Pellegrini-Stieda Syndrome of Left Knee. **A.** *Anterior blood pool image of left knee demonstrates minimal to mildly increased activity in the medial aspect of the knee.* **B.** *High-resolution anterior delayed images of both knees demonstrate asymmetry. Mildly increased uptake on both sides of the left knee joint is seen when compared with the opposite (right) knee. Focal area of increased activity is seen adjacent to the left medial femoral condyle (arrow).* **C.** *Magnified high-resolution delayed anterior image better identifies focal medial activity (arrow) corresponding to the insertion of the medial collateral ligament. M = medial; L = lateral; F = femur; T = tibia.*

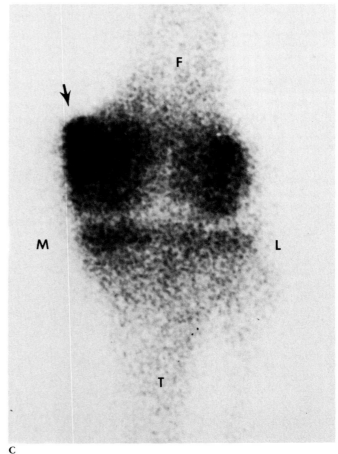

C

Pellegrini-Stieda disease (Fig. 1-30)

Avulsion of the medial collateral ligament of the knee with associated hemorrhage may be followed by ligamentous calcification. On TPBS, an active lesion will show nuclide uptake adjacent to the proximal aspect of the medial femoral condyle reflecting avulsion or tearing at that site.[88] Magnetic resonance scanning is a sensitive tool for visualizing acute tear of the superficial and deep layers of the medial collateral ligament.

Jumper's knee—infrapatellar tendinitis (Fig. 1-31)

Avulsion or strain of the patellar tendon in athletes has been termed *jumper's knee* and was first reported in a volleyball player.[89–90] Magnetic resonance imaging clearly depicts the structure of the patellar ligament. Sprain and mucoid degeneration are characterized by edema, hemorrhage, and tendon swelling. Prepatellar bursitis presents with a focal fluid collection anterior to the patellar tendon. TPBS demonstrates increased activity of the lower pole of the patella in patellar tendinitis.[91–93] The radiograph is usually normal in this condition.

Osgood-Schlatter disease (Fig. 1-32)

Microavulsions off the anterior tibial tubercle are caused by repeated trauma,[81] resulting in localized pain at that site.[94] TPBS shows increased nuclide activity at the anterior tibial tubercle in children between the ages of 10 and 15 years. Other more serious causes of knee pain in adolescents can be excluded (Drawing I). TPBS can also help identify and differentiate the following causes of chronic knee pain: painful bipartite patella[95–97]; reflex sympathetic dystrophy of the knee[67,98]; patellar stress fracture[51–53]; and tibial plateau stress fracture.[54–56]

Figure 1-31   Infrapatellar Tendinitis (Jumper's Knee).
A. *High-resolution delayed lateral image.* **B.** *High-resolution delayed anterior image. Arrow identifies increased activity localized to the inferior pole of the patella consistent with diagnosis of jumper's knee. In a patient with chronic knee pain, this very typical pattern of jumper's knee helps to identify this as the cause of the knee pain. The pattern is distinctly different from other causes of chronic knee pain. M = medial; L = lateral; F = femur; T = tibia.*

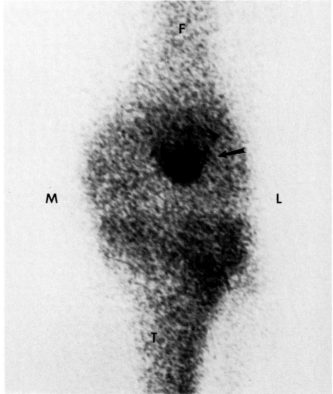

B

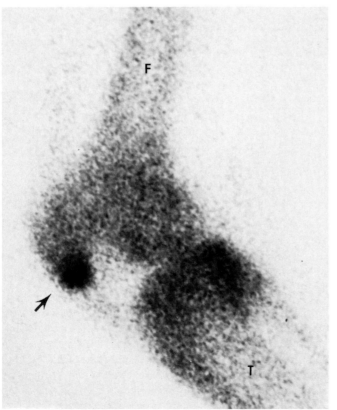

A

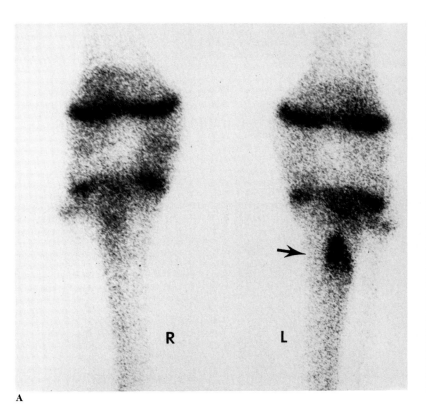

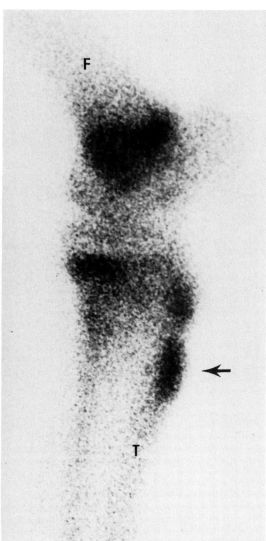

A

B

Figure 1-32 Osgood-Schlatter Disease in Teenage Lacrosse Player/Runner. One Month History of Anterior Knee Pain without Trauma. **A.** *High-resolution de-* *layed anterior images of both knees.* **B.** *High-resolution lateral image of left knee. Focal and asymmetric nuclide ac-* *tivity is noted in the anterior tibial tuber-* *cle of the left knee (arrow) consistent with clinical diagnosis. F = femur; T = tibia.*

Meniscal, capsular, and synovial cysts (Figs. 1-33 to 1-35)

Meniscal, capsular, and synovial cysts[99] frequently present as masses about the knee. Most meniscal cysts are located laterally, although cysts of the medial meniscus also occur. In a large majority of patients, meniscal cysts are associated with horizontal tears of the meniscus.[100] These tears allow the communication of synovial fluid through the meniscus to the periphery where the meniscal cyst develops. Cysts of the joint capsule are usually associated with normal underlying menscii.[101] Cysts of the meniscus, capsule, and synovium can all be identified with magnetic resonance imaging.

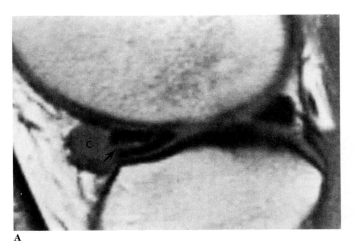

A   B

Figure 1-33   Lateral Meniscal Cyst. **A.** *Sagittal image at T1-weighted sequence demonstrates a horizontal cleft within the anterior horn of the lateral meniscus. A mass of intermediate signal intensity lies adjacent to that cleft.* **B.** *Sagittal MR image at T2-weighted sequence demonstrates high signal within a cyst of the lateral meniscus. The adjacent meniscus is torn. C = cyst; arrow = torn lateral meniscus.*

Figure 1-34   Communicating Capular Cyst. *CT examination of the left knee before (above) and after (below) intraarticular contrast administration shows the accumulation of contrast within a cystic space adjacent to the left medial femoral condyle. This represents a communicating cyst. The right knee is normal. Arrows = unopacified cyst prior to contrast administration; C = opacified cyst after intraarticular injection.*

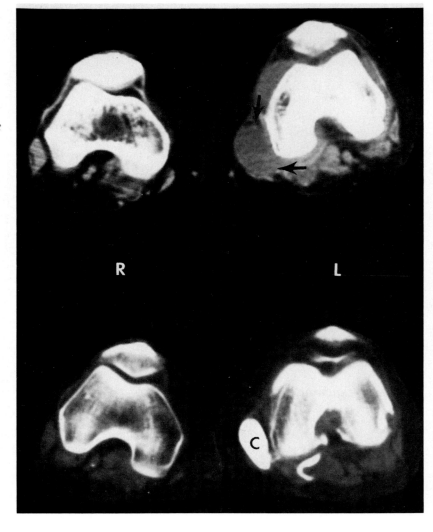

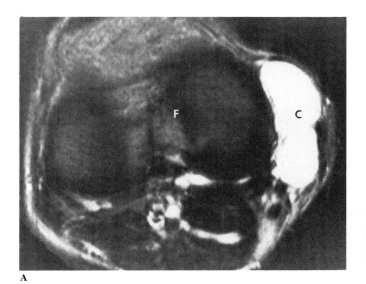

A

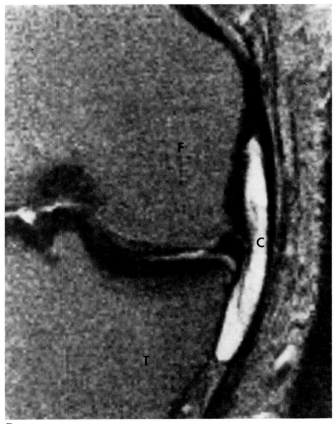

B

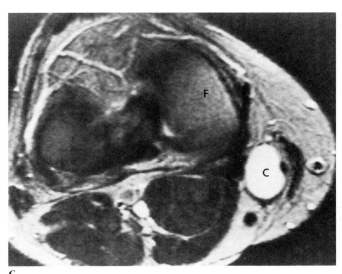

C

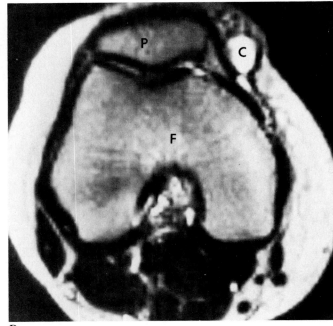

D

Figure 1-35   Noncommunicating Capsule Ganglion.
*A. Axial image at T2-weighted sequence demonstrates a multi-loculated cystic collection originating off the medial joint capsule and projecting superficially. **B.** Coronal MR image at T2-weighted sequence shows fluid collection within the medial collateral ligament from old collateral ligament injury. **C.** Axial MR image at T2-weighted sequence shows homogenous high-signal collection beneath the sartorius muscle representing a cyst. [From Levinsohn EM: MR imaging of extremities excels in knee evaluation, Diagnostic Imaging 11(5):103, 1989. Reproduced with permission.] **D.** Axial MR image at T2-weighted sequence shows a cyst originating from the superficial aspect of the medial patellar retinaculum. C = cyst; P = patella; F = femur; T = tibia.*

Discoid meniscus (Fig. 1-36)

This entity most frequently causes painful snapping in a young child. The characteristic appearance on magnetic resonance scanning is of a thickened and widened meniscus in both the sagittal and coronal planes,[102] producing the characteristic ''bow tie'' appearance on sequential images.

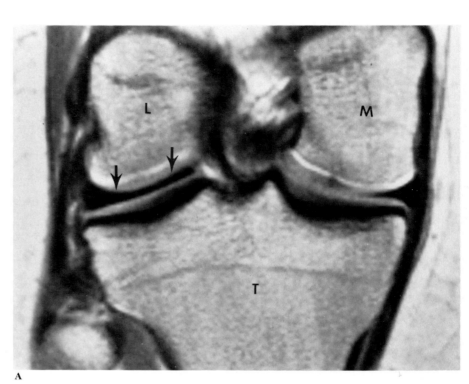

Figure 1-36   Discoid Lateral Meniscus. **A.** *Coronal image at proton density sequence demonstrates elongation of the lateral meniscus centrally with loss of the usual triangular appearance. This appearance, if present across the meniscus from front to back and from side to side, is characteristic for discoid meniscus. The medial meniscus is normal.* **B.** *Sagittal image at proton density sequence demonstrates a ''bow tie'' appearance to the lateral meniscus characteristic for discoid meniscal abnormality. L = lateral femoral condyle; M = medial femoral condyle; arrows = discoid lateral meniscus; T = tibia.*

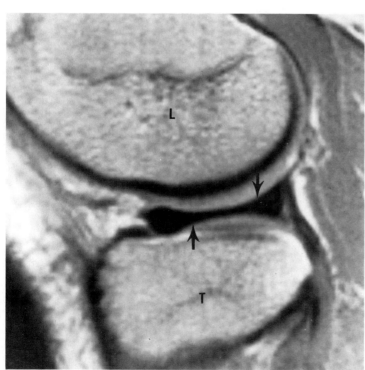

Additional pathologic entities (Figs. 1-37 to 1-40)

Magnetic resonance imaging and, to a lesser extent, CT are useful in the following additional conditions which cause chronic knee pain: popliteal cyst (Figs. 1-37 and 1-38); infrapatellar fat pad abnormality (Fig. 1-39); plica syndrome[103-105] (Fig. 1-40); pigmented villonodular synovitis[106-108]; meniscal evaluation following partial meniscectomy[109]; and meniscal evaluation following conservative management for tear.[110] CT and/or fluoroscopic examination may be necessary to visualize and identify intraarticular loose bodies.[111,112]

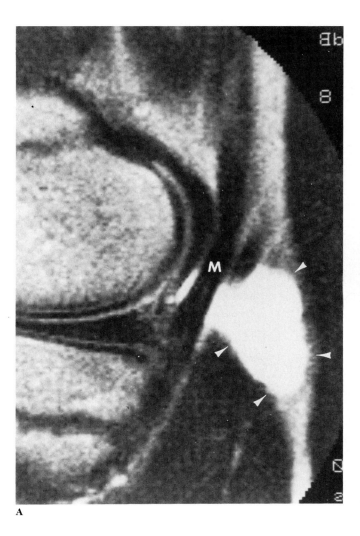

A

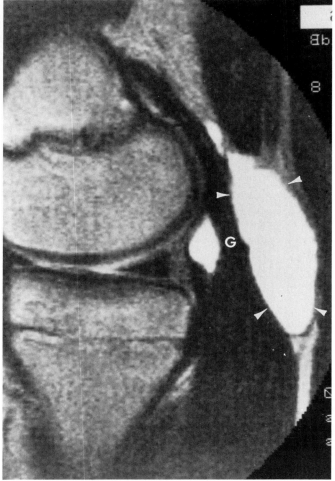

B

Figure 1-37 Popliteal Cyst. **A.** *Sagittal image through the medial aspect of the knee at T2-weighted sequence show a high signal collection projected around the semimembranosus tendon.* **B.** *At a slightly more central level, a sagittal image demonstrates high signal representing fluid within a popliteal cyst projected adjacent to the gastrocnemius tendon. These features are characteristic for a popliteal cyst. Arrowheads = popliteal cyst; M = semimembranosus tendon; G = gastrocnemius tendon.*

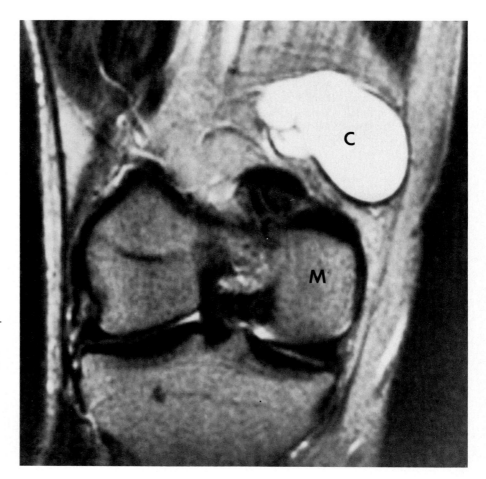

Figure 1-38 Atypical Popliteal Cyst. *Coronal image at T1-weighted sequence demonstrates a cystic collection proximal to the medial femoral condyle. This represents a popliteal cyst which is dissecting proximally rather than distally. C = popliteal cyst; M = medial femoral condyle.*

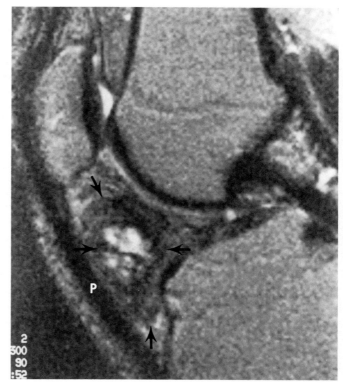

Figure 1-39 Fat Pad Abnormality. *Sagittal MR image at T2-weighted sequence shows a mixed signal pattern within the normally homogeneous infrapatellar fat pad. This represents hemorrhage with fluid and hemosiderin from previous fat pad injury. Arrows = abnormality within fat pad; P = patellar tendon.*

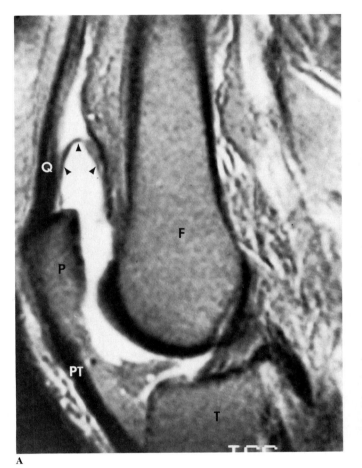

A

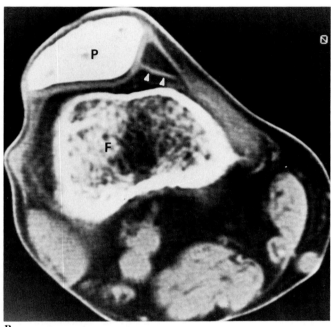

B

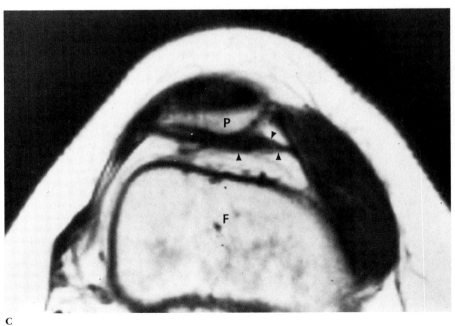

C

Figure 1-40 Plica. **A.** *Sagittal image at T2-weighted sequence through the medial aspect of the knee demonstrates fluid within the suprapatellar bursa. An arcuate structure represents normal suprapatellar plica.* **B.** *CT scan at the level of the distal metaphysis of the femur shows a normal plica.* **C.** *Axial scan at T1-weighted sequence shows thickened plica consistent with plica syndrome. Q = quadriceps tendon; PT = patellar tendon; F = femur; T = tibia; P = patella; arrowheads = plica.*

DIAGNOSTIC PROBLEMS

In the evaluation of the athlete complaining of pain about the knee, it is important to remember that primary disease not related to athletics may be the culprit. The knee is the single most common area in the body for the development of malignant bone tumors. Soft tissue tumors, arthritis, and neurovascular abnormalities should be considered in those individuals with atypical presentation or failure to respond to management (Figs. 1-41 to 1-44).

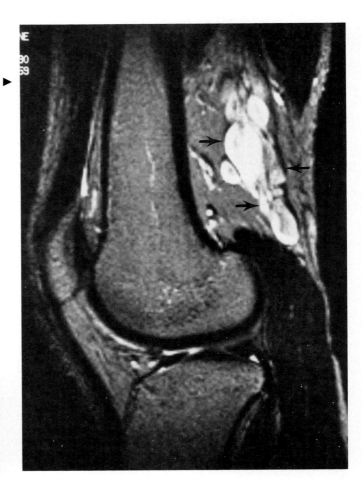

Figure 1-41   Neurofibromatosis. *Sagittal image at T2-weighted sequence shows a lumpy area of high-signal intensity (arrows) posterior to the distal femoral metaphysis representing plexiform neurofibromas.* ▶

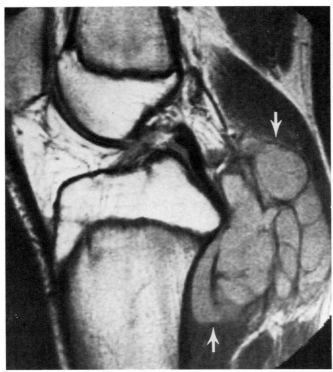

◀ **Figure 1-42**   Synovial Sarcoma. *Sagittal MR image at T1-weighted sequence through the midportion of the knee demonstrates multiloculated structure (arrows) with intermediate signal intensity behind the knee. Although the appearance of this closely resembles popliteal cyst, biopsy showed it to be synovial sarcoma. The signal inhomogeneity should arouse concern that a tumor is present.*

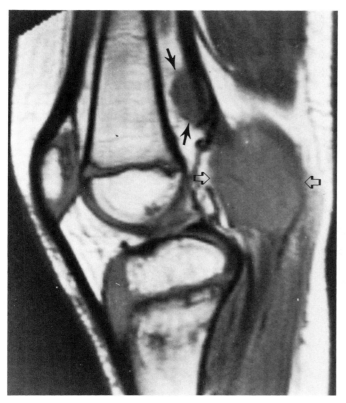

Figure 1-43   Recurrent Rhabdomyosarcoma. *Sagittal image at T1-weighted sequence through the knee demonstrates soft tissue mass posterior to the joint representing tumor. The appearance is quite different from popliteal cyst. No joint effusion is present. Also noted is an enlarged popliteal lymph node. Open arrow = neoplasm; arrows = lymph node.*

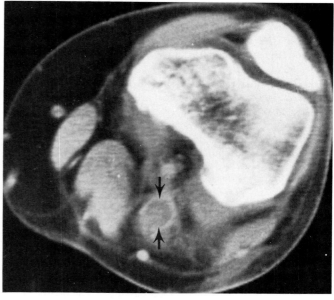

Figure 1-44   Thrombophlebitis. *Axial CT scan at the level of the distal femur after intravenous contrast injection shows a radiolucent structure with peripheral contrast enhancement characteristic for thrombophlebitis. Arrows = lucent thrombus.*

REFERENCES

1. Crues JV III, Ryu R: MRI of the knee: part I. Appl Radiol 19(7):18–24, 1990.
2. Gallimore GW Jr., Harms SE: Knee injuries: high-resolution MR imaging. Radiology 160:457–461, 1986.
3. Ghelman B: Meniscal tears of the knee: evaluation by high-resolution CT combined with arthrography. Radiology 157:23–27, 1985.
4. Manco LG, Kavanaugh JH, Fay JJ, Bilfield BS: Meniscus tears of the knee: prospective evaluation with CT. Radiology 159:147–151, 1986.
5. Mink JH, Deutsch AL: Magnetic resonance imaging of the knee. Clin Orthop 244:29–47, 1989.
6. Passariello R, Trecco F, de Paulis F, et al.: Meniscal lesions of the knee joint: CT diagnosis. Radiology 157:29–34, 1985.
7. Reicher MA, Bassett LW, Gold RH: High-resolution magnetic resonance imaging of the knee joint: pathologic correlations. AJR 145:903–909, 1985.
8. Reicher MA, Rauschning W, Gold RH, et al.: High-resolution magnetic resonance imaging of the knee joint: normal anatomy. AJR 145:895–902, 1985.
9. Levinsohn EM: MR imaging of extremities excels in knee evaluation. Diagn Imaging 11(5):100–104, 1989.
10. Mink JH, Reicher MA, Crues JV III, Fox JM: *Magnetic Resonance Imaging of the Knee*. Raven Press, New York, 1987.
11. Munk PL, Helms CA, Genant HK, Hold RG: Magnetic resonance imaging of the knee: current status, new directions. Skeletal Radiol 18:569–577, 1989.
12. Manco LG, Berlow ME, Czajka J, Alfred R: Bucket-handle tears of the meniscus: appearance at CT. Radiology 168:709–712,1988.
13. Selby B, Richardson ML, Montana MA, et al.: High resolution sonography of the menisci of the knee. Invest Radiol 21:332–335, 1986.

14. Mooar P, Gregg J, Jacobstein J: Radionuclide imaging in internal derangements of the knee. Am J Sports Med 15:132–137, 1987.
15. Collier BD, Johnson RP. Carrera GF, et al.: Chronic knee pain assessed by SPECT: comparison with other modalities. Radiology 157:795, 802, 1985.
16. Mesgarzadeh M, Schneck CD, Bonakdarpour A: Magnetic resonance imaging of the knee and correlation with normal anatomy. Radiographics 8:707–733, 1988.
17. De Smet AA: Meniscal tears on knee arthrography: patterns of arthrographic abnormalities. Skeletal Radiol 14:280–285, 1985.
18. Dumas JM, Edde DJ: Meniscal abnormalities: prospective correlation of double-contrast arthrography and arthroscopy. Radiology 160:453–456, 1986.
19. Glashow JL, Katz R, Schneider M, Scott WN: Double-blind assessment of the value of magnetic resonance imaging in the diagnosis of anterior cruciate and meniscal lesions. J Bone Joint Surg 71(A):113–119, 1989.
20. Gundry CR, Schils JP, Resnick D, Sartoris DJ: Arthrography of the post-traumatic knee, shoulder, and wrist: current status and future trends. Radiol Clin North Am 27:957–971, 1989.
21. Langer JE, Meyer SJF, Dalinka MK: Imaging of the knee. Radiol Clin North Am 28:975–990, 1990.
22. Levinsohn EM, Baker BE: Prearthrotomy diagnostic evaluation of the knee: review of 100 cases diagnosed by arthrography and arthroscopy. AJR 134:107–111, 1980.
23. Manco LG, Berlow ME: Meniscal tears—comparison of arthrography, CT and MRI. Crit Rev Diagn Imaging 29:151–179, 1989.
24. Selesnick FH, Noble HB, Bachman DC, Steinberg FL: Internal derangement of the knee: diagnosis by arthrography, arthroscopy, and arthrotomy. Clin Orthop 198:26–30, 1985.
25. Suman RK, Stother IG, Illingworth G: Diagnostic arthroscopy of the knee in children. J Bone Joint Surg 66(B):535–537, 1984.
26. Tegtmeyer CJ, McCue FC III, Higgins SM, Ball DW: Arthrography of the knee: a comparative study of the accuracy of single and double contrast techniques. Radiology 132:37–41, 1979.
27. Thijn CJP: Accuracy of double-contrast arthrography and arthroscopy of the knee joint. Skeletal Radiol 8:187–192, 1982.
28. Vahey TN, Bennett HT, Arrington LE, Shelbourne KD: MR imaging of the knee: pseudotear of the lateral meniscus caused by the meniscofemoral ligament. AJR 154:1237–1239, 1990.
29. Watanabe AT, Carter BC, Teitelbaum GP, et al.: Normal variations in MR imaging of the knee: appearance and frequency. AJR 153:341–344, 1989.
30. Kornick J, Trefelner E, McCarthy S, et al.: Meniscal abnormalities in the asymptomatic population at MR imaging. Radiology 177:463–465, 1990.
31. Kursunoglu-Brahme S, Schwaighofer B, Gundry C, et al.: Jogging causes acute changes in the knee joint: an MR study in normal volunteers. AJR 154:1233–1235, 1990.
32. Hajek PC, Gylys-Morin VM, Baker LL, et al.: The high signal intensity meniscus of the knee: magnetic resonance evaluation and in vivo correlation. Invest Radiol 22:883–890, 1987.
33. Stoller DW, Martin C, Crues JV III, et al.: Meniscal tears: pathologic correlation with MR imaging. Radiology 163:731–735, 1987.

34. Grover JS, Bassett LW, Gross ML, et al.: Posterior cruciate ligament: MR imaging. Radiology 174:527–530, 1990.
35. Bassett LW, Grover JS, Seeger LL: Magnetic resonance imaging of knee trauma. Skeletal Radiol 19:401–405, 1990.
36. Turner DA, Prodromos CC, Petasnick JP, Clark JW: Acute injury of the ligaments of the knee: magnetic resonance evaluation. Radiology 154:717–722, 1985.
37. Lee JK, Yao L, Phelps CT, et al.: Anterior cruciate ligament tears: MR imaging compared with arthroscopy and clinical tests. Radiology 166:861–864, 1988.
38. Bodne D, Quinn SF, Murray WT, et al.: Magnetic resonance images of chronic patellar tendinitis. Skeletal Radiol 17:24–28, 1988.
39. King JB, Perry DJ, Mourad K, Kumar SJ: Lesions of the patellar ligament. J Bone Joint Surg 72(B):46–48, 1990.
40. Matin P: Basic principles of nuclear medicine techniques for detection and evaluation of trauma and sports medicine injuries. Semin Nucl Med 18:90–112, 1988.
41. Matin PM: Appearance of bone scans following fractures including immediate and long term studies. J Nucl Med 20:1227–1231, 1979.
42. Matin PM: Bone scintigraphy in the diagnosis and management of traumatic injury. Semin Nucl Med 13:104–122, 1983.
43. Wahner HW: Radionuclides in the diagnosis of fracture healing. J Nucl Med 19:1356–1358, 1978.
44. Crues JV III, Lynch TCP: MR effective in detecting traumatic bone injuries. Diag Imaging 12(10):118–121, 1990.
45. Lynch TCP, Crues JV III, Morgan FW, et al: Bone abnormalities of the knee: prevalence and significance at MR imaging. Radiology 171:761–766, 1989.
46. Mink JH, Deutsch AL: Occult cartilage and bone injuries of the knee: detection, classification, and assessment with MR imaging. Radiology 170:823–829, 1989.
47. Martire JR: The role of nuclear medicine scans in evaluating pain in athletic injuries. Clin Sports Med 6:713–737, 1987.
48. Heckman JD, Alkire CC: Distal patellar pole fractures. Am J Sports Med 12:424–428, 1984.
49. Holder LE, Matthews LS: The nuclear physician and sports medicine, in Freeman L and Weissman H (eds): *Nuclear Medicine Annual 1984.* Raven Press, New York, 1984, pp 88–140.
50. Shelbourne KD, Fisher DA, Rettig AC, et al.: Stress fractures of the medial malleolus. Am J Sports Med 16:60–63, 1988.
51. Devas MB: Stress fractures of the patella. J Bone Joint Surg 42(B):71–74, 1960.
52. Dickason JM, Fox JM: Fracture of the patella due to overuse syndrome in a child—a case report. Am J Sports Med 10:248–249, 1982.
53. Iwaya T, Takatori Y: Lateral longitudinal stress fracture of the patella. Report of three cases. J Pediatr Orthop 5:73–75, 1985.
54. Engber WB: Stress fractures of the medial tibial plateau. J Bone Joint Surg 59(A):767–769, 1977.
55. Harolds JA: Fatigue fracture of the medial tibial plateau. South Med J 74:578–581, 1981.
56. Manco LG, Schneider R, Pavlov H: Insufficiency fractures of the tibial plateau. AJR 140:1211–1215, 1983.
57. Yao L, Lee JK: Avulsion of the posteromedial tibial plateau by the semimembranosus tendon: diagnosis with MR imaging. Radiology 172:513–514, 1989.

58. Nicholas JA, Friedman MJ: Orthopedic problems in middle-aged athletes. Phys Sports Med 7(12):53–64, 1979.

59. Ahuja SC, Bullough PG: Osteonecrosis of the knee. A clinicopathological study in 28 patients. J Bone Joint Surg 60(A):191–197, 1978.

60. Solomon L: Mechanisms of idiopathic osteonecrosis. Orthop Clin North Am 16:655–657, 1985.

61. Daffner RH, Martinez S, Gehweiler JA: Stress fractures in runners. JAMA 247:1039–1041, 1982.

62. Greyson ND, Lotem NM, Gross AE, et al.: Radionuclide evaluation of spontaneous femoral osteonecrosis. Radiology 142:729–735, 1982.

63. Bjorkengren AG, AlRowaih A, Lindstrand A, et al: Spontaneous osteonecrosis of the knee: value of MR imaging in determining prognosis. AJR 154:331–335, 1990.

64. Pollack MS, Dalinka MK, Kressel HY, et al.: Magnetic resonance imaging in the evaluation of suspected osteonecrosis of the knee. Skeletal Radiol 16:121–127, 1987.

65. Lotke PA, Ecker ML, Alavi A: Painful knees in older patients. Radionuclide diagnosis of possible osteonecrosis with spontaneous resolution. J Bone Joint Surg 59(A):617–621, 1977.

66. Goodfellow J, Hungerford DS, Zindel M: Patello-femoral joint mechanics and pathology. J Bone Joint Surg 58(B):287–290, 1976.

67. Hungerford DS, Barry M: Biomechanics of the patello-femoral joint. Clin Orthop 144:9–15, 1979.

68. Insall J: Patellar pain. J Bone Joint Surg 64(A):147–152, 1982.

69. Percy EC, Strother RT. Patellalgia. Phys Sports Med 13(7):43–59, 1985.

70. Dye SF, Boll DA: Radionuclide imaging of the patello-femoral joint in young adults with anterior knee pain. Orthop Clin North Am 17:249–262, 1985.

71. Fulkerson JP: The etiology of patellofemoral pain in young active patients: a prospective study. Clin Orthop 179:129–133, 1983.

72. Hayes CW, Sawyer RW, Conway WF: Patellar cartilage lesions: in vitro detection and staging with MR imaging and pathologic correlation. Radiology 176:479–583, 1990.

73. Boven F, Bellemans MA, Geurts J, et al.: The value of computed tomography scanning in chondromalacia patellae. Skeletal Radiol 8:183–185, 1982.

74. Delgado-Martins H: A study of the position of the patella using computerised tomography. J Bone Joint Surg 61(B):443–444, 1979.

75. Ihara H: Double-contrast CT arthrography of the cartilage of the patellofemoral joint. Clin Orthop 198:50–55, 1985.

76. Shellock FG, Mink JH, Deutsch AL, Fox JM: Patellar tracking abnormalities: clinical experience with kinematic MR imaging in 130 patients. Radiology 172:799–804, 1989.

77. Yulish BS, Montanez J, Goodfellow DB, et al.: Chondromalacia patellae: assessment with MR imaging. Radiology 164:763–766, 1987.

78. Reiser MF, Bongarts GP, Eriemann R, et al.: Gadolinium-DTPA in rheumatoid arthritis and related diseases: first results with dynamic magnetic resonance imaging. Skeletal Radiol 18:591–597, 1989.

79. DiStefano VJ: How I manage osteochondritis dissecans. Phys Sports Med 14(2):135–142, 1986.

80. Gray WJ, Bassett FH: Osteochondritis dissecans of the patella in a competitive fencer. Orthop Rev 1(19):96–98, 1990.

81. Ogden JA, Southwick WD. Osgood-Schlatter's disease and tibial tuberosity development. Clin Orthop 116:180–189, 1976.

82. Mubarak S, Carroll N: Juvenile osteochondritis dissecans of the knee. Clin Orthop 157:200–211, 1981.

83. Steiner ME, Grana WA: The young athlete's knee: recent advances. Clin Sports Med 3:527–546, 1988.

84. De Smet AA, Fisher DR, Graf BK, Lange RH: Osteochondritis dissecans of the knee: value of MR imaging in determining lesion stability and the presence of articular cartilage defects. AJR 155:549–553, 1990.

85. Gilley JS, Gelman MI, Edson DM, Metcalf RW: Chondral fractures of the knee. Radiology 138:51–54, 1981.

86. Cahill BR, Berg BC: 99m-technetium phosphate compound joint scintigraphy in the management of juvenile osteochondritis dissecans of the femoral condyles. Am J Sports Med 11:329–335, 1983.

87. D'Ambrosia RD, Shoji H, Riggins RS, et al.: Scintigraphy in the diagnosis of osteonecrosis. Clin Orthop 130:139–143, 1978.

88. Tehranzadeh J, Serafini AN, Pais MJ: *Avulsion and Stress Injuries of the Musculoskeletal System.* Karger, Basel, 1989.

89. Blazina ME, Kerlin RK, Jobe FW, et al.: Jumper's knee. Orthop Clin North Am 4:665–678, 1973.

90. Maurizio E: La Tendinite rotulea del giocatore di pallavolo. Arch Soc Tosco Umbra Chir 24:443–452, 1963.

91. Ferretti A, Ippolito E, Mariani P, et al.: Jumper's knee. Am J Sports Med 11:58–62, 1983.

92. Kahn D, Wilson MA: Bone scintigraphic findings in patellar tendinitis. J Nucl Med 28:1768–1770, 1987.

93. Roels J, Martens M, Mulier JC, et al.: Patellar tendinitis (jumper's knee). Am J Sports Med 6:362–368, 1978.

94. Baker BE: Current concepts in the diagnosis and treatment of musculotendinous injuries. Med Sci Sports Exerc 16:323–327, 1984.

95. Green WT: Painful bipartite patella. Clin Orthop 110:197–200, 1975.

96. Ogden JA, McCarthy SM, Jokl P: The painful bipartite patella. J Pediatr Orthop 2:263–269, 1982.

97. Weaver JK: Bipartite patella as a case of disability in the athlete. Am J Sports Med 5:137–143, 1977.

98. Rupani HD, Holder LE, Espinola DA, et al.: Three phase radionuclide bone imaging in sports medicine. Radiology 156:187–196, 1985.

99. Schwimmer M, Edelstein G, Heiken JP, Gilula LA: Synovial cysts of the knee: CT evaluation. Radiology 154:175–177, 1985.

100. Coral A, van Holsbeeck M, Adler RS: Imaging of meniscal cyst of the knee in three cases. Skeletal Radiol 18:451–455, 1989.

101. Burk DL Jr., Dalinka MK, Kanal E, et al.: Meniscal and ganglion cysts of the knee: MR evaluation. AJR 150:331–336, 1988.

102. Silverman JM, Mink JH, Deutsch AL: Discoid menisci of the knee: MR imaging appearance. Radiology 173:351–354, 1989.

103. Aprin H, Shapiro J, Gershwind M: Arthrography (plica views): a noninvasive method for diagnosis and prognosis of plica syndrome. Clin Orthop 183:90–95, 1984.

104. Kinnard P, Levesque RY: The plica syndrome: a syndrome of controversy. Clin Orthop 183:141–143, 1984.

105. Thijn CJP, Hillen B: Arthrography and the medial compartment of the patello-femoral joint. Skeletal Radiol 11:183–190, 1984.

106. Jelinek JS, Kransdorf MJ, Utz JA, et al.: Imaging of pigmented villonodular synovitis with emphasis on MR imaging. AJR 152:337–342, 1989.

107. Kottal RA, Vogler JB III, Matamoros A, et al.: Pigmented villonodular synovitis: a report of MR imaging in two cases. Radiology 163:551–553, 1987.

108. Mandelbaum BR, Grant TT, Hartzman S, et al.: The use of MRI to assist in diagnosis of pigmented villonodular synovitis of the knee joint. Clin Orthop 231:135–139, 1988.

109. Smith DK, Totty WG: The knee after partial meniscectomy: MR imaging features. Radiology 176:141–144, 1990.

110. Deutsch AL, Mink JH, Fox JM, et al.: Peripheral meniscal tears: MR findings after conservative treatment or arthroscopic repair. Radiology 176:485–488, 1990.

111. Hudson TM: Joint fluoroscopy before arthrography: detection and evaluation of loose bodies. Skeletal Radiol 12:199–203, 1984.

112. Sartoris DJ, Kursunoglu S, Pineda C, et al: Detection of intra-articular osteochondral bodies in the knee using computed arthrotomography. Radiology 155:447–450, 1985.

Orthopedic overview

The development of diagnostic imaging in the lower extremity has grown immensely over the past 15 years through advances made in triple-phase bone scanning (TPBS), computed tomography (CT), and magnetic resonance imaging (MRI). These tools have enhanced our ability to accurately and rapidly diagnose a multiplicity of lower extremity injuries. By utilizing these noninvasive modalities, an early diagnosis can be made, minimizing the time lost by the highly competitive athlete from training and competition.

As the population of North America has increasingly pursued both recreational and competitive athletics, the incidence of overuse syndromes in the lower extremity has changed markedly. Since the initial description of lower leg stress fracture in the late 1930s until the present time, there has been a dramatic increase in overuse syndromes of the lower extremity, reflecting the generalized increase in participation in athletic activities.

In my experience as a team physician at professional, college, high school and recreational levels, I derive significant helpful information from TPBS. This imaging modality gives a physiologic, or "dynamic," perspective of lower extremity stress injury in contradistinction to the "static" image provided by the radiograph. Plain roentgenography provides us with a "snapshot" view of pathologic processes. TPBS, on the other hand, provides a metabolically oriented image of the overused extremity. The ability of TPBS to help us to visualize the spectrum of stress injury, from bone remodeling to fracture, as well as to separate shin splints from stress fracture has been enlightening and clinically valuable. Overall, TPBS provides for the team physician information regarding site of stress injury, degree of bony metabolic activity, and estimate of chronicity of injury. This adds tremendously to our diagnostic acumen. Armed with this information, the physician can more accurately identify the serious stress injuries and prescribe treatment and activity accordingly.

The addition of CT and MRI to our imaging armamentarium provides significant helpful information in the evaluation of lower extremity injuries. The ability of MRI to demonstrate soft tissue structures with high contrast as well as the ability of conventional and three-dimensional computed tomography to depict bony detail and soft tissue calcification have been very helpful. The shape, size, and content of soft tissue masses and their relationship to adjacent osseous and neurovascular structures are important information obtainable with CT and MRI.

Finally, the advent of conventional ultrasound and of Doppler sonography can help the team physician to diagnose unusual soft tissue injury or swelling not responsive to routine therapy. These noninvasive techniques can help quickly establish the diagnosis of fluid collection in the lower leg, distinguishing that entity from ruptured popliteal cyst, hematoma, or post-operative abscess, when symptoms simulating compartment syndrome are present.

This chapter reviews the spectrum of sports-related injuries to the lower extremity. These range from direct trauma to overuse syndromes and include

CHAPTER 2

LOWER LEG

shin splints, stress fracture, and myositis ossificans. Differential considerations are presented which include bone cyst, fibrous cortical defect, and osteoid osteoma. In the vigorous athlete with a painful lower extremity, the diagnosis of these lesions often requires advanced imaging techniques which are available in the modern sports medicine center and the orthopedic hospital. The relative advantages of these modalities and the findings that they display in the spectrum of athletic injuries are presented.

KENNETH GERTSEN, M.D.
Director, Towson Sports Medicine Center, Towson, Maryland
Team Physician, Towson State University and Loyola University
Clinical Instructor, Orthopedic Surgery, The Johns Hopkins School of Medicine
Baltimore, Maryland

THE MOST COMMON utilization of triple-phase bone scanning (TPBS) involves sports injuries of the lower leg. This is due to the frequency of overuse problems usually associated with running. The ability of TPBS to simultaneously yield information about bones and soft tissue makes it the most versatile imaging tool for this region[1-5] (Fig. 2-1).

Sonography is gaining popularity and acceptance in the lower leg as a valuable imaging tool for assessing both acute and chronic soft tissue abnormality.[6-8] Computed tomography (CT) and magnetic resonance imaging (MRI) are both called upon for those diagnostic entities that require superior anatomic detail and multiplanar capability.[9-12] The broad spectrum of "sports tumors" found in the lower leg adds to the diagnostic challenge facing clinicians and radiologists.[13]

ACUTE PROBLEMS

Soft tissue injuries

Acute and subacute lower leg soft tissue injuries invariably present with pain, swelling, and negative radiographs. The diagnostic spectrum includes deep venous thrombosis, compartment syndrome, posttraumatic ossification, abscess, hematoma, and popliteal cyst. In addition to that which may be seen on the plain film, ultrasound, TPBS, CT, and MRI each offers unique information in the assessment of soft tissue abnormalities in this region.[2,7,14,15]

Plain films are of limited value in soft tissue evaluation because of the intrinsic low contrast they provide. They should, however, be performed prior to other imaging tests to exclude bony abnormality or soft tissue calcification. CT and MR provide information on soft tissue masses and their relationship to adjacent osseous and neurovascular structures.[16] MR, however, is the best tool available to visualize soft tissue masses.[17] Its intrinsic high contrast and multi-

planar capability are unsurpassed.[18,19] Sonography is useful to characterize lesions by distinguishing cystic masses from solid masses. Doppler is most useful in assessing venous and arterial flow and in demonstrating possible deep venous thrombosis and arterial abnormality.

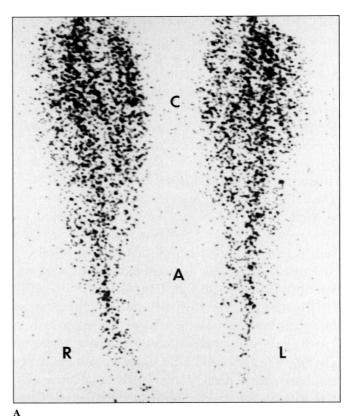

A

Figure 2-1   Normal. **A.** *Anterior blood flow image showing symmetric blood flow to the lower leg most prominent in the muscular calves. C = calf; A = ankle. (Fig. 2-1B and C continues on the opposite page.)*

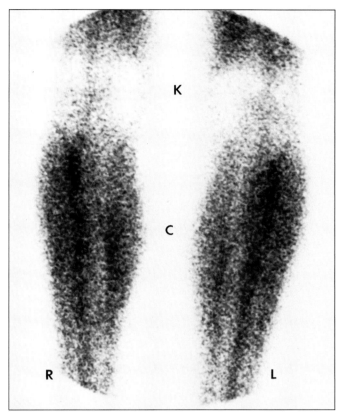

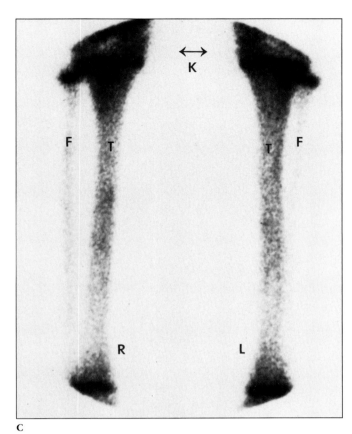

Figure 2-1 Normal (Continued).
B. *Anterior blood pool image of lower legs. Relative hypovascularity is noted in the knee region owing to the patella and knee joint. Predominance of blood pool uptake is in the large muscles. K = knee; C = calf.* **C.** *High-resolution delayed anterior view of lower leg. Predominance of uptake is always in the shaft of the tibia. In many patients, the activity in the fibula is minimal to barely perceptible. In this adolescent, increased activity (linear/horizontal uptake) is noted in the epiphyses of the proximal and distal portions of the long bones. K = knee; F = fibula; T = tibia.*

Myositis ossificans/interosseous membrane calcification (Figs. 2-2 to 2-5)

Severe muscle/tissue contusion or rotational injury of the lower leg can lead to bleeding and swelling followed by abnormal calcification or ectopic ossification.

Pain comes from the initial swelling and bleeding. Later, the calcified mass causes pain by direct mechanical irritation or increased compartment pressure. CT accurately demonstrates the margins and extent of the myositis ossificans.[11,20] The TPBS will reveal the hyperemia of the lesion, reflecting the metabolic state of the heterotopic bone formation, i.e., the degree of metabolic activity present.[21] This is critical, since any contemplated excision of a calcified mass should be done only with mature, or nonactive, lesions as determined by TPBS[22,23] (Fig. 2-2).

Severe ankle injuries can result in rotational forces tearing the interosseous membrane, which is located between the tibia and fibula. The resulting swelling and ectopic calcification can be a diagnostic problem unless one waits weeks or months for the calcification to become evident on radiographs. TPBS displays the characteristic flame-shaped area of nuclide uptake corresponding to the injured interosseous membrane[2] (Figs. 2-3 and 2-4). CT demonstrates the extent of exuberant new bone formation within the region of the interosseous membrane. The identification of this calcification allows separation of interosseous membrane injury from intramedullary disease[24] (Fig. 2-5). Severe or recurrent injuries of the interosseous membrane can eventually lead to bony tibiofibular synostosis[25] (Drawing I).

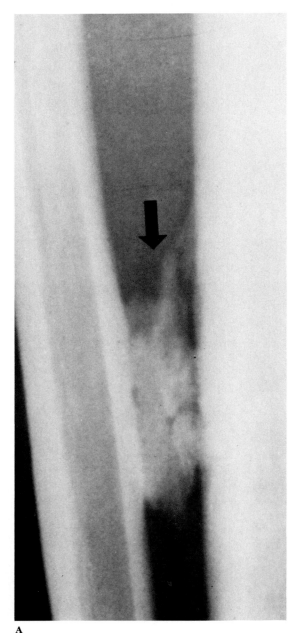

A

Figure 2-2 Myositis Ossificans. **A.** *Coned-down view of the lower leg shows calcification in muscles of the midcalf consistent with myositis ossificans. Arrows = muscle calcification.* **B.** *Anterior view of lower leg during blood pool phase of TPBS shows intense focus of activity in the area of myositis ossificans indicating that calcification is still metabolically active and not yet mature. Arrow = myositis ossificans uptake. (From Martire JR: The role of nuclear medicine scans in evaluating pain in athletic injuries.* Clinics in Sports Medicine *6:713–737, 1987. Reproduced with permission.)*

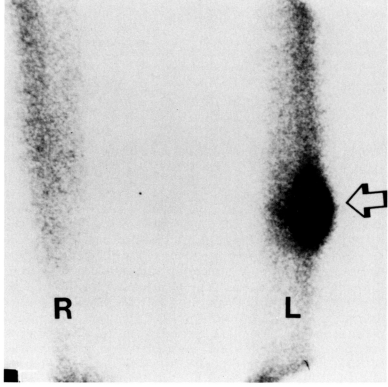

B

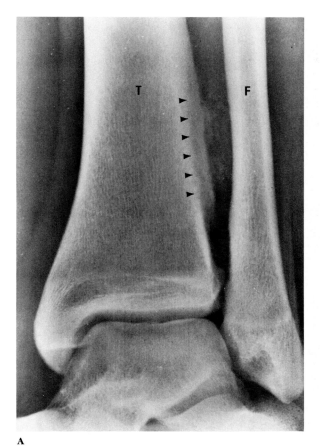

A

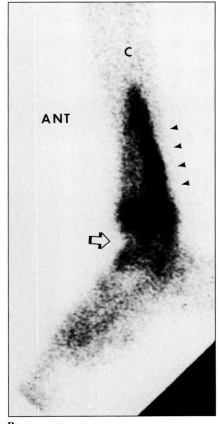

B

C

Figure 2-3 Interosseous Membrane Calcification.
A. *Coned-down mortise view of the ankle shows faint
calcification between the distal tibia and fibula
consistent with ossification of the interosseous
membrane following hemorrhage. Arrowheads =
calcification; T = tibia; F = fibula.* **B.** *High-
resolution delayed lateral image of lower leg/ankle
shows increased nuclide activity in the lower leg
corresponding to the area of interosseous membrane
calcification. C = calf; arrowheads = nuclide uptake
in calcification; open arrow = ankle.* **C.** *High-
resolution delayed anterior image of lower leg and
ankle. Linear/vertical nuclide activity between tibia
and fibula corresponds to interosseous membrane
calcification. Note the characteristic tapered or flame-
shaped appearance seen in this entity. C = calf;
arrowheads = nuclide uptake in calcification; open
arrow = ankle.*

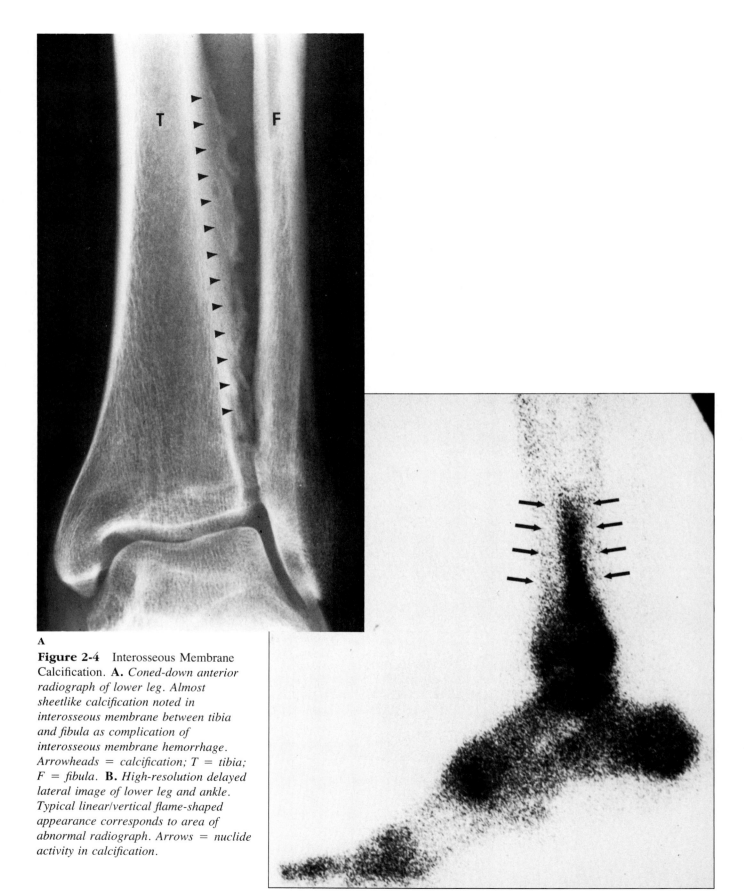

Figure 2-4 Interosseous Membrane Calcification. **A.** *Coned-down anterior radiograph of lower leg. Almost sheetlike calcification noted in interosseous membrane between tibia and fibula as complication of interosseous membrane hemorrhage. Arrowheads = calcification; T = tibia; F = fibula.* **B.** *High-resolution delayed lateral image of lower leg and ankle. Typical linear/vertical flame-shaped appearance corresponds to area of abnormal radiograph. Arrows = nuclide activity in calcification.*

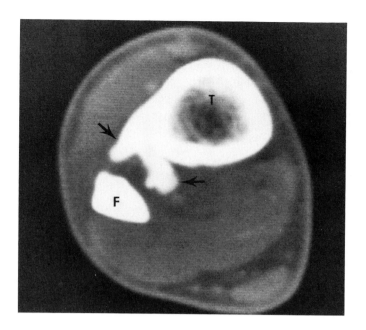

Figure 2-5   Interosseous Membrane Calcification. *CT image just proximal to the ankle joint shows exuberant new bone filling the distal tibiofibular joint space. T = tibia; F = fibula; arrows = posttraumatic calcification.*

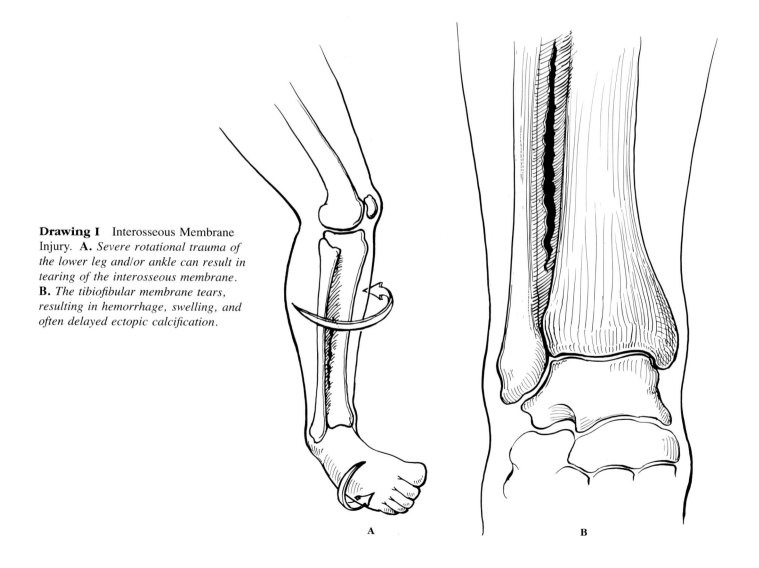

Drawing I   Interosseous Membrane Injury. **A.** *Severe rotational trauma of the lower leg and/or ankle can result in tearing of the interosseous membrane.* **B.** *The tibiofibular membrane tears, resulting in hemorrhage, swelling, and often delayed ectopic calcification.*

A   B

Evaluation of soft tissue masses

The two modalities of choice for evaluating soft tissue fluid collection or swelling/masses in the calf are sonography and MRI. Sonography offers the advantage of being easier to perform and quicker and less expensive than MR. It does not compare to MR for anatomic detail. The development of color flow Doppler sonography allows for the detection of deep venous thrombosis as a cause of calf pain and swelling.[6,7] Deep venous thrombosis in athletes can be a serious if not potentially lethal problem if diagnosis is delayed.[8,26] It is widely accepted that MRI is the modality of choice in visualizing the soft tissue structures of the lower leg. Because of MR's high soft tissue contrast and multiplanar imaging capability, it is the best modality for determining the location, extent, and tissue characteristics of a lesion.[16,27,28] Depending on the patient's clinical history, both sonography and MR contribute to the evaluation of calf swelling, pain, and masses.

Ruptured popliteal cyst (Figs. 2-6 and 2-7)

Space-occupying fluid collections in the calf cannot usually be seen by TPBS unless the photon-deficient area is large enough. TPBS usually detects these collections incidentally while testing for another problem, i.e., stress fractures or shin splints[2] (Fig. 2-6). Hemorrhage into a ruptured popliteal cyst demonstrates, on MRI, a variety of signal patterns that vary over time.[29,30] A rapidly changing pattern evolves as oxyhemoglobin is converted to deoxyhemoglobin over the first few hours, methemoglobin during the first week, and hemosiderin after several weeks. The presence of free blood and later edema also affects signal characteristics. The appearance of hemorrhage in the extremities usually shows a mixed signal pattern on T2-weighted sequences with areas of high-signal and low-signal intensity both present[31,32] (Fig. 2-7).

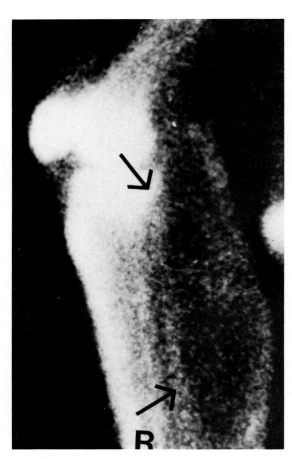

Figure 2-6 Ruptured Popliteal Cyst. *High-resolution delayed phase of TPBS. Lateral view of lower leg/calf demonstrates a rather well-circumscribed area of decreased photon activity in the proximal midposterior calf. Arrows = ruptured popliteal cyst. (From Martire JR: The role of nuclear medicine scans in evaluating pain in athletic injuries.* Clinics in Sports Medicine *6:713–737, 1987. Reproduced with permission.)*

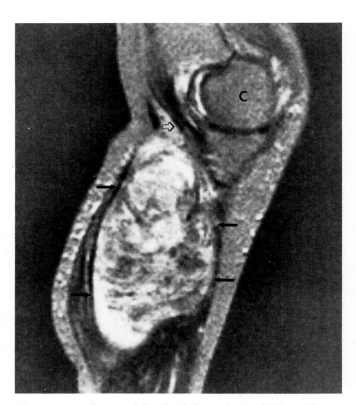

Figure 2-7 Ruptured Popliteal Cyst. *Sagittal MR at T2-weighted sequence shows a soft tissue mass containing regions of high and low signals within the posterior compartment. The mixed signal pattern represents blood at various stages of decomposition as well as clot and fluid. Extension upward around the semimembranosus tendon and into the knee joint is seen. Overlying muscles are displaced. Arrows = ruptured popliteal cyst; open arrow = semimembranosus tendon; C = medial femoral condyle). (Reprinted with permission from Levinsohn EM: MR imaging of extremities excels in knee evaluation.* Diagnostic Imaging *11:102, 1989.)*

Hematoma/abscess (Figs. 2-8 and 2-9)

Posttraumatic hematoma and/or abscess, as well as deep venous thrombosis (DVT), can cause symptoms similar to compartment syndrome. Whether as a result of direct trauma or surgery, acute or chronic fluid collections need to be properly evaluated to exclude the more serious problems, which may require hospitalization and/or surgery (Fig. 2-8). Finally, with the popularity of arthroscopy, postoperative collections of fluid in the calf have become increasingly reported.[33] Postoperative calf abscesses as well as joint effusions can be identified with sonography (Fig. 2-9).

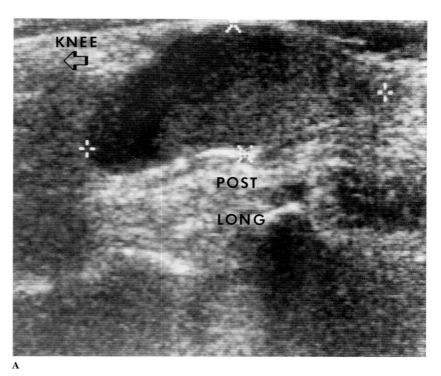

A

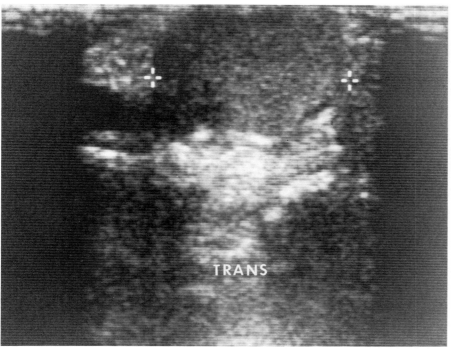

B

Figure 2-8 Posttraumatic Calf Hematoma. **A.** *Sonogram of lower leg in sagittal plane. Reasonably well-defined mass in central popliteal space with sonographic characteristics consistent with hematoma. Measures 7.0 cm × 3.6 cm on two longest dimensions in this projection. Open arrow = direction toward knee.* **B.** *Sonogram of lower leg/calf in transverse plane. Rather well-circumscribed hematoma measures 4.0 cm in widest dimension in this projection.*

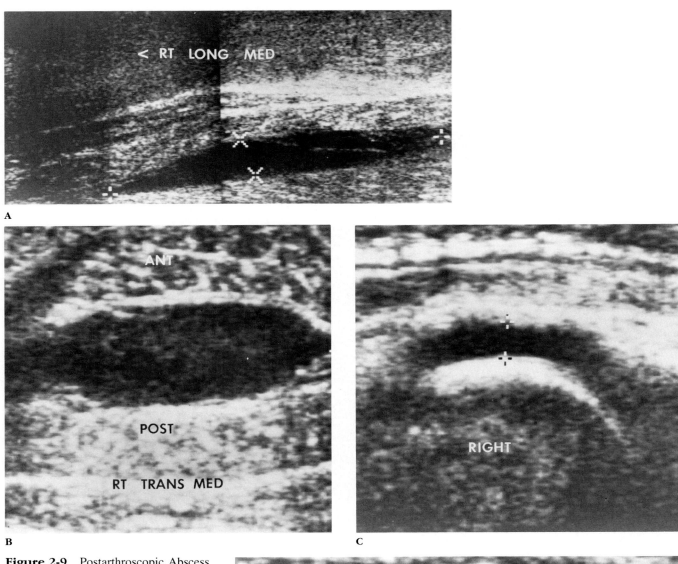

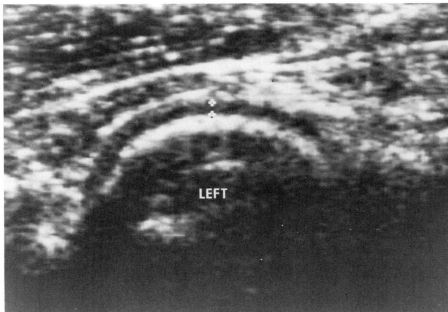

Figure 2-9 Postarthroscopic Abscess of Calf. **A.** *Sonogram of right calf in sagittal plane demonstrates rather well-marginated, oval-shaped mass consistent with a fluid collection such as abscess/hematoma. Measurements in longest dimensions were 16.2 cm × 20.0 cm· × 5.5 cm.* **B.** *Magnified image of ultrasound of calf in transverse plane demonstrates well-marginated collection described above.* **C.** *Sonogram of swollen right knee/femoral condyle demonstrates joint effusion measuring 5.4 mm.* **D.** *Sonogram of normal left knee/femoral condyle demonstrates a normal measurement of 1.5 mm.*

CHRONIC PROBLEMS

Overuse injuries

From a nuclear medicine point of view, TPBS is utilized most often in sports medicine to evaluate suspected lower leg stress injuries. Ever since the first reported tibial stress fracture in 1939, this problem has drawn a great deal of attention and controversy.[34] The following general concepts are important to remember with regard to stress fractures and shin splints:

1. Shin splints and stress fractures are distinct clinical and scintigraphic entities that can be differentiated by TPBS[2,35,36] (Table 2-1).

2. Shin splints and stress fractures can both be present and visualized simultaneously in the same patient using TPBS.[2,21]

3. Varying degrees of shin splint and stress fracture activity seen in a single patient reflects the spectrum or continuum of the different stages which are the preclinical (presymptomatic), acute, and healing stages.[2,5,37]

4. From an activity and therapy point of view, it is important to differentiate among shin splints, stress fracture, and compartment syndrome.[2,38]

Shin splints (Figs. 2-10 and 2-11)

The concept of *medial tibial stress* relates to a nonspecific diagnostic entity used to explain dull lower leg pain in athletes. The term *shin splint* was both misapplied and misused without any specific imaging or clinical criteria.[2,38,39] Recent studies rather clearly show distinct biomechanical causes, clinical findings, and TPBS appearance.[35,40] The typical linear/vertical uptake in the midposterior tibia seen on delayed images only corresponds to the periostitis along the origin of the soleus muscle and its investing fascia. The cause appears to be excessive pronation of the forefoot resulting in tearing of Sharpey's fibers between the muscle and bone.[35,40] Unlike stress fractures, shin splints are always associated with negative radiographs (Figs. 2-10 and 2-11, Table 2-2).

TABLE 2-1

Bone scan appearance[a]

Stress fracture	Versus	Shin splints
Any phase can be positive	TPBS	Only positive on delayed phase
Can be 1+ or 4+	Intensity	Usually 1+ or 3+
Round/fusiform	Shape	Linear/vertical
Anywhere in lower leg	Location	Midposterior tibia

[a] *Adapted from Martire JR: The role of nuclear medicine scans in evaluating pain in athletic injuries. Clinics in Sports Medicine 6:713–737, 1987; with permission.*

TABLE 2-2

Clinical and imaging characteristics of shin splints

Pain induced by exercise; relieved by rest
Dull ache to intense pain
Tenderness posterior-medial border of the tibia
No sensory, motor, or vascular abnormalities
Pronated feet
Probably caused by soleus muscle periostitis
TPBS positive on delayed images only
Linear/vertical activity in midposterior tibia; best seen on lateral view
Rarely seen anteriorly, corresponding to anterior tibialis periostitis
Radiographs always normal even at end stage

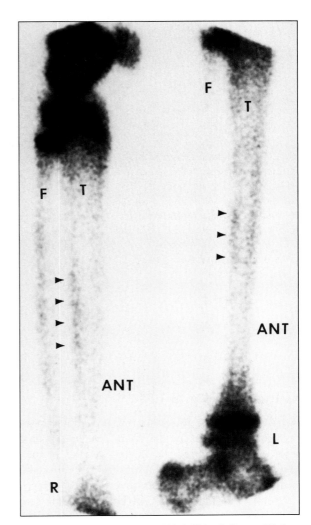

Figure 2-10 Bilateral Mild Tibial Shin Splints. *High-resolution delayed images of TPBS. Lateral views of both lower legs show minimal to mildly increased linear/vertical nuclide activity along the posterior middle third of each tibia consistent with shin splints. Arrowheads = increased nuclide activity in area of tibial periostitis.*

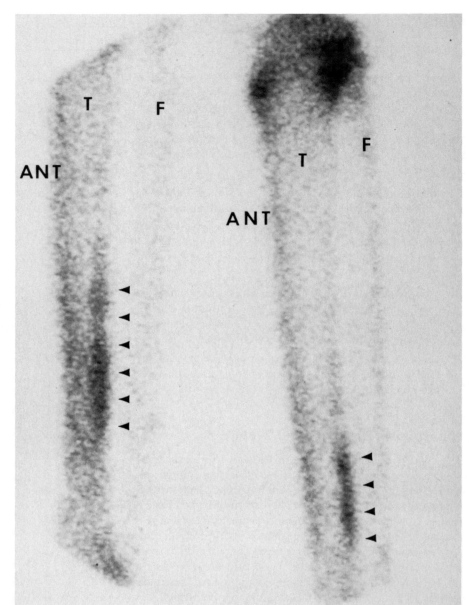

Figure 2-11 Bilateral Severe Tibial Shin Splints. *High-resolution delayed images of TPBS. Lateral views of bilateral lower legs show intense linear/ vertical nuclide accumulation in the posterior margin of both tibias consistent with shin splints. Arrowheads = increased nuclide activity in area of tibial periostitis.*

Stress fractures (Fig. 2-12)

Stress fractures of the lower leg are the most frequently reported stress fractures in the sports medicine literature. Matheson et al.[41] reported that stress fractures of the tibia account for one-half of all stress fractures in athletes. McBryde[42] reported 1000 consecutive cases of stress fractures in runners, with tibia (34 percent) and fibula (24 percent) being the most common sites.

Although the main modalities used to diagnose overuse injuries are the plain radiograph and TPBS, characteristic features of stress fractures have been reported with both CT and MRI.[10,12,43–46] Typically on CT examination, the fracture line in the cortex and endosteal sclerosis, callus, and soft tissue swelling are seen. Without visualizing the fracture line, however, the CT findings are nonspecific. When visualized with MR, stress fractures demonstrate areas of low-signal intensity in the marrow space on T1-weighted sequences and, after approximately 3 weeks, high-signal intensity on T2-weighted sequences. This signal pattern indicates hemorrhage and/or edema in the marrow and subperiosteal spaces. These changes, when visualized on MR, indicate trabecular microfracture. Some physicians suggest restricting sports activity from 4 to 6 weeks to prevent the development of an insufficiency or completed fracture[44,45] (Fig. 2-12).

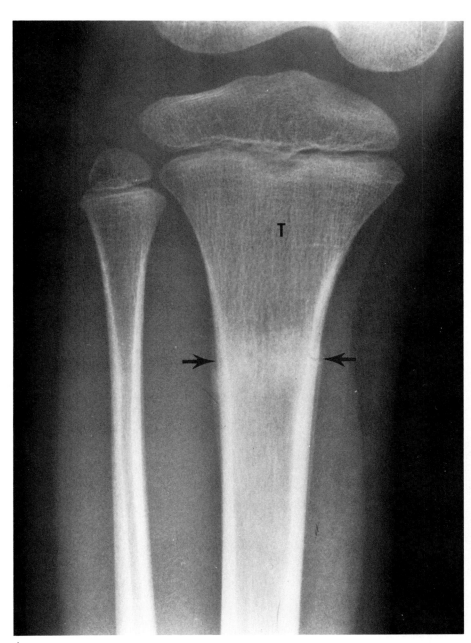

A

Figure 2-12   Tibial Stress Fracture. *A. Anteroposterior radiograph of the proximal left tibia shows a radio-dense band with periosteal response typical of a healing stress fracture. B. Axial MR image at T2-weighted sequence through this region shows a ring of cortical bone elevated from the cortex. Edema is present between periosteum and cortex and also superficial to the periosteum. T = tibia; arrows = stress fracture; open arrows = region of high signal indicating soft tissue edema.*

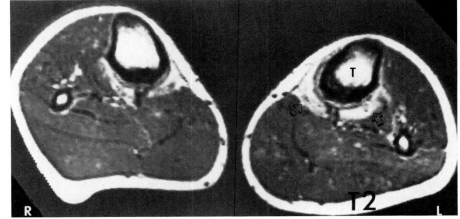

B

Tibial stress fracture (Figs. 2-13 to 2-17)

There are 10 useful observations to remember about tibial stress fractures:

1. Distribution is related to type and extent of activity and can be multifocal in nature[47] (Fig. 2-13).

2. The most common tibial site for stress fracture is the proximal third followed by the distal third, with the mid-tibia being the least likely site (less than 5 percent)[48–52] (Fig. 2-14).

3. Anterior midtibial and medial malleolar stress fractures are uncommon and often require surgical intervention.[53,54]

4. TPBS can estimate the age of tibial stress fractures[5] (Table 2-3).

5. Healed or healing stress fractures can still be positive on follow-up TPBS for a year or more.[2]

6. False-negative nuclide studies with stress fractures are exceedingly rare and may be most likely due to varying technical factors.[55]

7. Thermography and CT are interesting modalities for the evaluation of stress fractures, but TPBS yields more useful information.[12,43,56,57]

8. The differential diagnosis of tibial stress fracture includes shin splints, popliteal artery entrapment syndrome, and exertional compartment syndrome.[58]

9. Focal, mild, asymptomatic sites of nuclide activity are frequently seen on TPBS representing "stress remodeling" or "bone strain" consistent with the continuum of bony stress changes.[59,60]

10. Not all intense "hot spots" are stress fractures. They can also represent other bony pathologies such as tumors, infection, and fibrous cortical defects.[2]

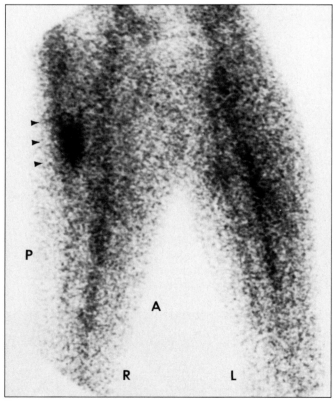

A

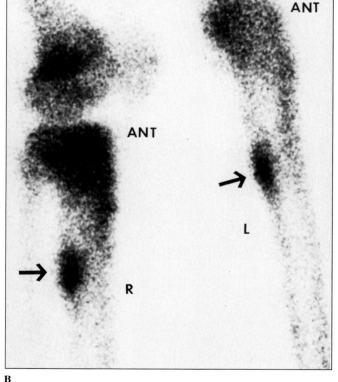

B

Figure 2-13 Proximal Right Tibial Stress Fracture. **A.** *Blood pool phase of TPBS. Oblique/lateral view of bilateral lower legs shows increased nuclide activity in proximal right tibia but none in the left. Arrowheads = increased nuclide activity, right tibia; A = anterior; P = posterior.* **B.** *High-* *resolution delayed images of TPBS. Lateral view of bilateral lower legs shows intense nuclide activity on the posterior border at the junction of proximal and middle third of each tibia consistent with stress fracture. Right tibial stress fracture (positive on blood pool and delayed images) is newer or* *more acute than that on the left, which shows a normal blood pool phase, i.e., multiple or bilateral stress fractures of different ages can exist in the same patient (see Table 2-3). Arrow = increased nuclide activity, posterior tibia. (Fig. 2-13C continues on the opposite page.)*

TABLE 2-3

Dating stress fractures by bone scan [a]

Phase	0 to 4 weeks	4 to 8 weeks	8 weeks to 12 months
Dynamic	+	−	−
Blood pool	+	+	Gradually decreases
Delayed	+	+	Intense (3+ or 4+) to about 12 weeks then decreases 3 to 8 months: can be positive up to 12 months

[a] *Adapted from Martire JR: The role of nuclear medicine scans in evaluating pain in athletic injuries.* Clinics in Sports Medicine *6:713–737, 1987; with permission.*

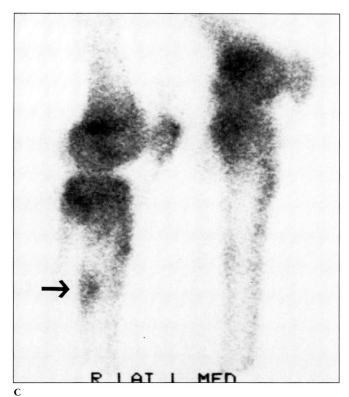

C

Figure 2-13   Proximal Right Tibial Stress Fracture (Continued). **C.** *High-resolution delayed images of TPBS. Follow-up study done 20 weeks since first exam (B) shows complete healing of left tibial stress fracture and only a minimal amount of residual activity on the right. Arrow = right posterior tibial nuclide activity.*

Figure 2-14   Right Posterior Midtibial Stress   ▶
Fracture. *High-resolution delayed image of TPBS. Lateral view demonstrates focal intense nuclide activity in midposterior shaft of tibia consistent with stress fracture. T = tibia; black arrow = increased activity, posterior tibia; open arrow = anterior ankle; post = posterior aspect of lower leg.*

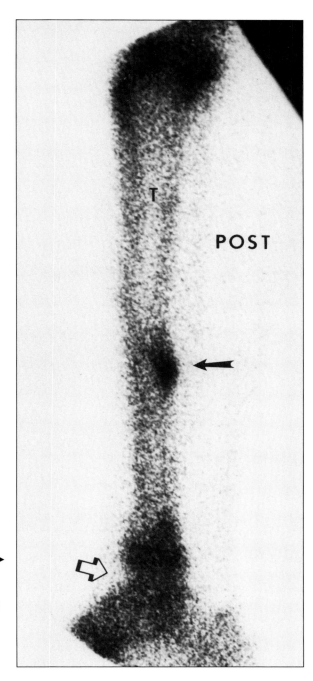

While stress fractures of the distal tibia are common, medial malleolar stress fractures are rare (Fig. 2-15). One report suggests that if radiographs of the medial malleolus are positive in addition to a positive bone scan, then open reduction and internal fixation would be advisable.[54] Stress fractures of the anterior midtibial shaft were first reported in ballet dancers.[53] Since that time, additional cases have been identified in other athletes who engage in significant jumping activity such as gymnasts and basketball players as well as a solitary case report in a professional football player.[61-63] Typically, these lesions have poor healing, often resulting in nonunion or incomplete fracture.[63-66] Treatment may involve electrostimulation or bony grafting of the lesion.[63,66] Radiographs reveal anterior cortical thickening and a horizontal fissure, or "black line." Of all the stress fractures of the lower legs, these are the most troublesome, often resulting in months to years of inactivity and follow-up. Adding to the difficulty, TPBS often shows only a minimally or mildly positive study despite obvious radiographic abnormalities. Negative TPBS in these cases has been thought to be possibly associated with bone infarct in the area of initial stress fracture[64,67] (Figs. 2-16 and 2-17).

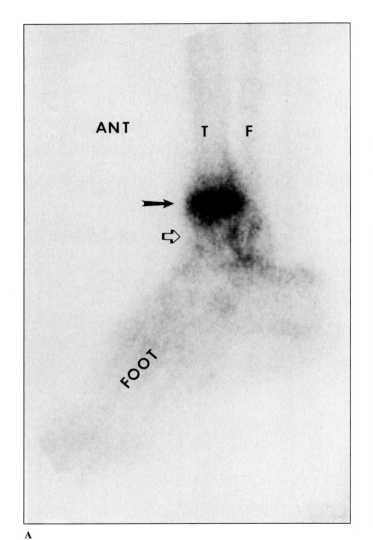

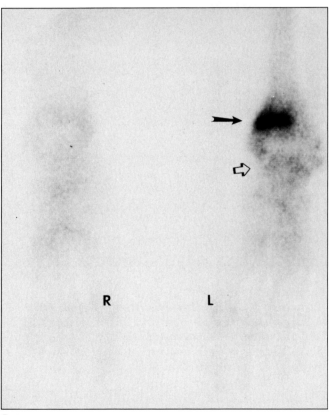

A

B

Figure 2-15 Left Distal Tibial/Medial Malleolar Stress Fracture. **A.** *High-resolution delayed image of TPBS. Lateral view of lower leg/ankle demonstrates increased linear/horizontal activity, distal tibia just at or above level of medial malleolus. Black arrow = increased tibial nuclide activity; open arrow = anterior aspect of ankle; T = tibia; F = fibula; ant = anterior.* **B.** *High-resolution delayed images of TPBS. Computer-subtracted anterior images of bilateral ankle and lower leg show linear/horizontal increased activity just above medial malleolus. Black arrow = increased tibial nuclide activity; open arrow = medial aspect of ankle.*

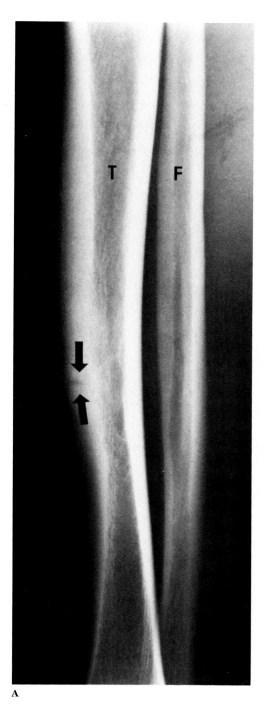

A

Figure 2-16 Right Anterior Midtibial Stress Fracture.
A. *Lateral radiograph of lower leg demonstrates faint, horizontal, linear, lucent line/fracture at anterior aspect of midtibia. Arrows = anterior tibial cortical fracture; T = tibia; F = fibula.* **B.** *High-resolution delayed image of TPBS done same day as radiograph. Lateral view of lower leg shows minimal focal activity in the anterior midtibia corresponding to radiographic abnormality. Arrow = anterior tibial nuclide activity.*

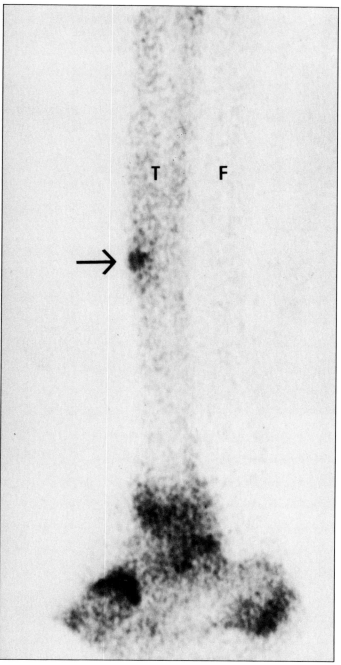

B

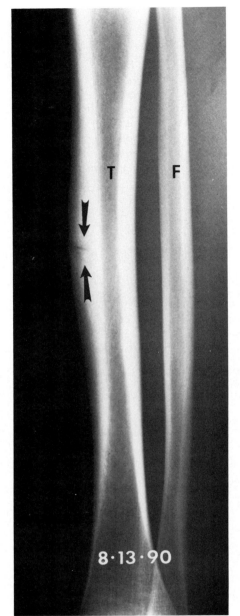

A

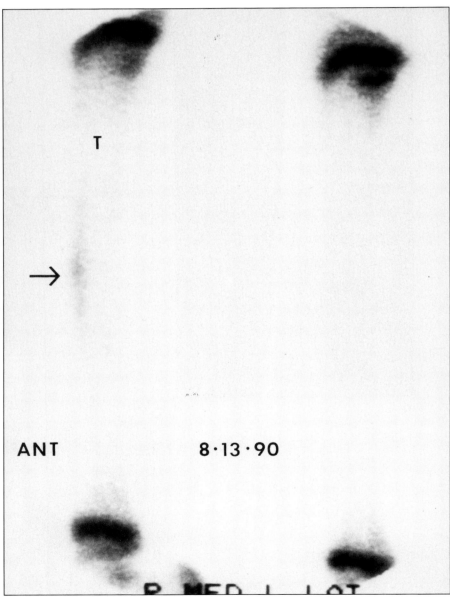

B

Figure 2-17   Right Anterior Midtibial Stress Fracture. **A.** *Lateral radiograph of lower leg demonstrates horizontal, linear, lucent line consistent with cortical fracture. Arrows = tibial fracture line; T = tibia; F = fibula.* **B.** *High-resolution delayed images of TPBS done same day as radiograph. Focal minimal increased nuclide activity, anterior tibia, corresponding to area of radiographic abnormality. Arrow = anterior tibial nuclide activity; T = tibia; ant = anterior aspect of right tibia.* (Fig. 2-17C continues on the opposite page.)

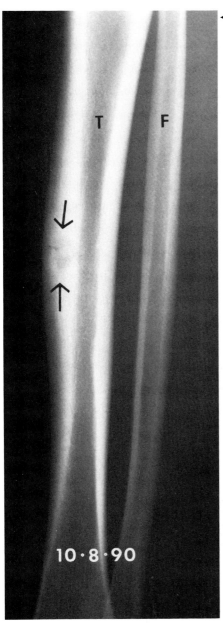

C

◄ Figure 2-17 Right Anterior Midtibial Stress Fracture (Continued). **C.** *Follow-up lateral radiograph of lower leg done after approximately 2 months of rest and no athletic activity. Worsening appearance of anterior tibial cortex with persistent horizontal, lucent line now surrounded by increasing area of bone resorption. Arrows = anterior tibial cortical fracture; T = tibia; F = fibula.*

Figure 2-18 Left Distal Fibular/Lateral Malleolar Stress Fracture. **A.** *Anteroposterior radiograph demonstrates very faint bone density at lateral aspect, distal left fibula, above level of lateral malleolus. Arrows = minimal focal bone density, fibular cortex, suggestive of stress fracture; T = tibia; F = fibula. (Fig. 2-18B and C continues on next page.)*

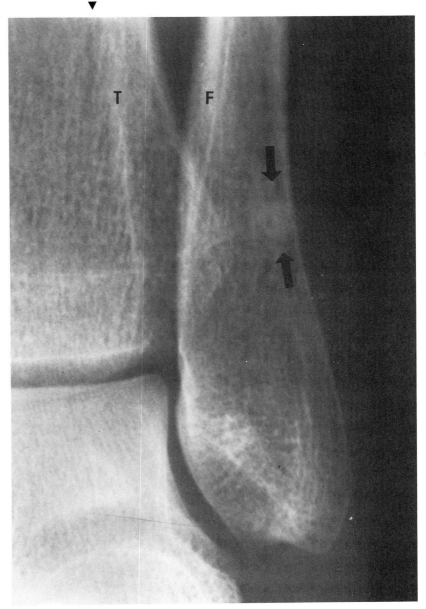

A

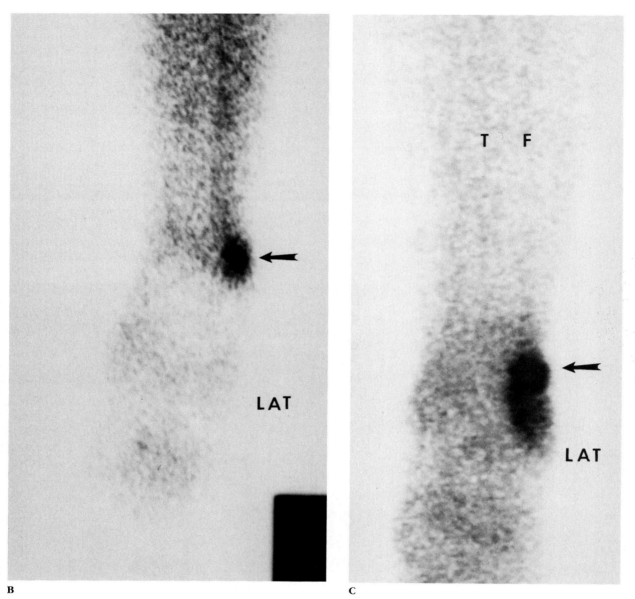

B

C

Figure 2-18 Left Distal Fibular/ Lateral Malleolar Stress Fracture (Continued). **B.** *Blood pool phase of TPBS. Anterior view demonstrates focal nuclide activity overlying distal left* *fibula. Arrow = increased blood pool nuclide accumulation; lat = lateral side of ankle/foot.* **C.** *High-resolution delayed image of TPBS. Anterior view of ankle demonstrates intense nuclide* *activity, distal fibula/lateral malleolus. Arrow = most intense activity in distal fibula corresponding to positive area seen on blood pool and radiograph; T = tibia; F = fibula.*

Fibular stress fractures (Figs. 2-18 to 2-20)

Fibular stress fractures are most commonly seen in the distal third, proximal to the lateral malleolus[68,69] (Figs. 2-18 and 2-19). Additionally, stress fractures of the lateral malleolus have also been noted especially in dancers, aerobic exercisers, gymnasts, and runners.[2] Radiographs are not usually positive until 3 to 4 weeks after the onset of symptoms, making TPBS the test of choice.[70] The differential diagnosis of fibular stress fracture includes biceps femoris tendinitis, peroneal nerve entrapment, and exertional compartment syndrome.[71] Proximal third fibular stress fractures are due to jumping injuries associated with powerful contraction of the flexor muscles of the ankle as they are exerted across the fibula (soleus, peroneus longus, and tibialis posterior)[70,72] (Fig. 2-20). Soldiers, hurdlers, basketball players, gymnasts, and ballet dancers are susceptible to this type of lesion. Less commonly, runners and older patients can be affected.[73]

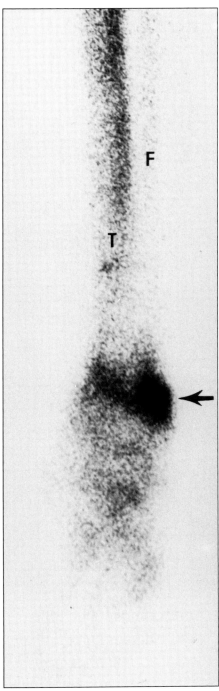

◄**Figure 2-19**   Left Distal Fibular/Lateral Malleolar Stress Fracture. *High-resolution delayed image of TPBS. Anterior view of distal lower leg and foot demonstrates intense nuclide activity overlying lateral malleolus. Arrow = increased nuclide activity; T = tibia; F = fibula.*

Figure 2-20   Proximal Right Fibular Stress Fracture and Right Tibial Shin Splints. **A.** *Blood pool phase of TPBS. Anterior view demonstrates focal, mildly increased nuclide activity, proximal lateral aspect of right lower leg. Arrows = increased nuclide activity overlying proximal right fibula.* (Fig. 2-20B and C continues on next page.)

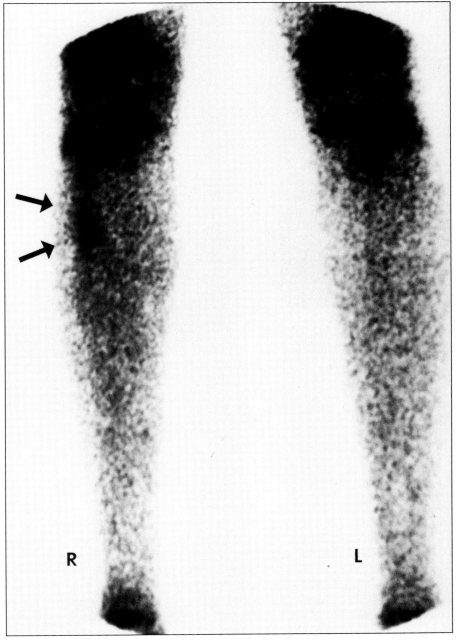

A

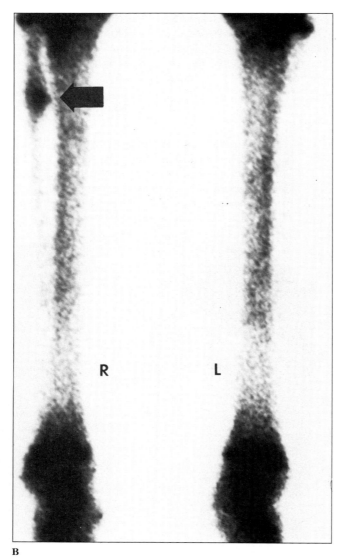

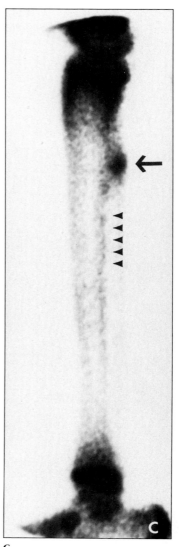

Figure 2-20   Proximal Right Fibular Stress Fracture and Right Tibial Shin Splints (Continued). **B.** *High-resolution delayed image of TPBS. Anterior view demonstrates focal nuclide activity, proximal right fibula, corresponding to area of abnormality on blood pool. Arrow = proximal right fibular stress fracture.* **C.** *High-resolution delayed image of TPBS. Lateral view of lower leg demonstrates focal oval-shaped area of increased activity in proximal right fibula and minimal area of increased activity, posterior third of tibia. Arrow = right fibular stress fracture; arrowheads = tibial shin splints; C = calcaneus.*

Muscle overuse

Magnetic resonance imaging may show changes associated with pain caused from heavy exertion without other injury as well as signal changes from recent muscle strain or tear.[9,74] The clinical appreciation of pain, either during the exercise or delayed for hours or days following the exercise, may indicate muscle strain. The magnetic resonance changes associated with strain include focal muscle enlargement with increased signal accentuated on gradient echo sequences and with perifascial enhancement on T2-weighted sequences.

Long-distance runners may show these abnormalities at the myotendinous junctions. With rhabdomyolysis, there is increased signal on T2-weighted sequences at 24 to 72 h after injury to the involved muscles. If a muscle tear has occurred, decreased muscle mass may be appreciated as well as low signal on T1-weighted sequences and linear zones of high signal at T2-weighted sequences likely representing the residua of dissecting blood.

DIAGNOSTIC PROBLEMS

Vascular lesions (Figs. 2-21 and 2-22)

Lower leg or calf discomfort can often mask vascular problems. Vascular narrowing, entrapment, aneurysm, and occlusion have all been reported in athletes.[75,76] The dynamic flow portion of the TPBS gives the radiologist vascular flow information that often reveals important and/or incidental pathology (Fig. 2-21).

Because of the flow void phenomenon on MR, blood in rapid motion demonstrates low-signal intensity on both T1- and T2-weighted sequences. This allows the demonstration of the arterial pattern (contrast-free arteriogram) without the necessity to inject radiographic contrast material (Fig. 2-22).

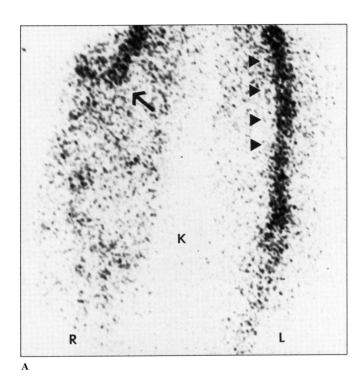

A

Figure 2-21 Peripheral Vascular Disease. **A.** *Early blood flow phase of TPBS. Anterior view of both legs centered over the distal thigh, knee, and proximal lower leg. On the left, the patent superficial femoral artery is noted along its entire course forming the popliteal artery at the level of the knee. On the right, there is abnormality with "cutoff" or occlusion of the superficial femoral artery at the level of the midthigh. Arrow = level of occlusion of right superficial femoral artery in midthigh; arrowheads = patent or normal left superficial femoral artery along its entire course; K = level of the knee.* **B.** *Late blood flow phase of TPBS. On the left, patent arterial system is seen including distal superficial femoral, and popliteal arteries, and runoff below the level of the knee. On the right, collateral blood flow distal to the level of blockage results in reconstitution of the right popliteal artery at the level of the knee with flow seen distal to this. Arrows = reconstituted popliteal artery at its origin; K = level of the knee.*

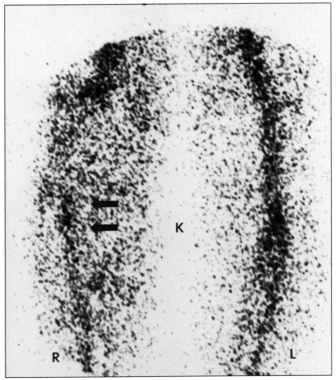

B

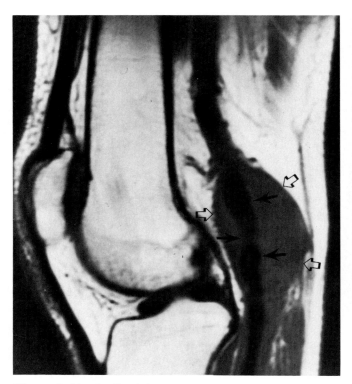

Figure 2-22 Popliteal Artery Aneurysm. *Midline sagittal MR image through the knee at T1-weighted sequence shows central arterial flow through a popliteal artery aneurysm. The arterial flow is black because of the signal void created by moving blood. Arrows = arterial flow; open arrows = aneurysm.*

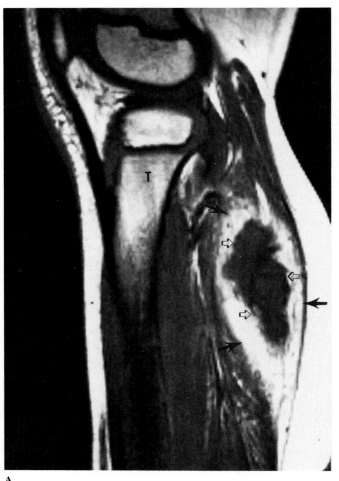

A

Figure 2-23 Benign Hemangioma. **A.** *Midline sagittal MR image through the calf at T1-weighted sequence shows a soft tissue mass in the upper portion of the gastrocnemius muscle. Low-signal intensity occupies the center of the mass, which is surrounded by a focus of high-signal intensity. Hemangiomas contain many tissue elements, including fat, smooth muscle, fibrous tissue, hemosiderin, and tortuous blood vessels. The different signal intensities seen here reflect those tissue differences. (Fig. 2-23B continues on the opposite page.)*

Soft tissue/muscle lesions (Figs. 2-23 to 2-25)

In athletes as well as in nonathletes, clinical suspicion of nontraumatic entities such as neoplasm, arthritis, or infection should be maintained, particularly in those individuals whose symptoms are atypical and/or unresponsive. Early imaging of the symptomatic region is indicated in those circumstances. In those situations where the abnormality involves the soft tissues, magnetic resonance is the modality of choice. Tumors, as with true sports injuries, can often present with soft tissue swelling and discomfort.

Hemangioma is the most common benign soft tissue neoplasm in infancy and childhood.[77–80] Although a variable appearance may be seen on MR, depending on the tissue makeup of the hemangioma, the features, size, and proximity to other structures can best be determined with this modality (Fig. 2-23). Similarly, malignant tumors can also be well defined anatomically with magnetic resonance (Fig. 2-24). Additionally, benign accessory muscles can often mimic tumors or masses presenting as a focal enlargement in the calf best evaluated by MR[81] (Fig. 2-25). Compartment syndromes as well as muscle injury have been demonstrated with MR.[9,74]

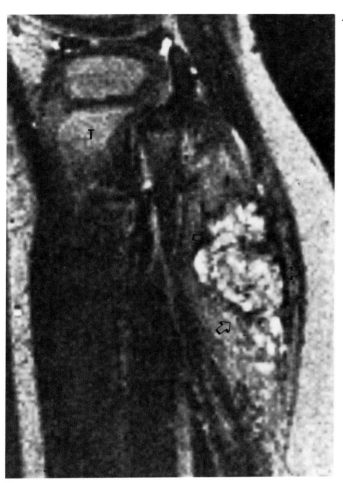

B

◀ **Figure 2-23** Benign Hemangioma (Continued). **B.** *Similar image at T2-weighted sequence shows serpiginous structures containing high signal in the center of the lesion. T = tibia; open arrows = vascular structures within the lesion; closed arrows = fat at the periphery of the lesion.*

Figure 2-24 Rhabdomyosarcoma of Right Calf. **A.** *Axial MR image at T2-weighted sequence demonstrates high-signal intensity within the right tibialis anterior muscle reflecting the high water content induced by tumor within that muscle. (Reprinted with permission from Levinsohn EM: MR imaging of extremities excels in knee evaluation.* Diagnostic Imaging *11:103, 1989.)* (Fig. 2-24B continues on next page.)
▼

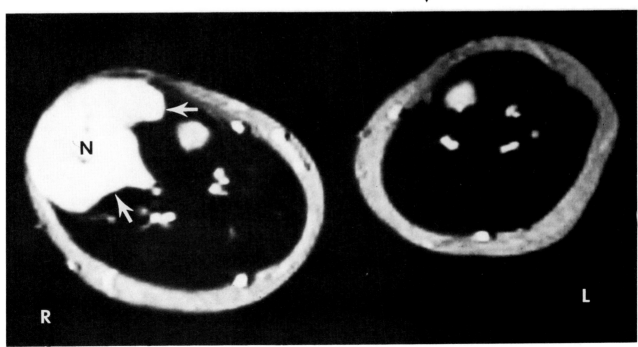

A

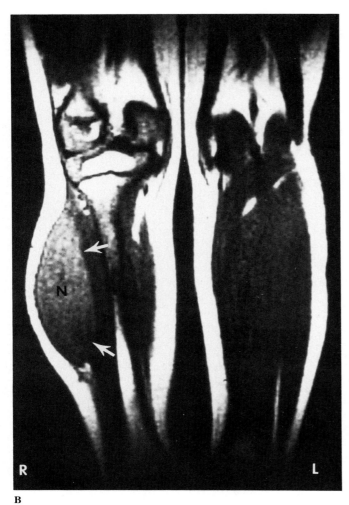

B

Figure 2-24 Rhabdomyosarcoma of Right Calf (Continued). **B.** *Image in the coronal plane at T1-weighted sequence shows the soft tissue mass and extent of tumor involvement. N = neoplasm within tibialis anterior muscle; arrows = extent of soft tissue mass.*

Figure 2-25 Accessory Muscle Simulating Mass. *Axial image through both lower legs demonstrates a soft tissue mass within the posterior compartment of the right leg with signal characteristics of normal muscle. Adjacent tendons, subcutaneous tissues, and bones are normal. T = tibia; F = fibula; arrows = accessory flexor muscle; A = achilles tendon; PT = posterior tibial tendon.*

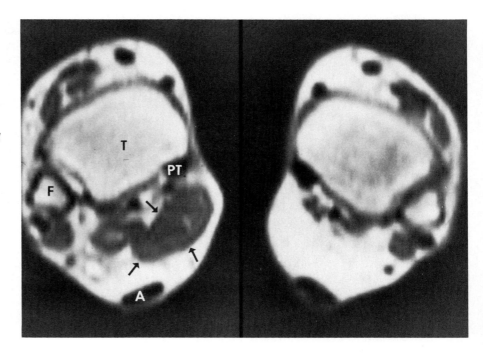

Bony lesions (Figs. 2-26 to 2-30)

Lower leg bone pain in athletes may be due to a sports injury or other bone pathology not associated with trauma[13] (Figs. 2-26 and 2-27). The initial radiographic evaluation after the clinical exam should begin with routine radiography of the area involved. That may provide sufficient diagnostic information to conclude the imaging evaluation. If not, the next most useful examination is the TPBS, since both benign and malignant bone lesions can accumulate nuclide activity[2] (Fig. 2-28). Finally, acute periostitis due to early acquired syphilis has been reported as having simulated shin splints.[82]

Osteoid osteoma is a unique, benign bone tumor that can create diagnostic problems for the radiologist and surgeon.[83–85] In the lower leg, osteoid osteoma can be found in the patella, tibia, or fibula. The TPBS appearance includes intense nuclide activity on all three phases.[2,86,87] The plain radiograph and/or multidirectional tomogram usually demonstrates a characteristic appearance. Occasionally, it is difficult to separate that appearance from stress fracture. In that circumstance, a CT scan through the area of abnormality often allows identification of the offending nidus. Finally, postoperative evaluation of osteoid osteoma utilizing TPBS and CT has been reported[88] (Figs. 2-29 and 2-30).

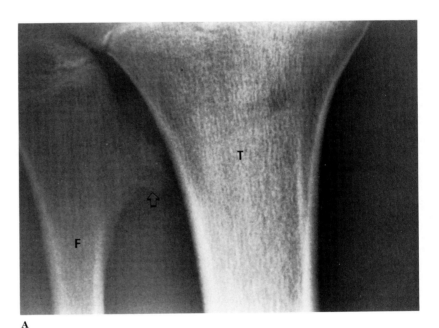

A

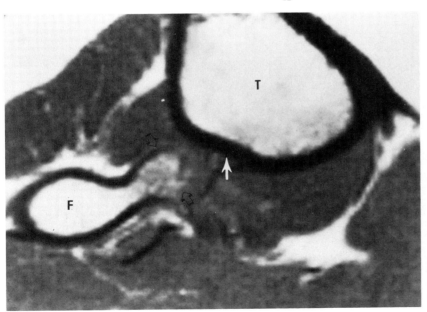

B

Figure 2-26 Impinging Osteochondroma of Proximal Fibula. *A snapping sensation just distal to the knee was caused by an osteochondroma projecting off the proximal metaphysis of the fibula and impinging upon the tibia.* **A.** *Anteroposterior radiograph demonstrates the proximity of the fibular osteochondroma to the proximal tibia.* **B.** *Axial MR scan at T1-weighted sequence shows the cartilage cap of the osteochondroma articulating with the posterolateral cortex of the tibia. Chronic tibial cortical resorption has resulted. T = tibia; F = fibula; open arrows = osteochondroma; arrow = tibial cortical remodeling.*

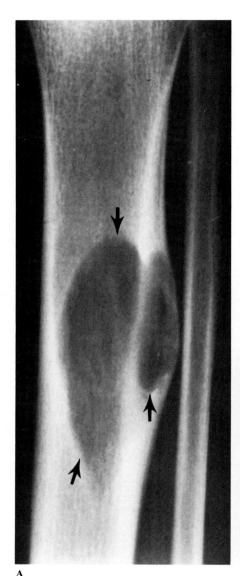

A

Figure 2-27   Unicameral Bone Cyst of the Tibia.
A. *Anteroposterior radiograph shows well-defined lucency representing a unicameral cyst.* **B.** *Axial image from a CT scan through the upper aspect of the cyst shows the intramedullary extent of that lesion. The surrounding soft tissues remain normal. Arrows = cyst.*

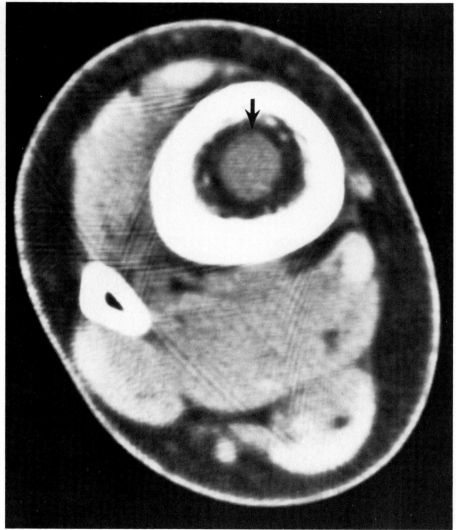

B

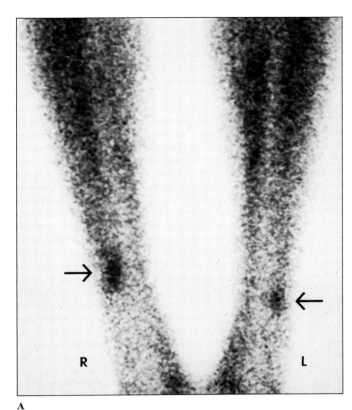

A

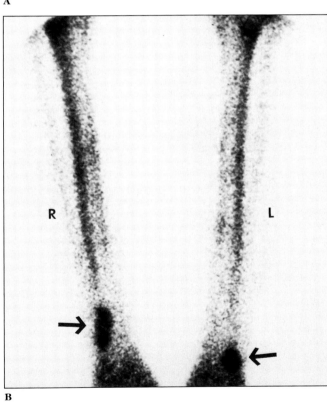

B

Figure 2-28 Bilateral Distal Tibial Fibrous Cortical Defect and Right Tibial Shin Splints. **A.** *Blood pool phase of TPBS. Anterior image of both lower legs shows mild nuclide activity distally. Arrow = increased nuclide activity overlying each lower leg.* **B.** *High-resolution delayed image of TPBS. Anterior view of both lower legs shows intense nuclide activity in both right and left distal tibias. Arrow = nuclide activity in both right and left tibias corresponding to abnormal area on blood pool.* **C.** *High-resolution delayed image of TPBS. Lateral view of right lower leg shows oval-shaped area of increased activity in distal right tibia and linear/vertical activity along posterior middle third of right tibia. Open arrow = distal right tibial activity (fibrous cortical defect); black arrows = posterior right tibial activity (shin splints).* (Fig. 2-28D and E continues on next page.)

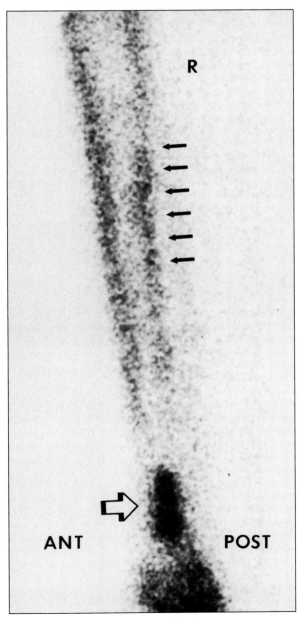

C

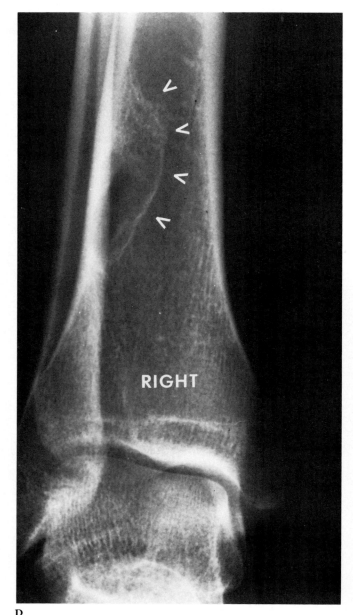

D

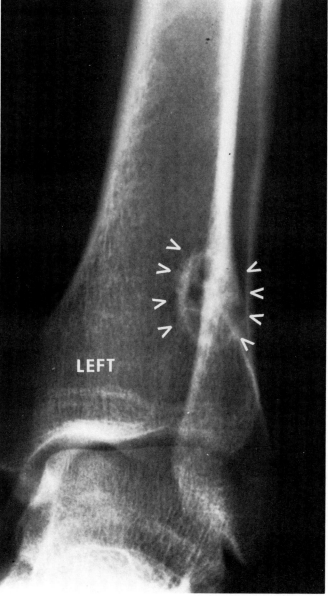

Figure 2-28   Bilateral Distal Tibial Fibrous Cortical Defect and Right Tibial Shin Splints (Continued). **D.** *Anteroposterior radiograph of distal right lower leg. Well-marginated, lucent bone lesion, distal lateral tibial shaft, consistent with fibrous cortical defect corresponding to abnormal areas of activity seen on blood pool and delayed images. White arrowheads = medial margin of bony lesion.* **E.** *Anteroposterior radiograph of distal left lower leg. Well-marginated, lucent bone defect, lateral aspect of tibia, corresponding to area of abnormal activity on blood pool and delayed images. White arrowheads = medial and lateral margins of fibrous cortical defect.*

E

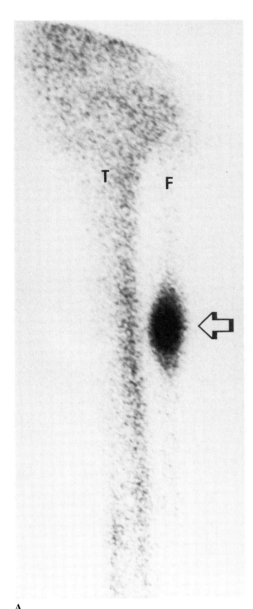

A

Figure 2-29   Osteoid Osteoma of Proximal Fibula.   **A.** *High-resolution delayed image of TPBS. Very intense nuclide activity, junction of proximal and middle thirds of the fibula. Open arrow = abnormal nuclide activity in fibula.* **B.** *Multidirectional tomography of left fibula demonstrates lytic, reasonably well-marginated bone lesion corresponding to abnormal area on bone scan shown in magnified view. Arrows demonstrate the superior and inferior aspects of bony lesion.* **C.** *High-resolution delayed image of TPBS following surgery of proximal fibula. Anterior view shows absent area of activity corresponding to removal of osteoid osteoma. Arrows = superior and inferior margin of resected fibula for osteoid osteoma. (T = tibia; F = fibula.)*

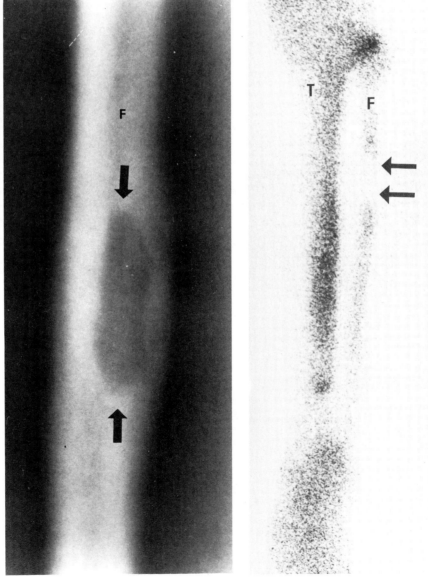

B   C

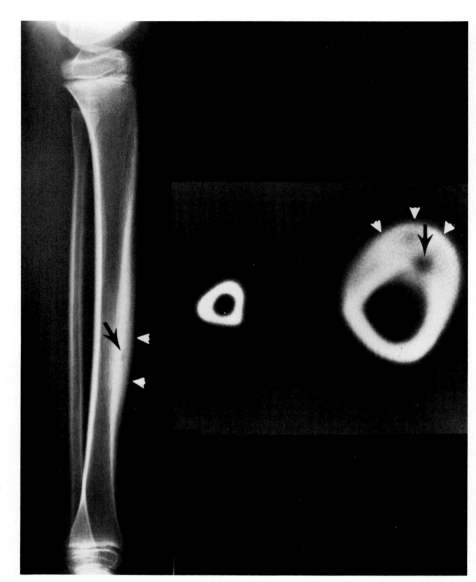

Figure 2-30 Osteoid Osteoma of Tibia. *Marked cortical thickening containing lucent nidus within the anterior cortex of the tibia. Black arrow = nidus; white arrowheads = chronic cortical thickening.*

REFERENCES

1. Holder LE: Clinical Radionuclide Bone Imaging, Radiology 176:607–614, 1990.
2. Martire JR: The role of nuclear medicine scans in evaluating pain in athletic injuries. Clin Sports Med 6:713–737, 1987.
3. Matin P: Basic principles of nuclear medicine techniques for detection and evaluation of trauma and sports medicine injuries. Semin Nucl Med 18:90–112, 1988.
4. Matin PM: Appearance of bone scans following fractures including immediate and long term studies. J Nucl Med 20:1227–1231, 1979.
5. Rupani HD, Holder LE, Espinola DA, et al.: Three phase radionuclide bone imaging in sports medicine. Radiology 156:187–196, 1985.
6. Aitken AG, Godden DJ: Real-time ultrasound diagnosis of deep vein thrombosis: a comparison with venography. Clin Radiol 38:309–313, 1987.
7. Cronan JJ, Dorfman GS, Grusmark J: Lower extremity deep venous thrombosis: further experience with and refinements of ultrasound assessment. Radiology 168:101–107, 1988.
8. Sidler GJ, Bugaieski SM, Sunderlin J, et al.: Case report: difficulty in diagnosing and treating deep vein thrombosis in a competitive basketball player. Phys Sports Med 13(7):113–118, 1985.
9. Fleckenstein JL, Weatherall PT, Parkey RW, et al.: Sports-related muscle injuries: evaluation with MR imaging. Radiology 172:793–798, 1989.

10. Lee JK, Yao L: Stress fractures: MR imaging. Radiology 169:217–220, 1988.

11. Levinsohn EM: Computerized tomography of the extremities. Contemp Diagn Radiol 7:1–6, 1981.

12. Yousem D, Magid D, Fishman EK, et al.: Computed tomography of stress fractures. J Comput Assist Tomogr 10:92–95, 1986.

13. Lewis MM, Reilly JF: Sports tumors. Am J Sports Med 4:362–365, 1987.

14. Alazraki N, Pye S: Myositis ossificans, in Nicholas JA, Holder LE (eds): *Bone Imaging in Orthopaedic Medicine: A Clinical Case Book*. Pro Clinical, New York, 1980, pp 30–31.

15. Ekelund L, Toolanen G: Low field (0.02T) magnetic resonance imaging of bone and soft tissue tumors. Skeletal Radiol 18:585–590, 1989.

16. Sundaram M, McGuire MH: Computed tomography or magnetic resonance for evaluating the solitary tumor or tumor-like lesion of bone? Skeletal Radiol 17:393–401, 1988.

17. Demas BE, Heelan RT, Lane J, et al.: Soft-tissue sarcomas of the extremities: comparison of MR and CT in determining the extent of disease. AJR 150:615–620, 1988.

18. Kalmar JA, Eick JJ, Merritt CRB, et al.: A review of applications of MRI in soft tissue and bone tumors. Orthopedics 11:417–425, 1988.

19. Kilcoyne RF, Richardson ML, Porter BA, et al.: Magnetic resonance imaging of soft tissue masses. Clin Orthop 228:13–19, 1988.

20. Weis L, Heelan RT, Watson RC: Computed tomography of orthopedic tumors of the pelvis and lower extremities. Clin Orthop 130:254–259, 1978.

21. Holder LE, Matthews LS: The nuclear physician and sports medicine, in Freeman L, Weissman H (eds): *Nuclear Medicine Annual 1984*. Raven, New York, 1984, pp 88–140.

22. Lipscomb AB, Thomas ED, Johnston RK: Treatment of myositis ossificans traumatica in athletes. Am J Sports Med 4:111–120, 1976.

23. Suzuki Y, Hisada K, Takeda M: Demonstration of myositis ossificans by 99mTc pyrophosphate bone scanning. Radiology 111:663–664, 1974.

24. Wetzel LH, Levine E, Murphey MD: A comparison of MR imaging and CT in the evaluation of musculoskeletal masses. Radiographics 7:851–874, 1987.

25. Whiteside LA, Reynolds FC, Ellsasser JC: Tibiofibular synostosis and recurrent ankle sprains in high performance athletes. Am J Sports Med 6:204–208, 1978.

26. Mackey JW, Webster JA: Deep vein thrombosis in marathon runners. Phys Sports Med 9(5):91–98, 1981.

27. Pettersson H, Gillespy T III, Hamlin DJ, et al.: Primary musculoskeletal tumors: examination with MR imaging compared with conventional modalities. Radiology 164:237–241, 1987.

28. Sundaram M, McLeod RA: MR imaging of tumor and tumor-like lesions of bone and soft tissue. AJR 155:817–824, 1990.

29. Grossman RI: MR highlights hemorrhage but can be misleading. Diagn Imaging 10(8):126–129, 1988.

30. Rubin JI, Gomori JM, Grossman RI, et al.: High-field MR imaging of extracranial hematomas. AJR 148:813–817, 1987.

31. Dooms GC, Fisher MR, Hricak H, Higgins CB: MR imaging of intramuscular hemorrhage. JCAT 9:908–913, 1985.

32. Pakter RL, Fishman EK, Zerhouni EA: Calf hematoma—computed tomographic and magnetic resonance findings. Skeletal Radiol 16:393–396, 1987.

33. Peek RD, Haynes DW: Compartment syndrome as a complication of arthroscopy. Am J Sports Med 6:464–468, 1984.

34. Roberts SM, Vogt EC: Pseudofracture of the tibia. J Bone Joint Surg 21:891–809, 1939.

35. Holder LE, Michael RH: The specific scintigraphic pattern of "shin splints" in the lower leg. J Nucl Med 25:865–869, 1984.

36. Orava S, Hulkko A: Stress fracture of the midtibial shaft. Acta Orthop Scand 55:35–37, 1984.

37. Collier BD, Johnson RP, Carrera GF, et al.: Scintigraphic diagnosis of stress-induced incomplete fractures of the proximal tibia. J Trauma 24:156–160, 1984.

38. Mubarak SJ, Gould RN, Lee YF, et al.: The medial tibial stress syndrome, a cause of shin splints. Am J Sports Med 10:201–205, 1982.

39. Devas MB: Stress fractures of the tibia in athletes or "shin soreness." J Bone Joint Surg 40(B):227–239, 1958.

40. Michael RH, Holder LE: The soleus syndrome. A cause of medial tibial stress (shin splints). Am J Sports Med 13:87–94, 1985.

41. Matheson GO, Clement DB, McKenzie DC, et al.: Stress fractures in athletes: a study of 320 cases. Am J Sports Med 15:46–58, 1987.

42. McBryde AM: Stress fractures in runners. Clin Sports Med 4:737–752, 1985.

43. Allen GJ: Longitudinal stress fractures of the tibia: diagnosis with CT. Radiology 167:799–801, 1988.

44. Crues JV III, Lynch TCP: MR effective in detecting traumatic bone injuries. Diagn Imaging 18(10):118–121, 1990.

45. Lynch TCP, Crues JV, Morgan FW, et al.: Bone abnormalities of the knee: prevalence and significance at MR imaging. Radiology 171:761–766, 1989.

46. Murcia M, Brennan RE, Edeiken J: Computed tomography of stress fracture. Skeletal Radiol 8:193–195, 1982.

47. Kinball PR, Savastano AA: Fatigue fractures of the proximal tibia. Clin Orthop 70:170–173, 1970.

48. Daffner RH, Martinez S, Gehweiler JA: Stress fractures in runners. JAMA 247:1039–1041, 1982.

49. Daffner RH, Martinez S, Gehweiler JA, et al.: Stress fractures of the proximal tibia in runners. Radiology 142:63–65, 1982.

50. Giladi M, Ahronson Z, Stein M, et al.: Unusual distribution and onset of stress fractures in soldiers. Clin Orthop 192:142–146, 1985.

51. Giladi M, Milgrom C, Simkin A, et al.: Stress fractures and tibial bone width: a risk factor. J Bone Joint Surg 69(B):326–329, 1987.

52. Meurman KO, Elfing S: Stress fractures in soldiers: a multifocal bone disorder. Radiology 134:483–487, 1980.

53. Burrows FJ: Fatigue infarction of middle of tibia in ballet dancers. J Bone Joint Surg 38(B):83–86, 1956.

54. Shelbourne KD, Fisher DA, Rettig AC, et al.: Stress fractures of the medial malleolus. Am J Sports Med 16:60–63, 1988.

55. Milgron C, Chisin R, Giladi M, et al.: Negative bone scans in impending tibial stress fractures. Am J Sports Med 12:488–491, 1984.

56. Goodman PH, Heaslett MW, Pagliano JW, et al.: Stress fracture diagnosis by computer-assisted thermography. Phys Sports Med 13(4):114–132, 1985.

57. Tehranzadeh J, Serafini AN, Pais MJ: *Avulsion and Stress Injuries of the Musculoskeletal System*. Karger, Basel, 1989.

58. Friedman MJ: Injuries to the leg in athletes, in Nicholas JA, Hershman EB (eds): *The Lower Extremity and Spine in Sports Medicine*. Mosby, St. Louis, 1986.

59. Matheson GO, Clement DB, McKenzie DC, et al.: Scintigraphic uptake of ^{99m}Tc at non-painful sites in athletes with stress fractures: the concept of bone strain. Sports Med 4:65–75, 1987.

60. Roub LW, Gumerman LW, Hanley EN, et al.: Bone stress: a radionuclide imaging perspective. Radiology 132:431–438, 1979.

61. Brahms MA, Fumich RM, Ippolito VD: Atypical stress fracture of the tibia in a professional athlete. Am J Sports Med 8:131–132, 1980.

62. Miller EH, Schneider HJ, Bronson JL, et al.: A new consideration in athletic injuries: the classic ballet dancer. Clin Orthop 111:181–191, 1975.

63. Rettig AC, Shelbourne KD, McCarroll JR, et al.: The natural history and treatment of delayed union stress fractures of the anterior cortex of the tibia, Am J Sports Med 16:250–255, 1988.

64. Blank S: Transverse tibial stress fractures: a special problem. Am J Sports Med 9:322–325, 1981.

65. Blank S: Transverse tibial stress fractures. Am J Sports Med 15:597–602, 1987.

66. Green NE, Rogers RA, Lipscomb AB: Nonunion of stress fractures of the tibia. Am J Sports Med 13:171–176, 1985.

67. Wilcox JR Jr., Moniot AL, Green JP: Bone scanning in the evaluation of exercise-related stress injuries. Radiology 123:699–703, 1977.

68. Blair WF, Manley SR: Stress fractures of the proximal fibula. Am J Sports Med 8:212–213, 1980.

69. Burrows FJ: Fatigue fractures of the fibula. J Bone Joint Surg 30(B):266–279, 1948.

70. Devas MB, Sweetnam R: Stress fractures of the fibula—a review of 50 cases in athletes. J Bone Joint Surg 38(B):818–829, 1956.

71. Hershman EB, Mailly T: Stress fractures. Clin Sports Med 10:183–214, 1990.

72. Symeonides PP: High stress fractures of the fibula. J Bone Joint Surg 62(B):192–193, 1980.

73. Newberg AH, Kalisher L: Case report: an unusual stress fracture in a jogger. J Trauma 18:816–817, 1978.

74. DeSmet AA, Fisher DR, Heiner JP, Keene JS: Magnetic resonance imaging of muscle tears. Skeletal Radiol 19:283–286, 1990.

75. Maguire DL, Ray RR, Zonnebelt SM: Case report: popliteal artery occlusion in a wrestler in the absence of known trauma. Phys Sports Med 13(8):139–141, 1985.

76. Rudo ND, Noble HB, Conn J, et al.: Popliteal artery entrapment syndrome in athletes. Phys Sports Med 5:105–114, 1982.

77. Buetow PC, Kransdorf MJ, Moser RP, et al.: Radiologic appearance of intramuscular hemangioma with emphasis on MR imaging. AJR 154:563–567, 1990.

78. Cohen EK, Kressel HY, Perosio T, et al.: MR imaging of soft-tissue hemangiomas: correlation with pathologic findings. AJR 150:1079–1081, 1988.

79. Hawnaur JM, Whitehouse RW, Jenkins JPR, Isherwood I: Musculoskeletal hemangiomas: comparison of MRI with CT. Skeletal Radiol 19:251–258, 1990.

80. Nelson MC, Stull MA, Teitelbaum GP, et al.: Magnetic resonance imaging of peripheral soft tissue hemangiomas. Skeletal Radiol 19:477–482, 1990.

81. Sartoris DJ: X-ray quiz. Appl Radiol 18(10):42–43, 1989.

82. Meier JL, Mollet E: Acute periostitis in early acquired syphilis simulating shin splints in a jogger. Am J Sports Med 14:327–328, 1986.

83. Sim FH, Dahlin DC, Beabout JW: Osteoid osteoma: diagnostic problems. J Bone Joint Surg 57(A):154–159, 1975.

84. Swee RG, McLeod RA, Beabout JW: Osteoid osteoma: detection, diagnosis and localization. Radiology 130:117–123, 1979.

85. Micheli LJ, Jupiter J: Osteoid osteoma as a cause of knee pain in the young athlete. Am J Sports Med 6:199–202, 1978.

86. Smith FW, Gilday DL: Scintigraphic appearance of osteoid osteoma. Radiology 137:191–195, 1980.

87. Winter PF, Johnson PM, Hilal SK, et al.: Scintigraphic detection of osteoid osteoma. Radiology 122:177–178, 1977.

88. Ghelman B, Vigorita VJ: Postoperative radionuclide evaluation of osteoid osteomas. Radiology 146:509–512, 1983.

Orthopedic overview

The percentage of the population that participates in athletic activities has increased dramatically over the past 20 years. It is becoming increasingly common for the physician to encounter an injured patient who, secondary to impatience or competition pressures, demands an immediate diagnosis of an athletic injury. It is estimated that 25 percent of these athletic injuries occur in the foot and ankle.

The physician's traditional skills of thorough history taking and comprehensive physical examination will yield an accurate diagnosis in the vast majority of athletic injuries. In difficult cases, imaging modalities may aid in making the diagnosis and establishing a treatment plan. The physician treating sports injuries in the foot and ankle makes use of plain and special view radiographs, tomographs, CT scans, TPBS, and MRI scans.

In my own practice, special imaging techniques have been very useful in treating athletic injuries to the ankle. Bone scans and, recently, MRI scans are used to evaluate osteochondritis dissecans and occult osteochondral fracture of the talus. Bone scans are used to evaluate whether an os trigonum is symptomatic when the clinical exam is equivocal. Computed tomographic scans can determine the adequacy of fragment reduction in triplane and other unusual ankle fractures. In the future, I suspect MRI will play an increasingly helpful role in evaluating ankle sprain, lateral synovitis, and lateral ankle impingement syndrome.

In the hindfoot, nuclear bone scans have been useful in differentiating between plantar fasciitis, heel pad syndrome, and stress fractures of the calcaneus. CT scans have been instrumental in diagnosing talocalcaneal coalition as a cause of pain and decreased hindfoot motion. If radiographs and physical examination are equivocal, nuclear bone scanning or MR scanning can be helpful in diagnosing bifurcate ligament injuries.

Injuries to the tarsal bones of the midfoot and to the Lisfranc and Chopart joints can be assessed with the aid of advanced imaging techniques. CT and MRI can both be helpful in making the diagnosis of a tarsal stress fracture. Triple-phase bone scans assist with the diagnosis and the determination of the age of this injury. In the patient with a midfoot sprain, CT scanning has been useful in defining subtle injuries to Lisfranc's joint that are not apparent on plain films.

The forefoot can also be a challenging diagnostic area for the sports medicine physician. Advanced imaging techniques can be used to aid in determining the exact diagnosis and age of the injury. Distinguishing between an early stress fracture or simply a stress reaction can be essential in the competitive runner. I have found the TPBS to be useful in this situation. Sesamoiditis, stress fracture of the sesamoid, or separation of a bipartite sesamoid can be difficult to diagnose without the aid of a TPBS. CT scanning can be useful in evaluating the severity of a hallux rigidus and as an aid in preoperative planning for this painful disorder. MRI or TPBS can be useful in evaluating an early Freiberg's infarction of the metatarsal head.

In summary, the physician treating athletic injuries in the foot and ankle has at his/her disposal an array of imaging techniques that aid in making a

CHAPTER 3

FOOT AND ANKLE

precise diagnosis. The ability to make an early diagnosis facilitates treatment and allows the athlete to return to competition safely and in a timely fashion.

JOHN B. O'DONNELL, M.D.
Orthopedic Surgery and Sports Medicine Center, The Union Memorial Hospital (Baltimore)
Clinical Instructor of Orthopedic Surgery, The Johns Hopkins School of Medicine
Baltimore, Maryland

THE ANKLE AND FOOT incur a wide spectrum of acute and chronic injuries,[1–4] which includes damage to the articular cartilage, subchondral bone, ligaments, tendons, and muscles. An extensive study of almost 17,000 patients at a large sports medicine center revealed that about 25 percent of all injuries seen involved the ankle and foot.[5] In a detailed review of injury pattern and biomechanical evaluation in ballet dancers, the ankle and foot sustained an injury rate as high as 38 percent of total sustained injuries.[1,6–8]

The phenomenal growth and development of modern imaging tools allow the evaluation of injury in this region with an extraordinary degree of accuracy. With the development of the CT scanner, it has become possible to accurately assess the bony and, to a lesser extent, the soft tissue elements of the ankle and foot in the cross-sectional plane.[9] Because of the complex curved nature of joint surfaces in this region, standard radiography has always been difficult and certain diagnostic entities have not lent themselves to assessment with plain film radiographs. CT's cross-sectional image, augmented by sagittal, coronal, and three-dimensional reconstructions, provides an optimal tool for visualizing fractures involving curved joints and for analyzing complicated anatomic regions such as the ankle and foot.[10] Magnetic resonance provides similar capability in visualizing the soft tissue structures in this region.[11] Its capability in depicting early marrow disease provides high sensitivity and accuracy in diagnosing osteomyelitis, marrow tumor, and avascular necrosis. The diagnosis of osteochondral fragments and the determination of possible loosening can now be achieved without resorting to invasive tests. Joint effusion is easily recognized with MR.[12]

Triple-phase bone scanning (TPBS) offers the opportunity to image both acute and chronic problems of the ankle and foot allowing an assessment of regional blood flow and of bony response to insult. The location and chronicity of abnormalities in this region can often be determined.[13–17] A normal TPBS of the ankle and foot is a misnomer. Virtually every scan performed shows minimal to mild foci of increased nuclide activity in one or more areas. These are foci of "nonspecific stress" in bones and joints, which usually reflect asymptomatic areas of bone remodeling.

ACUTE PROBLEMS

Fractures (Figs. 3-1 to 3-11)

Complicated fractures that occur in multiple planes are evaluated with great difficulty by standard radiographs and often require the cross-sectional image provided by CT or MR for adequate assessment. The triplane fracture of the distal tibia[18] (Fig. 3-1) and occult intraarticular fractures (Fig. 3-2) are such examples. Whenever a fracture involves a curved articular surface or propagates into a series of different planes,

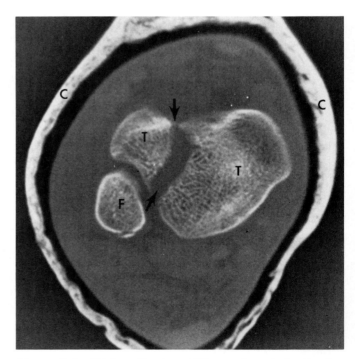

Figure 3-1   Triplane Fracture. *CT scan through the distal metaphyses of the tibia shows a metaphyseal fracture extending from anterior to posterior entering the tibiofibular joint space. Complex fractures about the ankle such as the triplane fracture are best evaluated with CT. T = tibia; F = fibula; arrows = fracture line; C = overlying cast.*

CT is indicated to demonstrate fracture features.[19] An acute fracture may be recognized on the magnetic resonance scan on T1-weighted sequences as a low-signal band representing the fracture line which becomes high signal at T2 weighting (Fig. 3-3). In the acute setting, edema of adjacent bone marrow also occurs.

Occult injury of the ankle and foot commonly presents with pain and/or swelling and often normal radiographs following inversion injury. The clinician usually takes a conservative approach treating an "ankle sprain." With persistence or recurrence of pain CT, MR, or TPBS is eventually utilized to evaluate the injury.

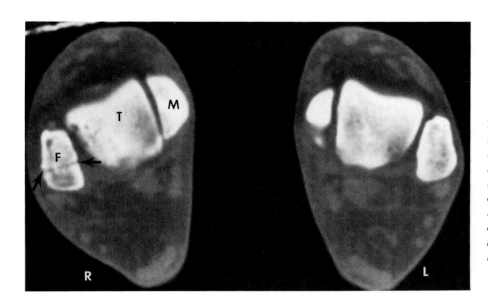

Figure 3-2   Occult Fracture. *CT scan through both ankles at the level of the upper talus shows a transverse fracture through the right fibula entering the tibiofibular joint space. The lateral margin of the talus shows posttraumatic deformity. These abnormalities were not visible on plain radiographs. T = talus; M = medial malleolus; F = distal fibula; arrows = fracture line.*

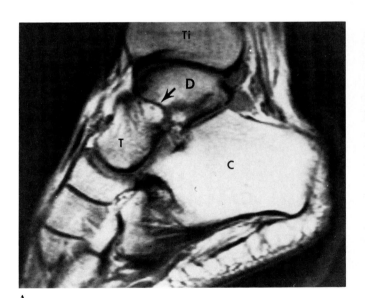

A

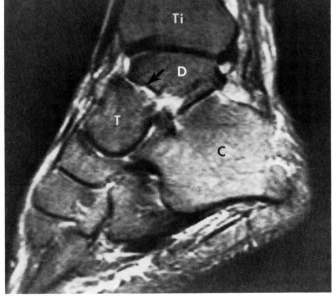

B

Figure 3-3   Talus Fracture. **A.** *MR scan at T1-weighted sequence shows a linear low-signal band crossing the neck of the talus representing an acute fracture.* **B.** *Sagittal image at T2-weighted sequence through the midtalus shows a* linear band of high signal traversing the talar neck representing blood within an acute talar fracture. Although avascular necrosis of the head of the talus later occurred in this patient, this scan was performed in the first 48 h following fracture and insufficient time had elapsed for the changes of early avascular necrosis to occur. Ti = tibia; D = dome of talus; T = distal talus; C = calcaneus; arrow = acute fracture.

The talus is a frequent site of undetected or occult fracture.[20] This may be diagnosed on either CT or MR examination.[21] Whether transcortical or of the osteochondral (osteochondritis dissecans) variety, the TPBS is positive and extremely sensitive[14,15] (Fig. 3-4). The identification of mobile loose bodies can often be accomplished with either fluoroscopic visualization[22] or MR.[23,24] Either MR or combined CT arthrography effectively shows the status of the articular cartilage (Figs. 3-5 and 3-6).[25,26] Multiple studies have concluded that osteochondral lesions probably have a traumatic origin.[27–29] Transchondral fractures almost always involve ankle inversion associated with either dorsal or plantar flexion.[30–32] With severe compression, as in weightlifting,

a transcondylar talar dome fracture may occur.[33] Some regions, such as the dome of the talus, are susceptible to developing posttraumatic avascular necrosis. Since the magnetic resonance findings of avascular necrosis depend on death of fat cells, which takes from 2 to 5 days to occur, magnetic resonance is useful in determining early avascular necrosis only after that period of time has elapsed.[34–36] Fractures of the navicular bone may be difficult to visualize on plain film radiographs but readily yield to CT assessment (Fig. 3-7). Fractures of the cuboid and cuneiform bones, although less frequently fractured, may be clearly identified on TPBS[15,37] (Figs. 3-8 and 3-9).

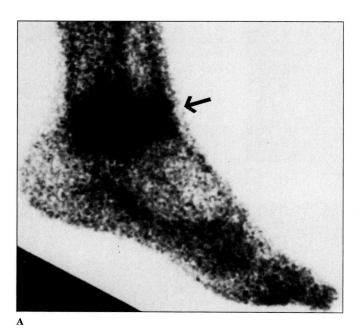

A

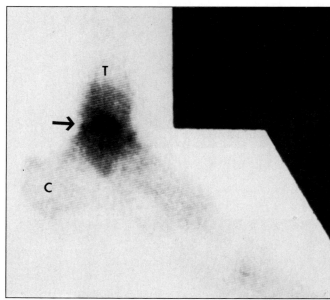

B

C

Figure 3-4 Osteochondral Fracture, Dome of Talus. *Twenty-year-old female cheerleader with right ankle pain and normal radiographs.* **A.** *Lateral blood pool image of right ankle demonstrates increased nuclide activity in the region of the talus (arrow).* **B.** *Computer-enhanced high-resolution delayed lateral image shows focally increased activity in the dome of talus (arrow).* **C.** *Computer-enhanced high-resolution anterior view demonstrates focally increased nuclide activity in the lateral portion of the dome of the talus (arrow). Computer enhancement allows the technologist and/ or radiologist to subtract out or "dial down" adjacent background to show the most focal or intense "hot spot." Preenhanced images showed intense activity in the entire tibiotalar joint not allowing for definite localization of the nuclide abnormality. T = tibia; C = calcaneus.*

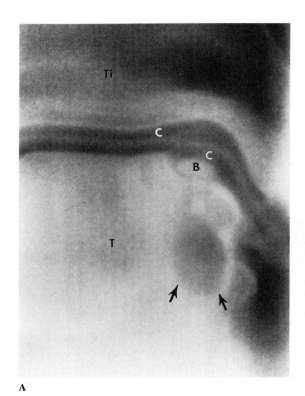

A

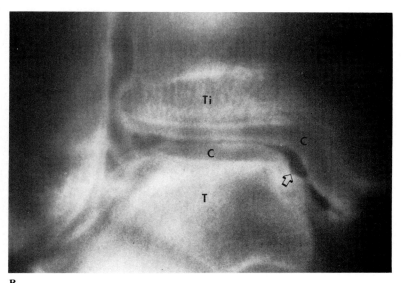

B

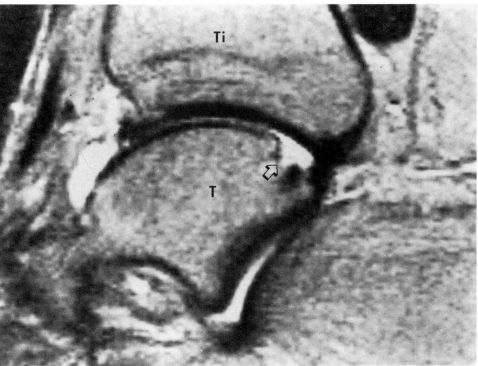

C

Figure 3-5   Osteochondritis Dissecans of Talus. **A.** *Anteroposterior radiograph following contrast injection into the ankle joint shows a bony fragment making up the medial dome of the talus. The overlying articular cartilage is smooth and intact. A large cyst has developed within the talus beneath the contained* *bony fragment.* **B.** *Anteroposterior radiograph following contrast injection into the ankle joint shows depression of the medial articular surface of the dome of the talus. The overlying articular cartilage is similarly depressed but remains intact.* **C.** *Sagittal image at T2-weighted sequence shows depression of the poste-* *rior cortex of the dome of the talus. Joint fluid fills that depressed region. Ti = tibia; T = talus; C = articular cartilage; B = bony fragment; open arrow = region of cortical depression; arrows = cyst.*

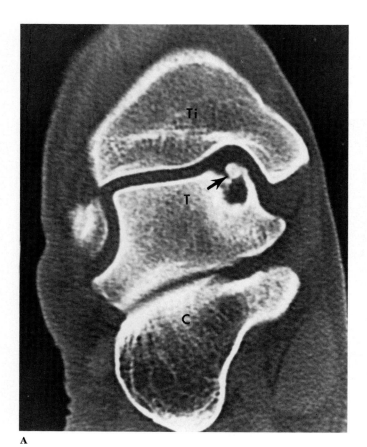

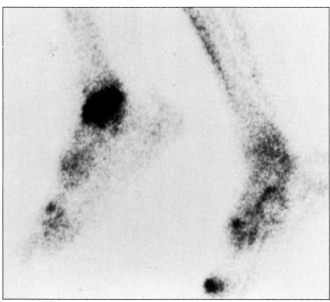

Figure 3-6 Osteochondritis Dissecans of Talus. **A.** *CT scan in the coronal plane shows a loose bony fragment making up the dome of the talus medially. An underlying cyst has developed.* **B.** *High-resolution delayed image (lateral view) demonstrates increased nuclide activity corresponding to the focus of osteochondritis dissecans and cyst formation. Ti = tibia; T = talus; C = calcaneous; arrow = bony fragment.*

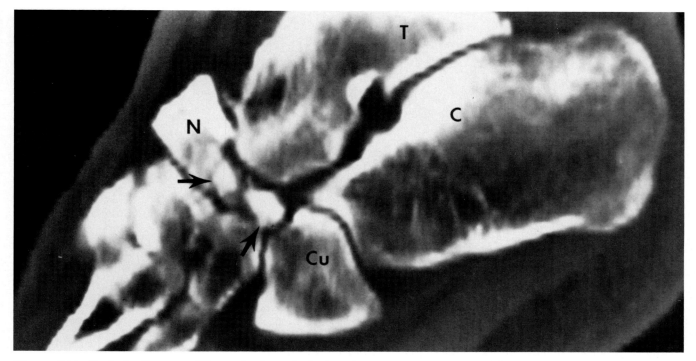

Figure 3-7 Navicular Fracture. *CT scan in the sagittal plane demonstrates a comminuted fracture of the inferior aspect of the navicular bone laterally. Several bony fragments are present. T = talus; C = calcaneus; Cu = cuboid; N = navicular; arrows = bony fragments.*

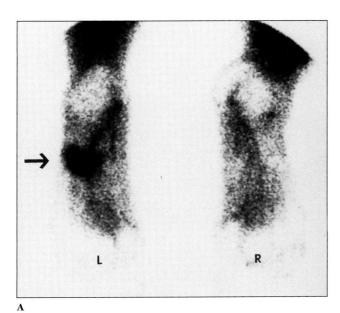

Figure 3-8   Left Cuboid Fracture. *Thirty-three-year-old female touch football player with sudden onset of pain and negative radiographs.* **A.** *Blood pool image of TPBS demonstrates increased activity in the lateral aspect of left midfoot (arrow).* **B.** *High-resolution delayed image demonstrates increased activity in left midfoot laterally corresponding to that area of abnormal nuclide activity demonstrated above.* **C.** *High-resolution delayed images (lateral view) demonstrate intense nuclide activity (open arrow) corresponding to the left cuboid bone. Note focal regions of minimally increased activity in several other areas of both feet representing physiologic "stress remodeling"; this type of incidental activity, which is most often asymptomatic, is very commonly seen on ankle and foot scans.*

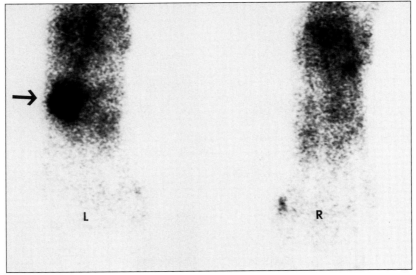

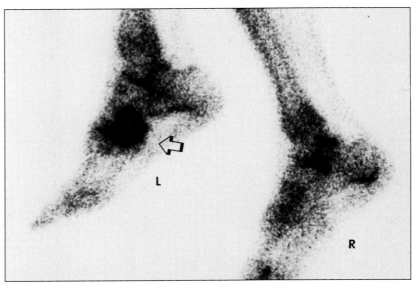

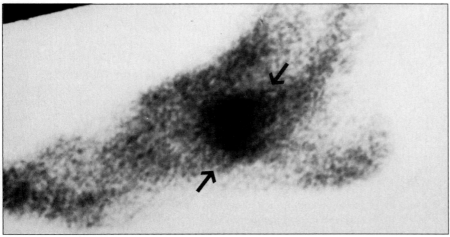

A

Figure 3-9   Cuboid Fracture. *Sixty-two year old female tennis player with right foot pain and negative radiographs.* **A.** *Magnified lateral blood pool image of TPBS demonstrates focal area of mildly increased activity in the region of the cuboid bone (arrows).* **B.** *Magnified lateral high-resolution delayed image shows focally increased nuclide activity in the region of the right cuboid (arrows).* **C.** *CT scan shows occult linear fracture (arrowheads) of the cuboid bone which was not apparent on plain film radiographs.*

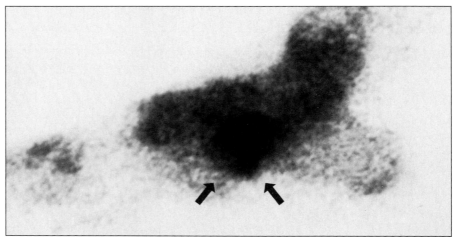

B

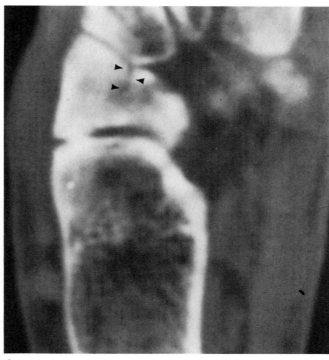

C

Calcaneal fractures account for from 33 to 51 percent of all tarsal fractures. The nuclear bone scan may be positive within 7 h. If negative by the third day, fracture can be excluded.[38] Two types of fracture involve the anterior calcaneal process, both of which may be positive on TPBS and CT scan.[39] The more common injury is the avulsion type (type 1) with severe inversion forcefully stretching the bifurcate ligament which connects the anterior calcaneal process to the adjacent cuboid and navicular bones. This force

causes avulsion of the anterior calcaneal process and tearing of the origin of the extensor digitorum brevis muscle[3,39–41] (Fig. 3-10, Drawing I). The compression type (type 2) involves forced abduction and dorsiflexion of the forefoot, which compresses the calcaneocuboid joint resulting in fracture of the anterior process of the calcaneus without avulsion of the bifurcate ligament.[40] Some fractures at this site may require operative management.[42] MR effectively shows the bifurcate ligament and can be used in assessing its injury.

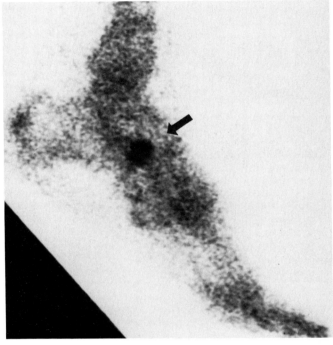

◄ **Figure 3-10** Fracture, Anterior Calcaneal Tubercle. *Severe inversion injury of the ankle with negative radiographs and persistent pain. High-resolution lateral delayed image of TPBS demonstrates focally increased nuclide activity corresponding to the anterior calcaneal tubercle or process (arrow). This area is difficult to identify on lateral radiographs of the foot because of proximity or overlapping of multiple bones. TPBS allows for localization of a focal abnormality. (See Drawing I.)*

Drawing I Anterior Calca- ► neal Process Fracture. *The most common injury of the anterior calcaneal process is an avulsion fracture with stretching of the bifurcate ligament (which connects the anterior calcaneal process to the cuboid and navicular bones) and avulsion of the extensor digitorum brevis muscle at its origin. This lateral drawing of the foot demonstrates the course of the extensor digitorum brevis muscle. The magnified drawing shows the avulsed calcaneal fragment, the stretched bifurcate ligament, and the torn extensor digitorum brevis muscle.*

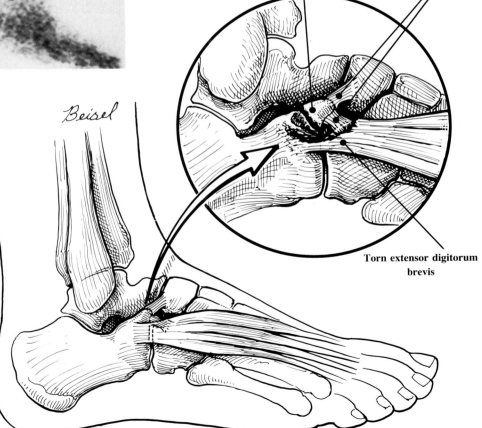

Avulsed fragment

Bifurcate ligament

Torn extensor digitorum brevis

Beisel

Fractures of the calcaneus with extension into either the subtalar joint or calcaneal-cuboid joint are particularly well assessed with CT scanning. Typically thin section axial scans are performed, which are then reformatted into the coronal and sagittal planes to assess the posterior facet of the subtalar joint as well as the anterior and middle calcaneal facets (Fig. 3-11). The CT scan is indicated in virtually all subtalar fractures with intraarticular extension to assess the congruence of the subtalar joint. Additionally, diagnosis of fibular impingement by calcaneal fragments can be made or excluded with CT evaluation.

Normal tendon anatomy

The lateral aspect of the ankle contains the peroneus longus and brevis tendons. These tendons run posteriorly and inferiorly to the fibula. The peroneus brevis tendon inserts at the proximal aspect of the fifth metatarsal, and the peroneus longus tendon inserts on the plantar aspect of the medial cuneiform and to the base of the first metatarsal. The flexor tendons to the foot and toes lie posteromedially. The most lateral is the flexor hallucis longus tendon. Just medially lies the flexor digitorum longus with the tibialis posterior positioned behind and inferior to the medial malleolus. The flexor hallucis longus tendon lies immediately below the suscentaculum with the flexor digitorum longus lying just medially to that structure.

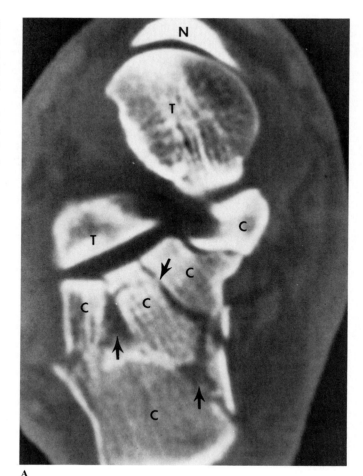

A

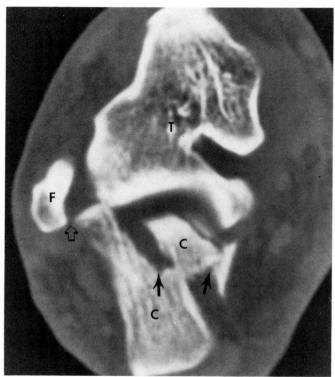

B

Figure 3-11   Calcaneus Fracture. **A.** *CT scan in the axial plane through the inferior aspect of the posterior facet shows a comminuted fracture of the calcaneus with extention of fracture lines into the joint space.* **B.** *Axial scan of same patient at a more proximal level shows displacement of calcaneal fragments with impingement of the lateral fragments against the fibula. The CT scan provides the most detailed images of the facet joints of the foot and is an indicated examination in all subtalar fractures. C = calcaneus; F = fibula; N = navicular bone; T = talus; arrows = calcaneal fractures; open arrow = region of fibular impingement.*

Avulsion injuries (Figs. 3-12 to 3-17)

The accessory navicular bone is usually an asymptomatic normal variant. It typically has a fibrous union with the parent navicular. Blunt or forceful inversion may cause injury or disruption to this union resulting in symptoms. Avulsion of the tibialis posterior tendon, which partially attaches to the accessory navicular bone, can occur. The combination of the tearing of the fibrous union and/or avulsion of the tibialis posterior tendon produces symptoms that require diagnostic evaluation. Surgery may be necessary to excise the accessory bone and to reattach the tibialis posterior tendon to the navicular bone. Avulsion injury to this small accessory bone is termed *accessory navicular syndrome* (Fig. 3-12).

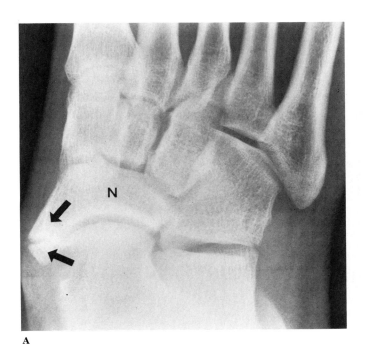

A

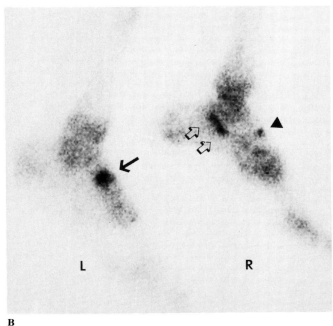

B

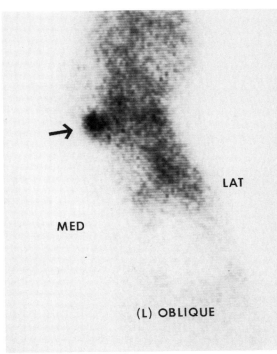

C

Figure 3-12 Accessory Navicular Syndrome. *College lacrosse player with inversion injury of the left foot and a 2-month history of left foot pain.* **A.** *Oblique radiograph of left foot demonstrates accessory navicular bone (arrows). N = navicular.* **B.** *High-resolution delayed lateral images of both ankles. Increased nuclide activity in the left foot is seen involving part of the tarsal navicular bone (long arrow). Incidental findings on the right side include linearly increased activity in the subtalar joint (open arrows) and probable dorsal spurring of right tarsal navicular bone (single arrowhead).* **C.** *Computer enhanced, magnified, delayed, high-resolution oblique image of the left foot shows increased activity in the medial aspect of the left foot proximally representing activity in the accessory navicular bone (fracture involving the body of the navicular bone would cover a larger area). This represents injury/ separation of the fibrous union between the accessory bone and the navicular bone. This injury is often associated with disruption of the tibialis posterior tendon.*

Another common injury about the ankle is avulsion of the insertion of the peroneus brevis tendon from the lateral (superficial) aspect of the fifth metatarsal bone. Radiographs may show only soft tissue swelling. Magnetic resonance scanning may show edema and hemorrhage at the insertion of the peroneus brevis tendon. The TPBS typically shows linear uptake on the periphery of the proximal aspect of the fifth metatarsal bone at the site of the avulsion injury. This injury commonly occurs in dancers who accidentally forcefully invert their foot while in the plantigrade position[6] (Fig. 3-13 and Drawing II). Peroneal tendon dislocation, usually secondary to ski injury,[43] may be reliably diagnosed with either CT or MR imaging.

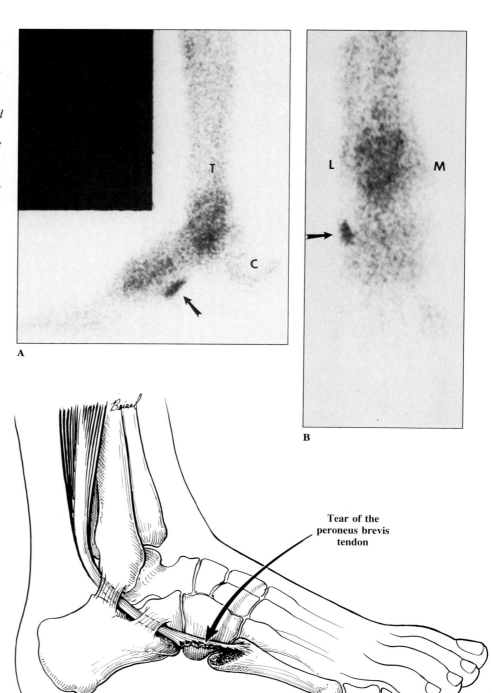

Figure 3-13   Avulsion of the Peroneus Brevis Tendon. *Twisting injury of the left foot with persistent pain and normal radiographs.* **A.** *High-resolution delayed lateral image of the left foot shows linear area of increased activity at the base of the left 5th metatarsal (arrow) where the peroneus brevis tendon normally attaches.* **B.** *High-resolution anterior view of the left foot shows increased nuclide activity in the same area (arrow). L = lateral; M = medial; T = tibia; C = calcaneus. (See Drawing II.)*

Drawing II   Tear of the Insertion of the Peroneus Brevis Tendon. *Lateral drawing of the foot and ankle demonstrates the distal course of the peroneus brevis tendon inserting at the base of the 5th metatarsal. Insertional injury may result in partial or complete tearing of the tendon. Although radiographs are most often normal unless an associated bony fragment is avulsed with the torn tendon, the TPBS demonstrates increased nuclide activity caused by hyperemia at the injury site.*

Tear of the peroneus brevis tendon

Magnetic resonance scanning is particularly valuable in determining avulsion of the tibialis posterior tendon. The tendon of the tibialis posterior muscle lies immediately anterior and superior to the flexor digitorum longus tendon and is directed along the posterior surface of the medial malleo-

lus. Avulsion of the tibialis posterior tendon (Fig. 3-14) and tendinitis with soft tissue injury adjacent to that tendon (Figs. 3-15 and 3-16) are important diagnostic entities which can be imaged both with MRI and CT scanning.[44]

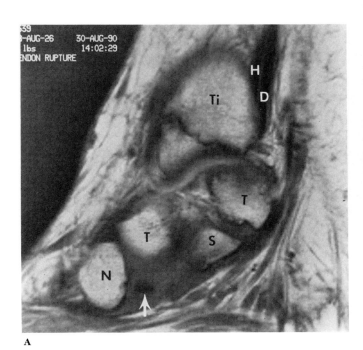

A

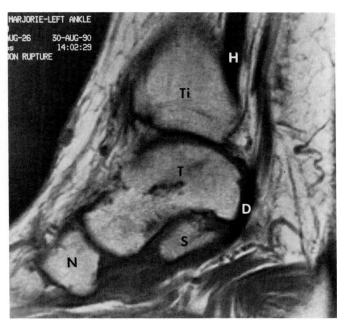

B

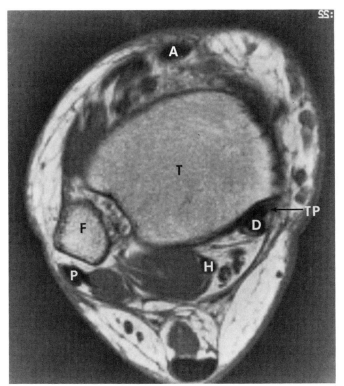

C

Figure 3-14   Avulsion of the Tibialis Posterior Tendon.
A. *Sagittal image medially at T1-weighted sequence shows the tibialis posterior tendon in its normal location posterior to the talus and inferior to the sustentaculum. A focus of low signal represents an avulsed fragment off the navicular. There is loss of continuity of the tibialis posterior tendon in this area.*
B. *Sagittal MR image at a slightly more lateral level shows discontinuity of the tibialis posterior tendon in the region between the sustentaculum and navicular bone. This indicates avulsion of the tibialis posterior tendon in this region.*
C. *Axial image at T1-weighted sequence at the level of the distal metaphysis of the tibia shows the tibialis posterior tendon to be in its normal location: anterior and medial to the flexor digitorum longus tendon. (Fig. 3-14D continues on next page.)*

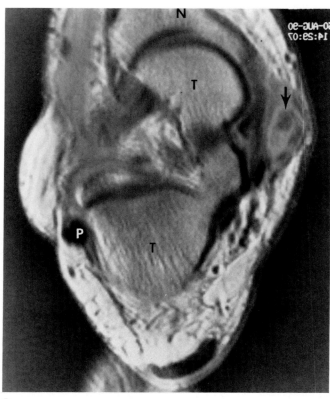

Figure 3-14   Avulsion of the Tibialis Posterior Tendon
(Continued). **D.** *Axial image at a more distal level shows
disruption of the tibialis posterior tendon. Ti = tibia; T =
talus; S = sustentaculum; TP = tibialis posterior tendon; D
= flexor digitorum longus tendon; H = flexor hallucis longus
tendon; P = peroneal tendons; A = tibialis anterior tendon;
arrow = avulsed bony fragment off the navicular; N =
navicular.*

D

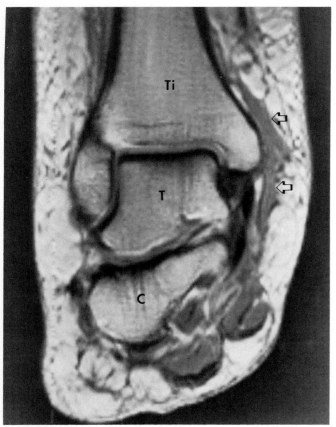

Figure 3-15   Tibialis Posterior Tendinitis, Soft-Tissue
Hemorrhage. **A.** *Coronal image at T1-weighted sequence
shows a diffuse area of intermediate signal intensity in the soft
tissues adjacent to the medial malleolus.* (Fig. 3-15B and C
continues on the opposite page.)

A

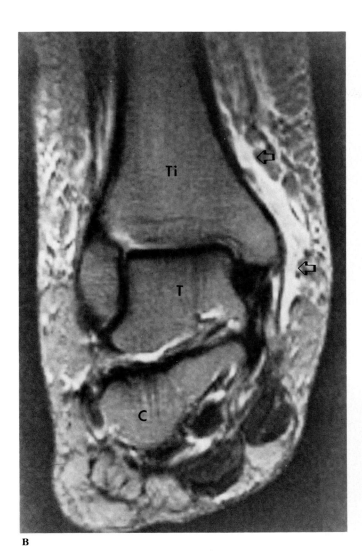

B

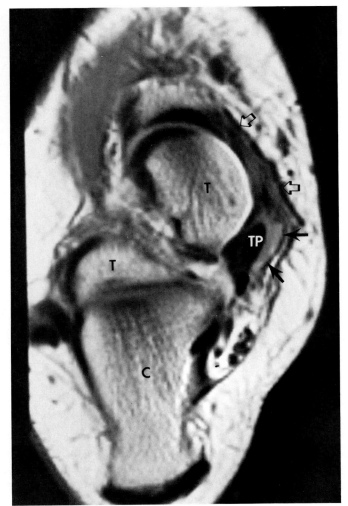

Figure 3-15   Tibialis Posterior Tendinitis, Soft-Tissue Hemorrhage (Continued). **B.** *Coronal image at T2-weighted sequence shows a region of high-signal intensity in the soft tissues adjacent to the medial malleolus. These changes, in association with acute ankle trauma, indicate hemorrhage into the medial soft tissues.* **C.** *Axial image at proton density sequence shows the tibialis posterior tendon to be surrounded by intermediate signal intensity. The tendon is intact. Intermediate signal within the medial soft tissues is present. These findings indicate subcutaneous hemorrhage and posttraumatic tendinitis of the tibialis posterior tendon. The flexor digitorum longus and flexor hallucis longus tendons are intact. Ti = tibia; T = talus; C = calcaneus; TP = tibialis posterior tendon; arrows = fluid surrounding tibialis posterior tendon; open arrows = soft tissue hemorrhage.*

C

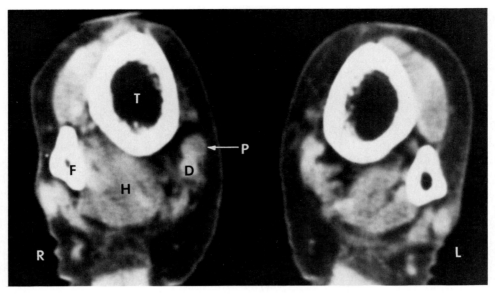

Figure 3-16   Tendinitis of Tibialis Posterior Tendon.   *CT scan in the axial plane at the level of the distal right tibia shows swelling of the tibialis posterior tendon sheath. T = tibia; F = fibula; H = flexor hallucis longus muscle; D = flexor digitorum longus tendon; P = swollen tibialis posterior tendon.*

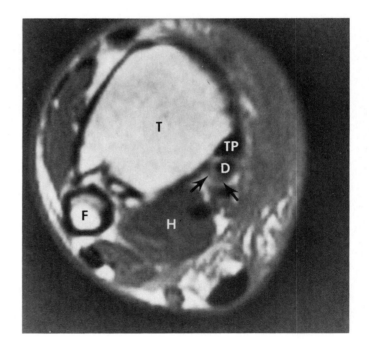

Figure 3-17   Soft Tissue Hemorrhage with Posttraumatic Tendinitis of the Flexor Digitorum Longus Tendon.   *Axial image at T1-weighted sequence shows a diffuse region of intermediate signal within the medial soft tissues indicating hemorrhage into that area. A small area of intermediate signal surrounds the flexor digitorum longus tendon indicating focal tendinitis. T = tibia; F = fibula; H = flexor hallucis longus muscle; D = flexor digitorum longus tendon; TP = tibialis posterior tendon; arrows = soft tissue hemorrhage.*

Chronic rupture of the posterior tibial tendon may result in progressive flat foot deformity. Although this may result from acute inversion, usually chronic degenerative change within the tendon is a predisposing factor. CT and MR are both highly accurate and sensitive tools for making this diagno-sis.[44,45] Tendinitis of the flexor digitorum longus tendon may similarly present with pain and swelling posterior to the medial malleolus. The flexor digitorum longus tendon lies dorsal and inferior to the tibialis posterior tendon and is clearly visualized on MRI and CT (Fig. 3-17).

Tibialis anterior tendon rupture (Fig. 3-18)

The extensor tendons lie along the dorsum of the foot and ankle. Positioned from medial to lateral are the tendons of the extensor tibialis anterior muscle, extensor hallucis longus muscle, and extensor digitorum longus muscle. These structures may be clearly seen on either CT or MR. Tear of the tibialis anterior tendon resulting from forcibly restricted extension is characterized by swelling, loss of tendinous continuity, and increased signal within the tendon at T2-weighted sequences (Fig. 3-18).

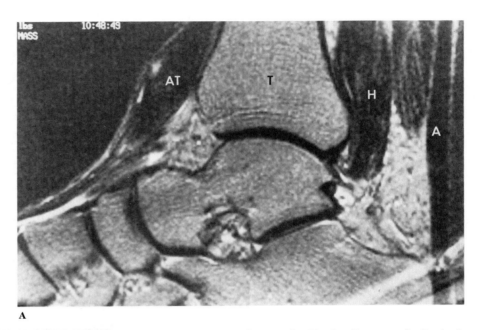

A

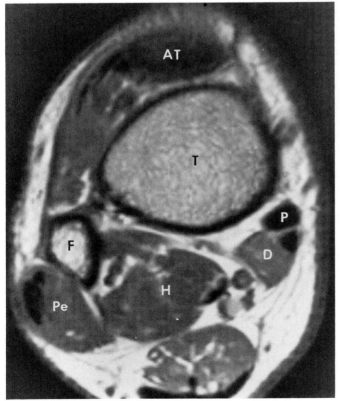

B

Figure 3-18   Tibialis Anterior Tendon Rupture. **A.** *Sagittal image at T2-weighted sequence shows enlargement of the tibialis anterior tendon with loss of distal continuity.* **B.** *Axial image at T1-weighted sequence demonstrates diffuse enlargement of the tibialis anterior tendon. H = flexor hallucis longus muscle; D = flexor digitorum longus muscle and tendon; P = tibialis posterior tendon; Pe = peroneal muscles and tendons; AT = swollen tibialis anterior tendon; T = tibia; F = fibula; A = Achilles tendon.*

Tear of the gastrocnemius-soleus muscle (Fig. 3-19)

Magnetic resonance scanning is very effective in demonstrating intramuscular hematoma following muscle tear (Fig. 3-19). Normal muscle typically shows intermediate-to-low signal intensity on both T1- and T2-weighted sequences. Acute hematoma tends to show low-to-intermediate signal intensity on T1-weighted sequences and high-signal intensity with T2 weighting. Chronic hematoma has a variable appearance because of breakdown of hemoglobin with conversion to hemosiderin and because of edematous change in the involved region.

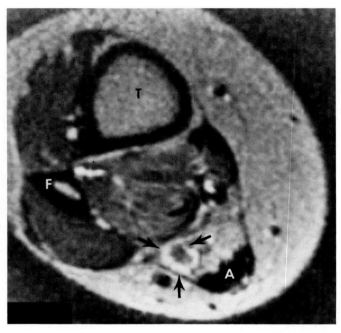

Figure 3-19   Tear of the Gastrocnemius-Soleus Muscle. *Axial image at T2-weighted sequence at the level of the distal tibia demonstrates a ring of increased signal within the soft tissues anterior to the Achilles tendon. This represents a focal area of intramuscular hematoma. The Achilles tendon remains intact. T = tibia; F = fibula; A = Achilles tendon; arrows = focal muscle tear.*

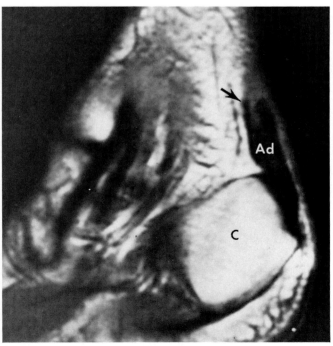

◀ **Figure 3-20**   Complete Tear of the Achilles Tendon. **A.** *Sagittal image at T1-weighted sequence shows disruption of the midportion of the Achilles tendon with loss of continuity of tendinous structures. (Fig. 3-20B continues on the opposite page.)*

A

MR is also a valuable tool when used to show acute strain associated with delayed onset muscle soreness which accompanies postmarathon myalgia. Typically the magnetic resonance scan demonstrates prolongation of T1 and T2 relaxation times within the muscle which is a self-limited finding lasting up to 3 weeks.

Achilles tendon abnormalities (Figs. 3-20 to 3-25)

Magnetic resonance and, to a lesser extent, CT provide accurate noninvasive tools to show the tendons about the foot.[46,47]

The Achilles tendon originates in the gastrocnemius-soleus muscle complex and inserts on the upper posterior aspect of the calcaneus. Normally, the Achilles tendon is uniformly hypointense on both T1- and T2-weighted sequences and is uniform in size. It tends to be flattened on its anterior border and is rounded medially, laterally, and posteriorly. Up to 25 percent of injuries to the Achilles tendon are incorrectly diagnosed clinically.[48] Tears of the extensor mechanism of the foot may involve the origin of the gastrocnemius and soleus muscles, the muscle bellies, the musculotendinous junction, or the site of tendon insertion. Achilles tendon tears occur most commonly in men who are in their third through fifth decade. The most usual site for tendon rupture is from 2 to 3 cm proximal to tendon insertion.[48] This injury occurs in either well-trained athletes or in men who are in poor physical tone and engaged primarily in weekend sports.

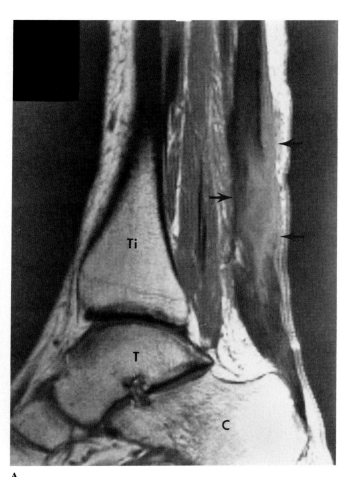

B

Figure 3-20 Complete Tear of the Achilles Tendon (Continued). **B.** *Sagittal image at a slightly more lateral position than above shows disruption of the Achilles tendon with proximal retraction of the proximal segment. Ti = tibia; T = talus; C = calcaneus; Ap = proximal tendon segment; Ad = distal tendon segment; M = gastrocnemius muscle; arrow = tendon tear.*

A

Figure 3-21 Achilles Tendon Tear at Musculotendinous Junction. **A.** *Sagittal image at T1-weighted sequence demonstrates a large area of intermediate signal intensity within the Achilles tendon near the musculotendinous junction. The involved segment shows diffuse thickening of the Achilles tendon. (Fig. 3-21B continues on next page.)*

Acute tears of the Achilles tendon are characterized by loss of continuity of tendinous structures (Figs. 3-20 and 3-21). Partial tears demonstrate high-signal intratendinous collections (Fig. 3-22). Tendinitis shows thickening of the tendon with foci of increased intratendinous signal (Figs. 3-23 and 3-24). With healing of a tendon tear, there is diffuse tendon thickening with uniformly low signal throughout both on T1- and T2-weighted sequences (Fig. 3-25).

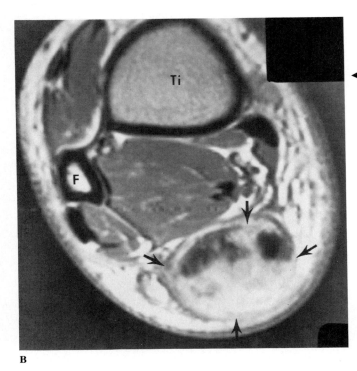

B

◀ **Figure 3-21**   Achilles Tendon Tear at Musculotendinous Junction (Continued). **B.** *Axial image at T1-weighted sequence shows diffuse enlargement of the Achilles tendon near the musculotendinous junction. Ti = tibia; T = talus; C = calcaneus; arrows = tendon tear.*

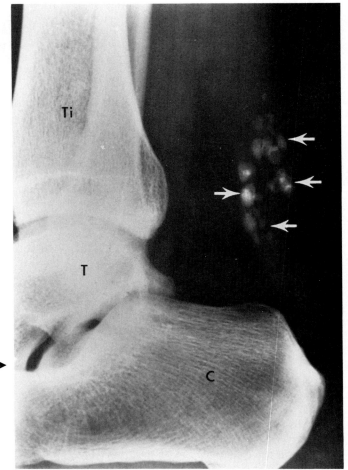

A

Figure 3-22   Partial Degenerative Tear of the Achilles Tendon. **A.** *Lateral radiograph demonstrates enlargement of the Achilles tendon with multiple focal calcifications noted within the tendinous structure.* (Fig. 3-22B, C, and D continues on the opposite page.)

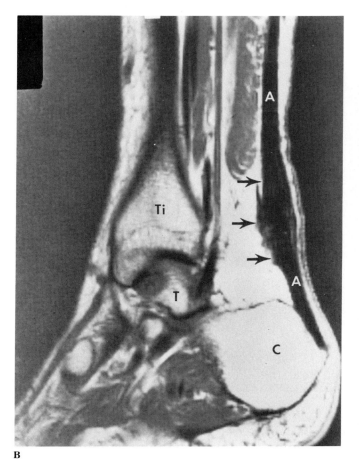

B

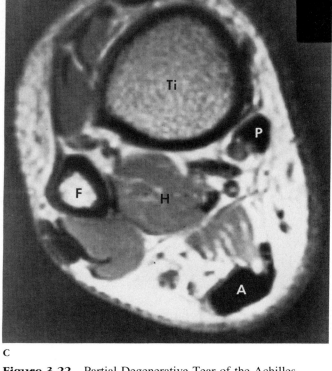

C

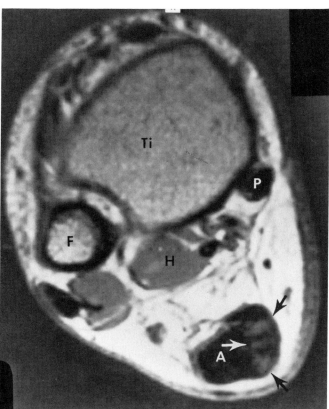

D

Figure 3-22   Partial Degenerative Tear of the Achilles Tendon (Continued). **B.** *Sagittal image at T1-weighted sequence shows enlargement of the midportion of the Achilles tendon. Focal areas of diminished signal are present within the tendon representing intratendinous ossifications, a degenerative phenomenon.* **C.** *Axial image at T1-weighted sequence near the musculotendinous junction shows the Achilles tendon to appear normal.* **D.** *Axial image at T1-weighted sequence through the midportion of the Achilles tendon demonstrates tendinous enlargement with focal areas of increased signal. These changes are often associated with an impending tear of the Achilles tendon.* (Fig. 3-22E and F continues on next page.)

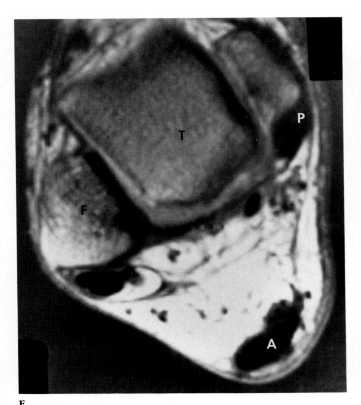

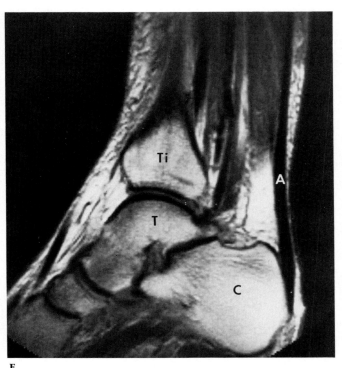

E

F

Figure 3-22 Partial Degenerative Tear of the Achilles Tendon (Continued). **E.** *Axial image at T1-weighted sequence near the attachment of the Achilles tendon to the calcaneus demonstrates a nor-* *mal appearing tendon.* **F.** *Sagittal image in another patient at T1-weighted sequence shows a normal-appearing Achilles tendon characterized by uniform thickness of the tendon and low signal* *throughout. Ti = tibia; F = fibula; T = talus; C = calcaneus; A = Achilles tendon; H = flexor hallucis longus muscle; P = tibialis posterior tendon; arrows = region of tendinous degeneration.*

Figure 3-23 Left Achilles Tendinitis. *Athlete with chronic left heel pain and normal radiographs. High-resolution delayed lateral image from TPBS shows intense tracer activity adjacent to the superoposterior aspect of the calcaneus which extends into the area of insertion of the Achilles tendon (multiple arrowheads). T = tibia; C = calcaneus.*

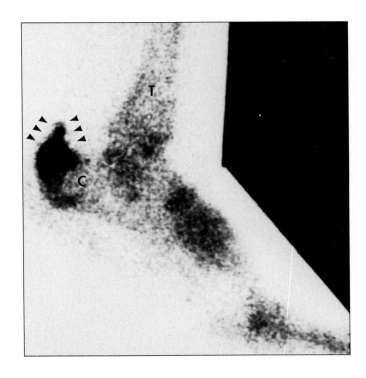

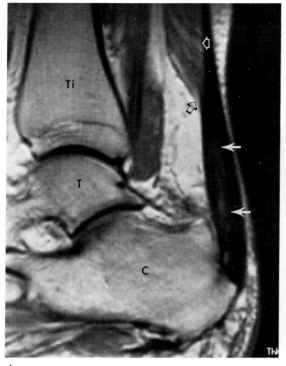

A

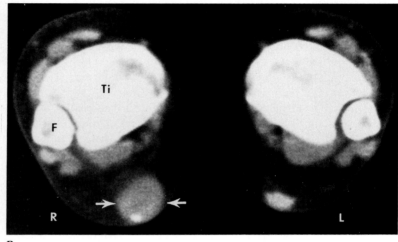

B

Figure 3-24 Achilles Tendinitis.
A. *Sagittal scan at T1-weighted se-quence shows diffuse widening of the Achilles tendon with a linear region of increased signal representing a focus of tendinitis. The musculotendinous junction*

is normal. **B.** *CT scan in the axial plane shows thickening of the right Achilles tendon which contains tiny punctate cal-cifications. This represents chronic de-generative change of the Achilles tendon which may precede tendon rupture. Ti =*

tibia; T = talus; C = calcaneus; F = fibula; arrows = abnormal region of Achilles tendon; open arrows = normal musculotendinous junction.

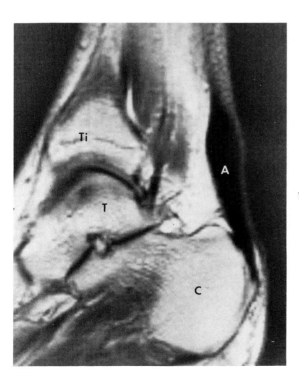

Figure 3-25 Healed Tear of the Achilles Tendon. *Sagittal image at T1-weighted sequence shows diffuse enlargement of the Achilles tendon. There remains low signal throughout the involved area indicating complete healing of a previous Achilles tendon tear. Ti = tibia; T = talus; C = calcaneus; A = Achilles tendon.*

CHRONIC PROBLEMS

Stress fracture (Figs. 3-26 to 3-34)

In McBryde's review of 1000 consecutive stress fractures in runners, 22 percent were in the ankle and foot, with 20 percent of those fractures being metatarsal stress fractures and only 2 percent occurring elsewhere in the foot.[49] It is very common to see a spectrum of subclinical as well as healing stress fractures reflecting the full continuum of stress injury.[15,50] With multiple views and magnification techniques, TPBS is able to define the anatomy of the ankle and the foot, including the specific stress fracture of individual bones.[15,51–54] On CT examination, one sees marrow edema, callous formation, soft tissue swelling, and fracture line visualization.[56,57] On magnetic resonance images a bandlike area of low signal may be present in the intramedullary space, which is continuous through to the cortex. There is decreased signal on T1-weighted sequences and increased signal with T2 weighting consistent with marrow edema. These findings become positive within 3 weeks. Standard

radiographs are notoriously insensitive in the detection of early stress fracture with only 28 percent of those fractures identified on first examination. Since the first report of tarsal navicular stress fracture in 1970, a great deal of effort has been directed at understanding the mechanism and toward detecting this condition.[58–62] Torg et al. reported the first large series and concluded that navicular stress fractures occur predominantly in young active male athletes (average age 21.8 years) and that from onset of symptoms to diagnosis the delay was approximately 7 months.[63] This is due to the insensitivity of standard radiographs in making this early diagnosis.[64] Navicular stress fractures occur because of repetitive longitudinal stress as the navicular is compressed between the head of the talus and the cuneiform bones[65] (Figs. 3-26 and 3-27). These occur predominantly in the middle third of the navicular and may be related to the relative avascularity of this region.[66,67]

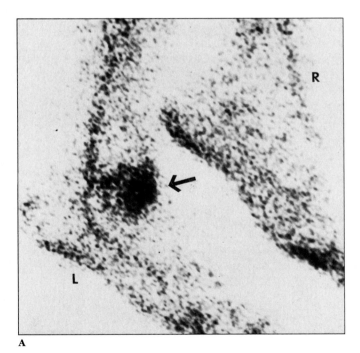

A

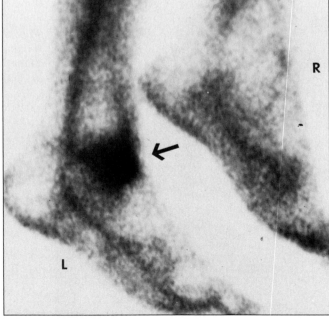

B

Figure 3-26 Navicular Stress Fracture. *Overuse injury with negative radiographs and persistent left foot pain.* **A.** *Blood flow lateral image of TPBS.* **B.** *Lateral view of blood pool.* (Fig. 3-26C continues on the opposite page.)

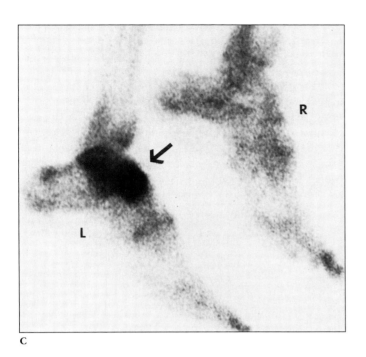

C

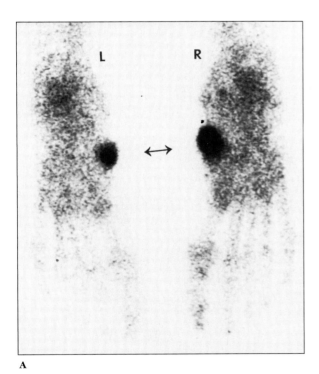

A

Figure 3-26   Navicular Stress Fracture (Continued). **C.** *High-resolution delayed lateral images. All three phases show focally intense activity with nuclide accumulation in the left navicular bone (arrow). (From Martire JR: The role of nuclear medicine scans in evaluating pain in athletic injuries.* Clinics in Sports Medicine *6:713–737, 1987. Reproduced with permission)*

Figure 3-27   Bilateral Tarsal Navicular Stress Fractures. *Nineteen-year-old female runner with bilateral foot pain and negative radiographs.* **A.** *High-resolution delayed TPBS plantar images of both feet show increased nuclide activity bilaterally in the same area (double-headed arrow).* **B.** *High-resolution delayed lateral images of both feet show increased activity in each tarsal navicular bone.*

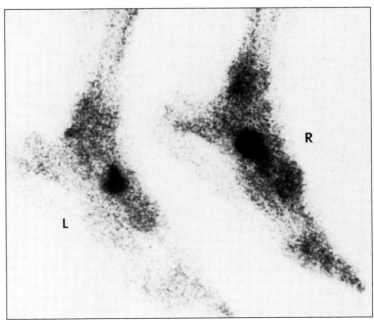

B

The second and third metatarsals, being the most immobile, represent the site of about 90 percent of metatarsal stress fractures[49,68] (Figs. 3-28 and 3-29). The first, fourth, and fifth metatarsals are the next in decreasing frequency of occurrence.[69–72] Stress fracture of the great toe is rarely reported.[73]

Since the sesamoid bones may be multipartite in from 5 to 30 percent of individuals, there is great difficulty in identifying stress fracture of the sesamoid[74–76] (Figs. 3-30 and 3-31). Dancers have been reported to be especially susceptible to sesamoid stress fracture.[77] The differential diagnosis of sesamoid stress injury includes tendinitis of the flexor hal-

lucis longus, synovitis of the metatarsal-phalangeal joint of the great toe, sesamoid bursitis, and sesamoid osteochondritis.[78] Stress fracture of the cuboid and malleoli are infrequent[15] (Fig. 3-32).

Calcaneal stress fracture results in a vertically oriented linear band of increased nuclide activity in the middle-to-upper portion of the body of the calcaneus without extension into the soft tissues (Figs. 3-33 and 3-34). This is clearly different from plantar fasciitis, retrocalcaneal bursitis, and Achilles tendinitis, in which the increased nuclide activity extends into the adjacent soft tissues.[15]

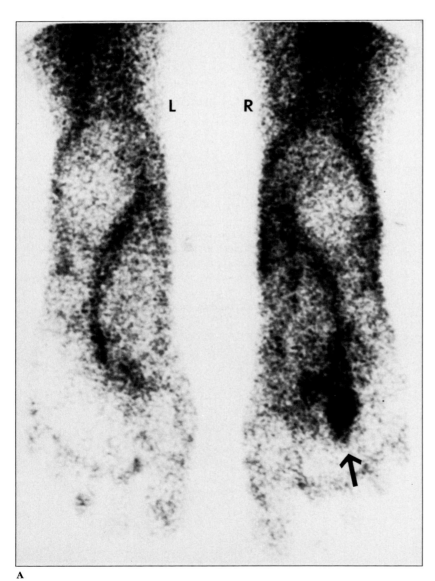

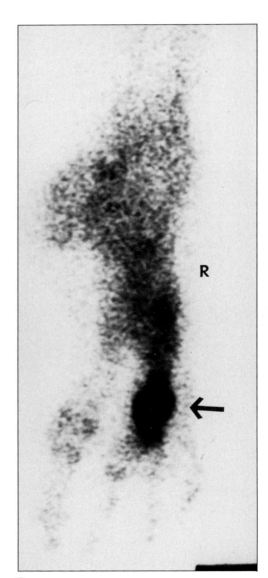

A

B

Figure 3-28 Metatarsal Stress Fracture. *Overuse injury of right foot with negative radiographs.* **A.** *Plantar view of blood pool images from TPBS of both feet shows focally intense nuclide activity overlying the right 3rd metatarsal (arrow).* **B.** *High-resolution delayed anterior oblique view shows intense nuclide activity corresponding to the shaft of the right 3rd metatarsal (arrow).*

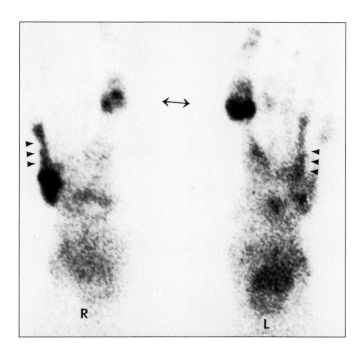

Figure 3-29   Bilateral Metatarsal and Sesamoid Stress Fractures. *College baseball player with acute and chronic bone pain bilaterally. High-resolution delayed plantar images of both feet from TPBS show stress fractures of varying ages and severity. Bilaterally increased activity in the sesamoids is seen (double-headed arrow) which is much more intense on the left side representing the chronic or healing phase. Increased activity in the left 4th metatarsal (mild) and right 5th metatarsal (severe) (multiple arrowheads) represents different ages of metatarsal stress fractures. This case illustrates how abnormal foot biomechanics may lead to multiple symptomatic areas with different degrees of TPBS abnormality.*

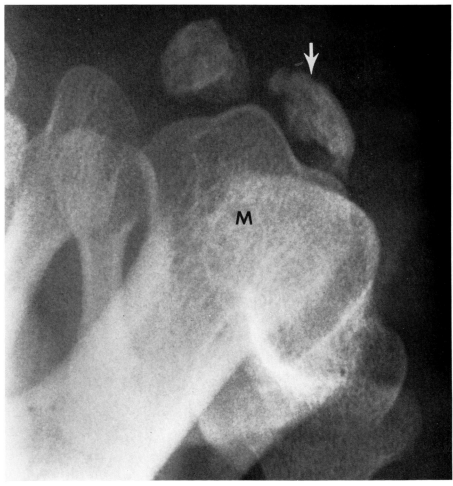

A

Figure 3-30   Sesamoiditis. **A.** *Axial radiograph of the sesamoids adjacent to the head of the first metatarsal shows irregularity of the articulating surface of the medial sesamoid and loss of continuity of its trabeculae.* (Fig. 3-30B and C continues on next page.)

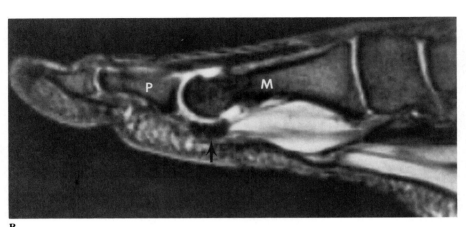

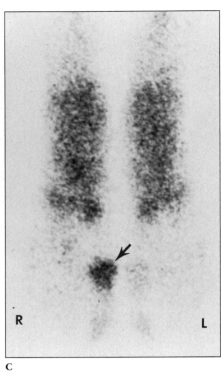

Figure 3-30 Sesamoiditis (Continued). **B.** *Sagittal MR scan at short TR gradient echo (FISP 20°) shows reduced signal diffusely involving the medial sesamoid.* **C.** *Delayed image derived from a radionuclide bone scan shows diffusely increased nuclide activity in the region of the right medial sesamoid. These findings all represent either stress fracture or avascular necrosis of the medial sesamoid. M = metatarsal; P = proximal phalynx; arrow = abnormal sesamoid.*

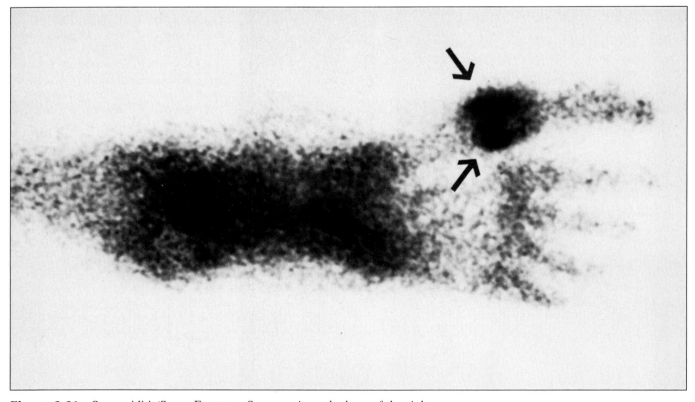

Figure 3-31 Sesamoiditis/Stress Fracture. *Severe pain at the base of the right great toe and first metatarsophalangeal joint with negative radiographs. High-resolution delayed anterior image of TPBS of the foot shows asymmetrically increased uptake in the medial and lateral sesamoid bones (arrows).*

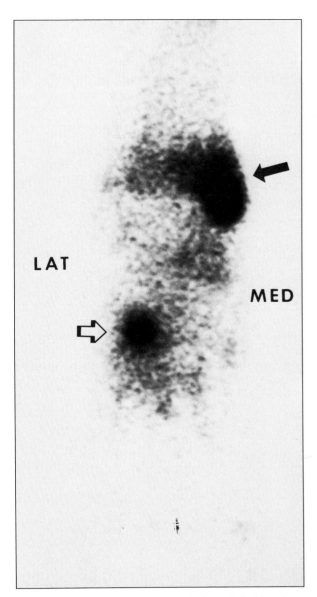

Figure 3-32   Stress Fracture of Right Cuboid and Right Medial Malleolus. *Female high school athlete with right ankle and foot pain and normal radiographs. High-resolution delayed anterior image of TPBS shows increased nuclide activity. Medial malleolus = black arrow; cuboid = open arrow; MED = medial; LAT = lateral.*

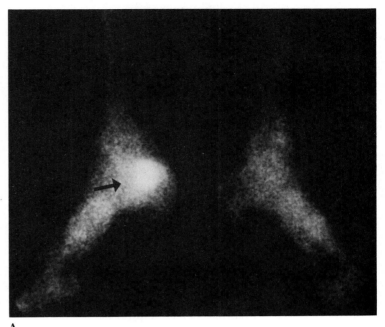

A

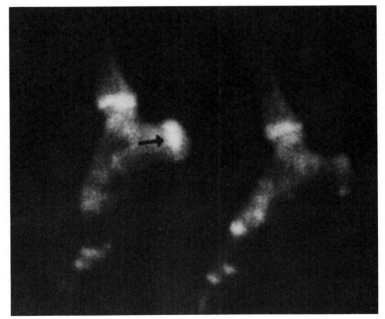

B

Figure 3-33   Left Calcaneal Stress Fracture. *Overuse injury with persistent left heel pain and normal radiographs.* **A.** *Lateral blood pool images from TPBS show nonspecific increased nuclide activity in the body of the calcaneus posteriorly (arrow).* **B.** *High-resolution delayed lateral images show focally increased nuclide activity in the posterior aspect of left calcaneus (arrow). Note that the activity is limited to the calcaneus proper and does not extend superiorly (as in Achilles tendinitis), posteriorly (as in retrocalcaneal bursitis), or plantarly (as in plantar fasciitis). This study was done with the older triple lens/Polaroid technique.*

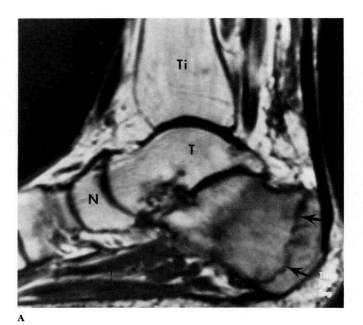

A

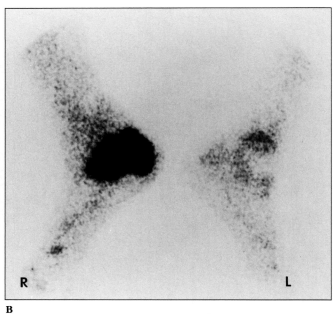

B

Figure 3-34 Calcaneal Stress Fracture. **A.** *Sagittal image at T1-weighted sequence shows a linear area of low signal within the posterior tuberosity of the calcaneus representing a stress fracture.* *Low signal indicating marrow edema surrounds the linear abnormality. Plain radiographs were inconclusive.* **B.** *Delayed image from a radionuclide bone scan shows intense nuclide activity in the* *right calcaneus corresponding to the stress fracture. Ti = tibia; T = talus; N = navicular; arrows = stress fracture.*

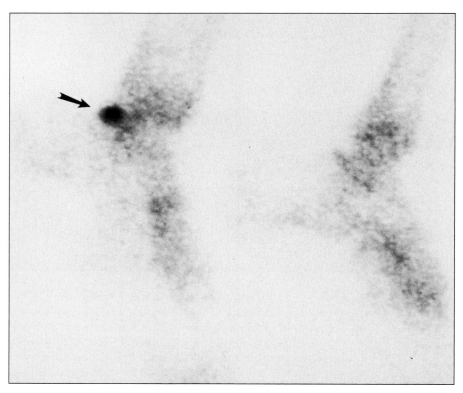

Figure 3-35 Stress Fracture of Left Os Trigonum (Posterior Impingement Syndrome). *High-resolution delayed lateral images of both ankles from TPBS show focally increased nuclide accumulation in the left os trigonum (arrow).*

Impingement syndromes (Figs. 3-35 to 3-39)

The *posterior impingement syndrome,* also called the *talar compression syndrome* and *os trigonum syndrome,* results from impaction of the os trigonum between the calcaneus and the posterior rim of the tibia.[6,79–82] This is the result of repeated plantar flexion which can be seen in ballet dancers, gymnasts, and downhill runners. This may result in a stress fracture of the os trigonum, which demonstrates a focal area of increased nuclide activity seen on the TPBS[15] (Figs. 3-35 and 3-36).

Quick, forceful, and repeated dorsiflexion of the ankle, as would occur in ballet dancing, high jumping, basketball,

and gymnastics, is the underlying mechanism of the *anterior impingement syndrome.*[83] The repetitive pulling of the ankle joint capsule added to impingement of the talus against the tibia can lead to the development of calcific deposits along the path of capsule fibers.[84] This eventually causes cartilaginous or osseous spurring on the dorsum of the tibia anteriorly, the tibiotalar joint, or the talonavicular joint.[85] These hypertrophic spurs cause potentially painful joint impingement that may require surgical excision.[83] If more than one spur is noted on radiographs, TPBS will be useful in identifying the active symptomatic focus (Figs. 3-37 to 3-39).

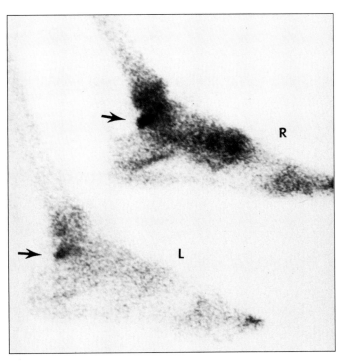

Figure 3-36 Bilateral Os Trigonum Stress Fracture (Posterior Impingement Syndrome). *Female gymnast with bilateral posterior ankle/heel pain and normal radiographs. High-resolution delayed lateral images from TPBS of both feet/ankles show increased nuclide activity in os trigonum (arrows) (right greater than left) consistent with stress fracture.*

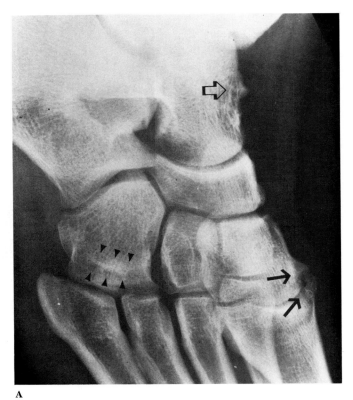

A

Figure 3-37 Hypertrophic Spur, Dorsum of Right Foot (Talus and First Metatarsophalangeal Joint). *All American college lacrosse player with severe, chronic right foot pain and positive radiograph.* **A.** *Oblique radiograph of the foot shows dorsal hypertrophic spurring of the talus (open arrow) and of the first metatarsophalangeal joint (black arrows). Additionally, linear bony sclerosis is present in the distal aspect of the cuboid bone (multiple arrowheads). Bone scan performed to identify which of these radiographic abnormalities was metabolically active.* (Fig. 3-37B continues on next page.)

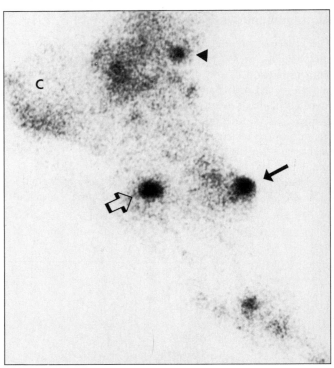

Figure 3-37 Hypertrophic Spur, Dorsum of Right Foot (Talus and First Metatarsophalangeal Joint) (Continued). **B.** *High-resolution delayed lateral image from TPBS shows that all three radiographic abnormalities show increased activity. Dorsal talus (arrowhead), first metatarsophalangeal joint (black arrow), and cuboid (open arrow) show varying degrees of nuclide activity. C = calcaneus. Painful spurs were surgically removed. Cuboid uptake represents a stress fracture.*

B

Figure 3-38 Dorsal Hypertrophic Spur/Anterior Impingement Syndrome. *Female athlete with chronic foot pain dorsally.* **A.** *Lateral radiograph of right foot demonstrates dorsal hypertrophic traction spurs (arrows) originating from talus and navicular. T = talus; N = navicular.* **B.** *High-resolution magnified delayed lateral image of right foot from TPBS shows nuclide activity at dorsal aspect of the talonavicular joint consistent with hypertrophic spurring (arrow).*

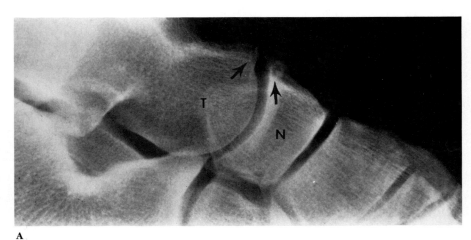

A

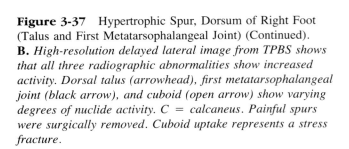

B

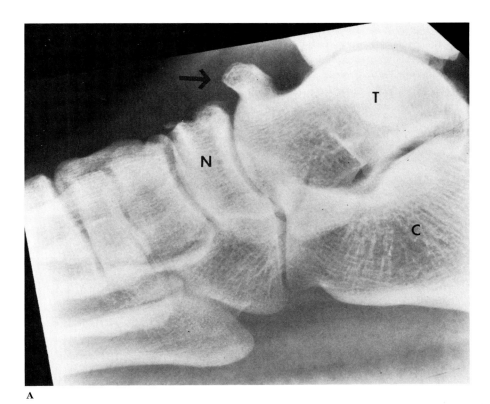

A

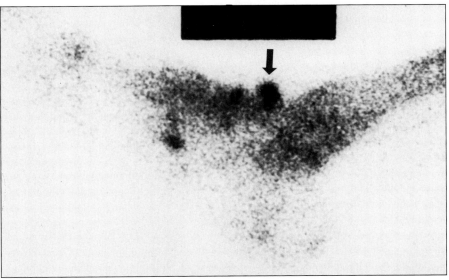

B

Figure 3-39   Dorsal Hypertrophic Spur/Anterior Impingement Syndrome of Talus. *Male college athlete with right foot pain and abnormal radiographs.* **A.** *Oblique radiograph of the foot shows a giant spur on the distal aspect of the talus dorsally (arrow). Some minimal irregularity is also noted on the dorsum of navicular bone. T = talus; C = calcaneus; N = navicular.* **B.** *High-resolution delayed lateral image of the foot shows focally increased nuclide activity (arrow) corresponding to the giant talar spur seen on radiograph.*

Tarsal coalition (Fig. 3-40)

This abnormality, inherited with autosomal dominant transmission, represents failure of complete joint formation in the hind and midfoot.[86,87] Coalitions occur in 1.8 to 2 percent of the population[88] and may involve the calcaneonavicular, talocalcaneal, talonavicular, or calcaneocuboid joints. The most common is the calcaneonavicular coalition, which oc-

curs in approximately 60 percent of patients. Usually this abnormality is asymptomatic in childhood and becomes symptomatic in early adolescence.[89] Initially, cartilaginous or fibrous coalition is present, which allows some motion to occur at the interface between the involved tarsal bones.

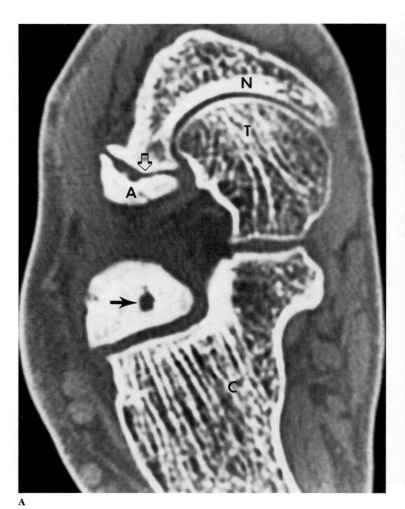

A

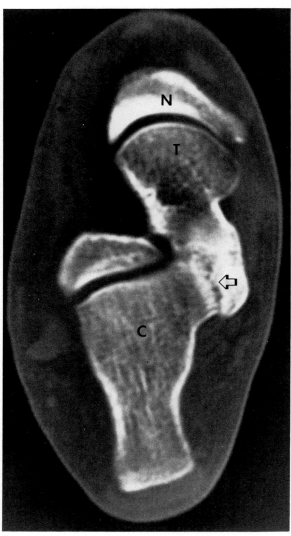

B

Figure 3-40 Calcaneonavicular Coalition with Degenerative Subtalar Cyst. **A.** CT scan in the axial plane through the lower aspect of the subtalar joint shows an irregular and narrowed joint space between the anterior process of the calcaneus and the navicular bone. This represents an incomplete bony coalition. Sclerosis and cyst formation within the inferior articular process representing premature degenerative arthritis has resulted. **B.** Subtalar coalition involving sustentaculum. Complete bony coalition of the sustentaculum tali and adjacent articulating process of talus is present. The inferior articular process of the talus and the adjacent subtalar joint remain normal. A = anterior process of calcaneus; C = calcaneus; T = talus; N = navicular; arrow = cyst within inferior articular process of talus; open arrow = subtalar coalition.

With maturation, there is a predisposition to ossification of that coalition. When ossification occurs, normal motion ceases and compensatory and excessive motion develops at other uninvolved joints.[90] Patients present with spastic flatfoot deformity. The condition is frequently bilateral, and more than one joint may be coalesced.[87] Plain radiographs may demonstrate the typical talar beak, which results from transient upward displacement of the navicular bone at the talonavicular junction and secondary osteophyte formation.[91] This condition becomes symptomatic in the adolescent with

pain attributed to early osteoarthritis (Fig. 3-40). Prior to the advent of CT, arthrography was used to demonstrate the subtalar joint.[92,93] Computed tomography currently is the most useful imaging tool to confirm the presence of coalition.[94,95] Nuclear bone scans typically show increased nuclide activity in the subtalar joint and in the region of the talar beak.[96] The pain is worsened by exercise and, unless treated, severely hampers an athlete's running ability.[97] A large os trigonum may cause a posterior bony block and lead to posterior talocalcaneal coalition.[98]

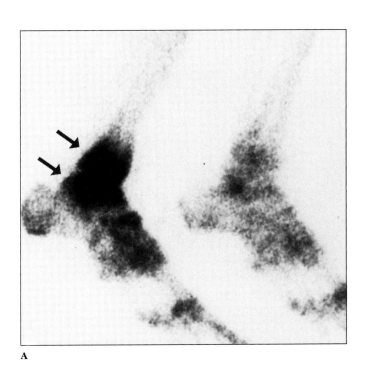

A

Figure 3-41 Posttraumatic Arthritis of the Ankle. *Thirty-seven-year-old male athlete with persistent left ankle pain and normal radiographs after injury.* **A.** *High-resolution delayed lateral images of both ankles from TPBS show nuclide asymmetry. Increased activity is seen on both sides of the left ankle joint within the talus and tibia (arrows).* **B.** *High-resolution dorsal images of both ankles and feet show diffusely increased nuclide activity on both sides of the tibiotalar joint (arrow). These nonspecific findings are consistent with posttraumatic arthritis of the tibiotalar joint. (Note increased activity incidentally present in the sesamoid bones of both feet.)*

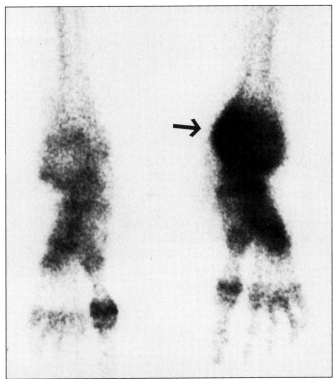

B

Posttraumatic arthritis (Figs. 3-41 to 3-46)

Sometimes, despite normal radiographs, the end result of an ankle sprain is residual pain that does not respond to usual management. In this setting, TPBS may show increased nuclide activity on both sides of one or more joints (Figs. 3-41 to 3-43). This is the typical appearance for posttraumatic arthritis. If inflammatory change is present, one sees increased activity on the blood flow and blood pool phases.

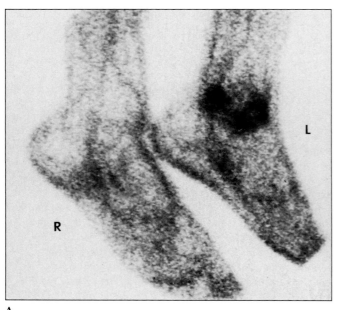

A

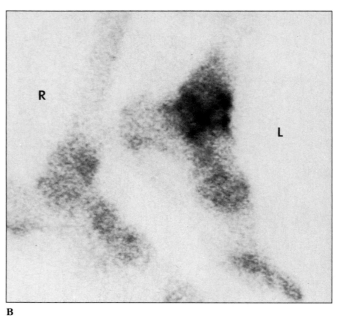

B

Figure 3-42 Posttraumatic Arthritis of the Left Ankle. *Continued left ankle pain with normal radiographs. A. Blood pool images in the lateral projection from* TPBS show diffusely increased activity in the left tibiotalar joint. *B. High-resolution delayed lateral images of both ankles show increased activity in the left* tibiotalar joint consistent with posttraumatic tibiotalar arthritis.

Figure 3-43 Posttraumatic Arthritis of the Ankle. *Severe ankle sprain with persistent pain and normal radiographs. A. Lateral blood pool image from TPBS demonstrates linear activity in the subtalar joint (open arrows) and talonavicular joint (black arrows). (Fig. 3-43B continues on the opposite page.)*

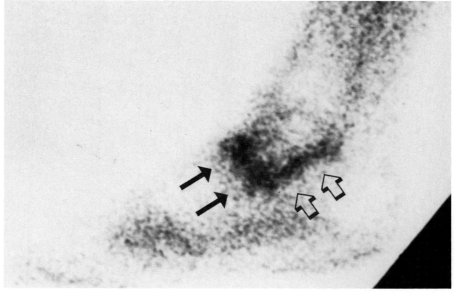

A

The magnetic resonance scan in posttraumatic arthritis shows low-signal intensity at both T1- and T2-weighted sequences involving both sides of the affected joint (Fig. 3-44).[99] Additionally, subcortical cysts may result from degenerative arthritis of posttraumatic origin. Although these cysts may be shown on MRI as intermediate signal structures on T1-weighted sequences and high-signal structures with T2 weighting,[100] (Fig. 3-45) the CT scan is an ideal tool for more clearly defining the margins of those cysts (Fig. 4-46). Sagittal and coronal reconstructions may effectively demonstrate a communicating tract between a subcortical cyst and the adjacent joint.

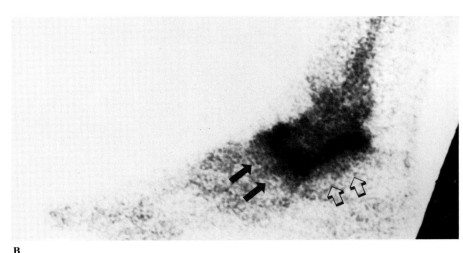

B

Figure 3-43 Posttraumatic Arthritis of the Ankle (Continued). **B.** *High-resolution delayed lateral image of the ankle shows increased nuclide activity in the same joints as above without evidence of focally increased activity elsewhere. The findings of increased nuclide activity on early and delayed images is consistent with a nonspecific, inflammatory (probably posttraumatic), arthritis as the cause for this patient's persistent pain. These findings exclude the likelihood of occult fracture.*

Figure 3-44 Subtalar Arthritis. *Coronal image at T1-weighted sequence shows low signal within the marrow spaces of the talus and calcaneus on both sides of the posterior facet representing reactive bony change from subtalar arthritis. The tibiotalar joint is normal. Ti = tibia; F = fibula; T = talus; C = calcaneus; arrows = subtalar joint.*

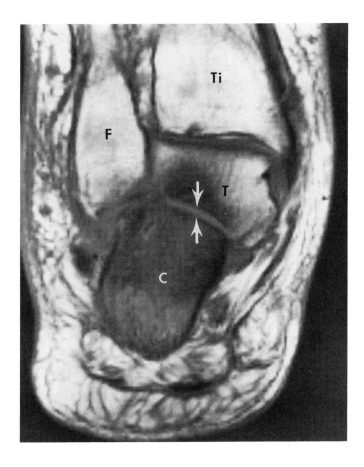

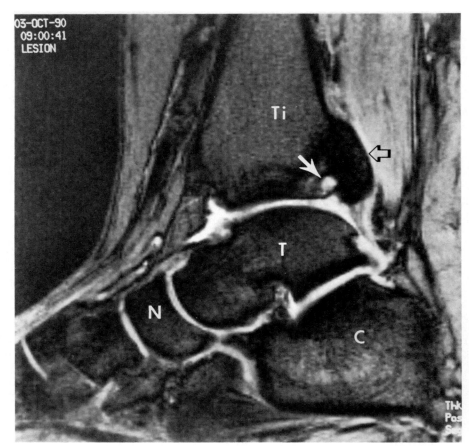

Figure 3-45 Posttraumatic Cyst of the Tibia. *Sagittal image at short TR gradient echo (FISP 20°) sequence shows deformity of the posterior malleolus of the tibia from a healed fracture. A focus of high signal within the subcortical region of the distal tibia represents a posttraumatic cyst. Ti = tibia; T = talus; N = navicular; C = calcaneus; open arrow = deformity from posterior malleolar fracture; arrow = posttraumatic cyst.*

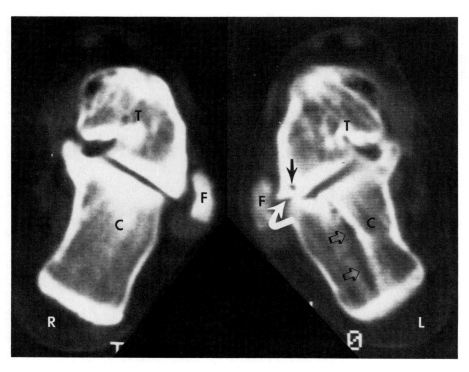

Figure 3-46 Posttraumatic Subtalar Arthritis. *Axial CT scan through the left midsubtalar joint shows irregular narrowing of the joint space with bony sclerosis and subcortical cyst. A healed fracture of the calcaneus is present. These changes represent subtalar arthritis from a previous calcaneus fracture. T = talus; C = calcaneus; F = fibula; arrow = degenerative cyst; curved arrow = region of posttraumatic arthritis; open arrows = healed calcaneal fracture.*

Posttraumatic fasciitis and bursitis (Figs. 3-47 and 3-48)

Plantar fasciitis and retrocalcaneal bursitis are common clinical overuse syndromes seen in athletes which may mimic calcaneal stress fracture.[102-105] These entities have distinguishing characteristics on TPBS.

Plantar fasciitis is a posttraumatic inflammatory abnormality involving the long plantar ligament.[106,107] On TPBS, this condition reveals focally intense curvilinear nuclide activity on the plantar surface of the calcaneus at the site of insertion of the plantar fascia[15] (Fig. 3-47). Retrocalcaneal bursitis and Achilles tendinitis show increased nuclide activity extending posteriorly and superiorly, respectively, beyond the margin of the calcaneus[15] (Fig. 3-48). Achilles tendinitis represents approximately 20 percent of ankle tendon problems in athletes.[108] Retrocalcaneal bursitis can result in severe heel pain and adjacent bony changes necessitating partial calcaneal osteotomy.[109,110] In patients with chronic, undiagnosed heel pain, TPBS is the imaging test of choice[15] (Table 3-1,[111] Drawing III).

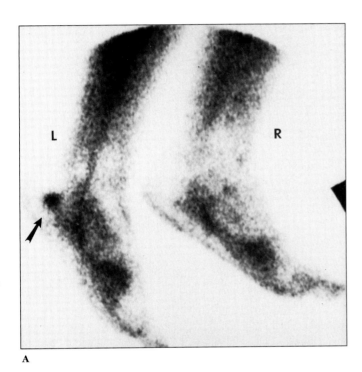

A

Figure 3-47 Left Plantar Fasciitis. *Thirty-six-year-old female athlete with chronic left heel pain and normal radiographs.* **A.** *Lateral blood pool images of both feet from TPBS demonstrate increased activity in the plantar surface of left heel (arrow).* **B.** *High-resolution delayed magnified lateral image of left foot shows focally intense nuclide activity on the plantar aspect of left calcaneus in the general area of the insertion of the plantar fascia representing plantar fasciitis (arrows).*

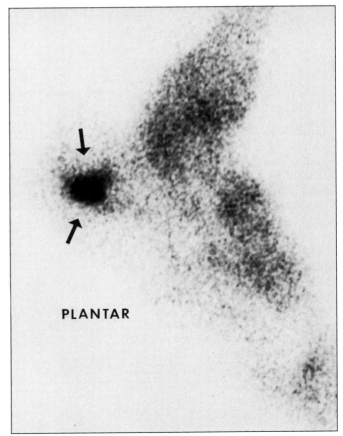

B

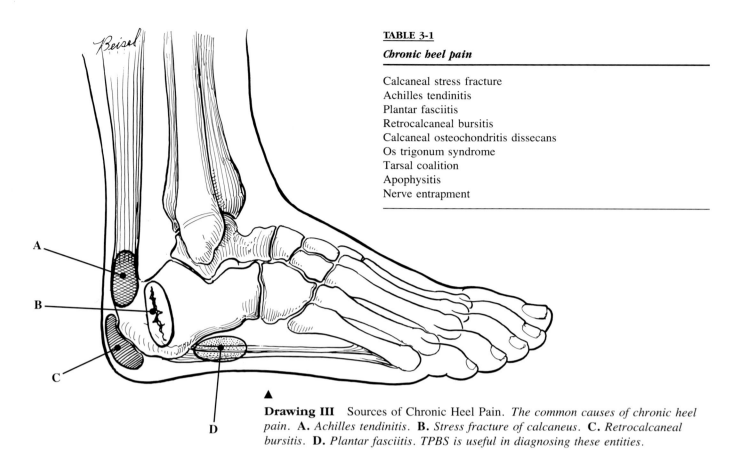

TABLE 3-1

Chronic heel pain

Calcaneal stress fracture
Achilles tendinitis
Plantar fasciitis
Retrocalcaneal bursitis
Calcaneal osteochondritis dissecans
Os trigonum syndrome
Tarsal coalition
Apophysitis
Nerve entrapment

▲

Drawing III   Sources of Chronic Heel Pain. *The common causes of chronic heel pain.* **A.** *Achilles tendinitis.* **B.** *Stress fracture of calcaneus.* **C.** *Retrocalcaneal bursitis.* **D.** *Plantar fasciitis. TPBS is useful in diagnosing these entities.*

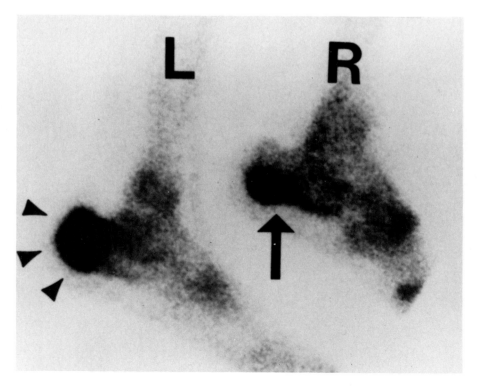

Figure 3-48   Right Plantar Fasciitis and Left Retrocalcaneal Bursitis. *Bilateral heel pain with normal radiographs. High-resolution delayed lateral images of both feet from TPBS show increased activity along the entire plantar aspect of right calcaneus (arrow) and in the posterior aspect of the tuberosity of the left calcaneus with extension into the retrocalcaneal bursa (arrowheads). Not only is there inflammatory component in the bursa but frequently the adjacent bone undergoes secondary changes which are positive on bone scan. (See Drawing III and Table 3-1.) (From Martire JR: The role of nuclear medicine scans in evaluating pain in athletic injuries.* Clinics in Sports Medicine *6:713–737, 1987. Reproduced with permission.)*

Tibiotalar instability (Figs. 3-49 and 3-50)

Ankle instability following sprain is a common problem. Numerous radiologic tests have been devised to assess the stability of the ankle in this setting. Forceful inversion, stressing the lateral ligaments, is a commonly used test. There is not good correlation, however, between positive talar tilt (or lack thereof) and surgically demonstrated ligamentous instability.[112] Although normally both ankles show symmetric laxity with inversion and eversion, this is not always the case. More than 10° of eversion is considered abnormal. Unfortunately, up to 25° of inversion may be considered normal, limiting the value of the inversion tilt test.[113] Arthrography, if performed within the first 7 days following ankle injury, is a reliable predictor of ligamentous tear.[113–116] Combined tenography and arthrography of the peroneal tendons has been reported to demonstrate a positive predictive value of 100 percent for diagnosis of lateral ligament tear.[117] These examinations are invasive and uncomfortable. Magnetic resonance effectively shows the ligaments stabilizing the ankle[118–120] (Figs. 3-49 and 3-50). The anterior and posterior tibiofibular ligaments and the anterior and posterior talofibular ligaments are best seen in the axial plane.[121] The calcaneofibular ligament and the deltoid ligament are more optimally seen in the coronal or oblique planes.[121] Some inhomogeneity and irregularity of the talofibular and deltoid ligaments are normally seen.

Magnetic resonance has also been shown to be useful in assessment of the tarsal tunnel syndrome caused by pressure on the posterior tibial nerve.[122] The posterior tibial nerve normally lies between the flexor hallucis and flexor digitorum muscles beneath the flexor retinaculum. Soft tissue masses in this region may compress the posterior tibial nerve resulting in a burning pain radiating to the toes, to the sole of the foot, and to the medial aspect of the heel. The ligaments of the sinus tarsi may also be clearly visualized with magnetic resonance imaging.

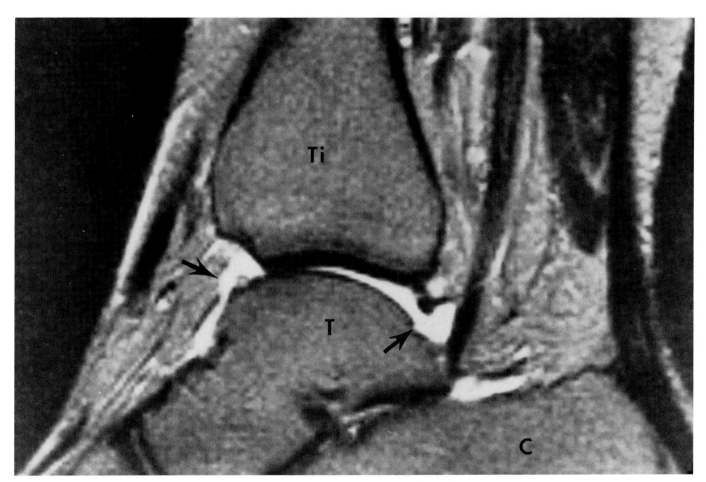

Figure 3-49   Tibiotalar Instability. *Sagittal image at T1-weighted sequence shows anterior subluxation of talus at the tibiotalar joint. A joint effusion is present. These findings indicate instability of the tibiotalar joint from previous sprain. Ti = tibia; T = talus; C = calcaneus; A = Achilles tendon; arrows = joint effusion.*

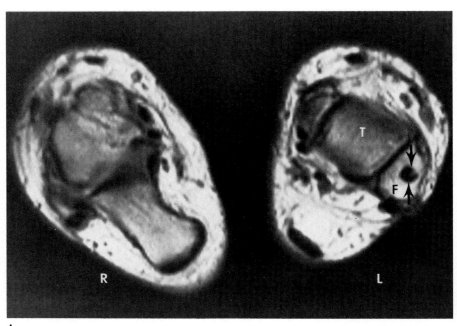

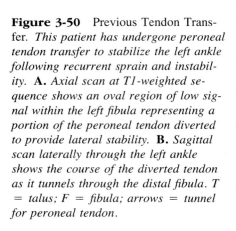

Figure 3-50   Previous Tendon Transfer. *This patient has undergone peroneal tendon transfer to stabilize the left ankle following recurrent sprain and instability.* **A.** *Axial scan at T1-weighted sequence shows an oval region of low signal within the left fibula representing a portion of the peroneal tendon diverted to provide lateral stability.* **B.** *Sagittal scan laterally through the left ankle shows the course of the diverted tendon as it tunnels through the distal fibula. T = talus; F = fibula; arrows = tunnel for peroneal tendon.*

A

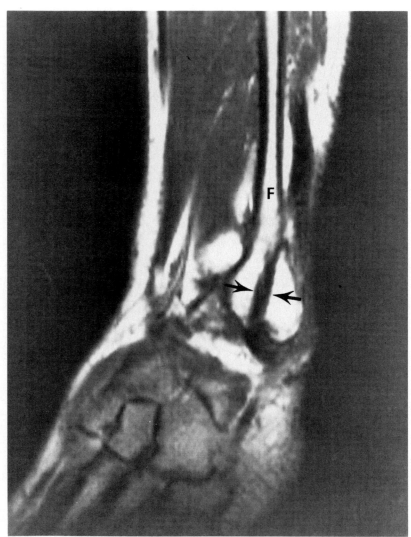

B

DIAGNOSTIC PROBLEMS

Figure 3-51 demonstrates the TPBS appearance of a soft tissue hemangioma. This vascular mass shows increased activity on the blood flow and blood pool images without increased nuclide activity on the delayed images. This indicates that the mass is in the soft tissues and is unrelated to underlying bony pathology. The magnetic resonance scan is particularly useful in depicting soft tissue masses. Neoplasms frequently show high-signal intensity on T2-weighted sequences. Just as MR may help to define the location and features of a neoplasm, absence of a neoplasm or presence of benign causes for soft tissue fullness or swelling can be demonstrated with MR imaging (Figs. 3-52 and 3-53).

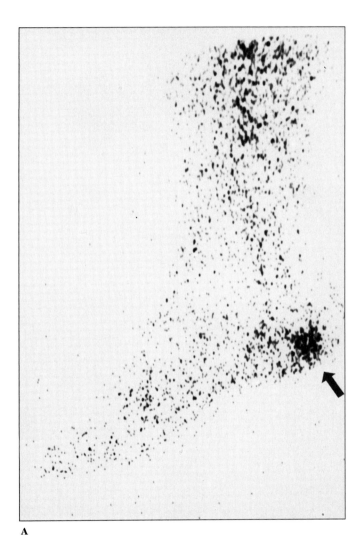

A

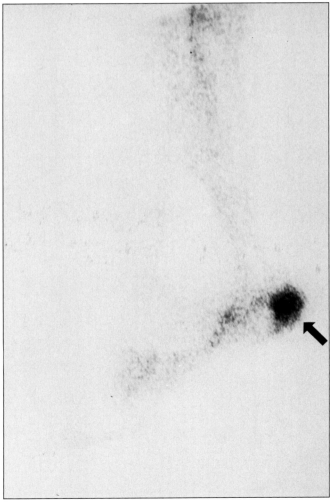

B

Figure 3-51 Hemangioma of Plantar Soft Tissues of Left Foot. *Thirty-year-old male with noticeable soft tissue mass on the plantar aspect of the foot beneath the calcaneus. Radiographs were normal.* **A.** *Lateral blood flow image from TPBS shows increased flow to the posterior plantar aspect of the calcaneus (arrow).* **B.** *Lateral blood pool image of the foot shows increased soft tissue activity on the plantar surface of the calcaneus (arrow).* (Fig. 3-51C and D continues on next page.)

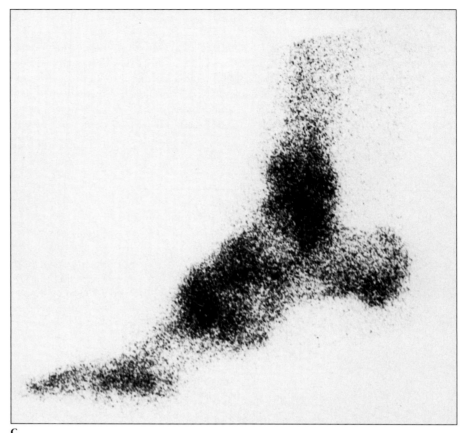

C

Figure 3-51 Hemangioma of Plantar Soft Tissues of Left Foot (Continued). **C.** *High-resolution lateral image of the foot shows no abnormal uptake in the calcaneus. (Blood flow and blood pool activity is in the soft tissues and, therefore, not identified on delayed images as abnormal bone activity.)* **D.** *Digital subtraction angiogram shows vascular blush (arrows) in the plantar soft tissues beneath the calcaneus. Surgical exploration showed this to be hemangioma. C = calcaneus; T = talus. TPBS demonstrates that the palpable mass represents a vascular soft tissue lesion without any bony involvement.*

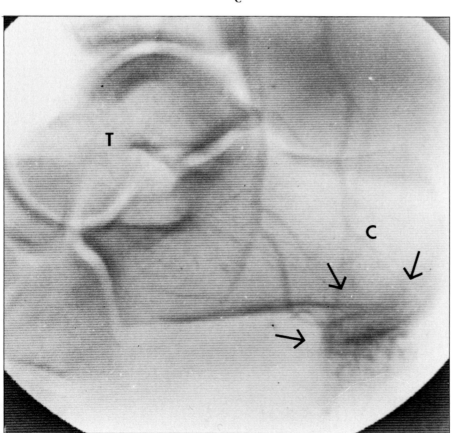

D

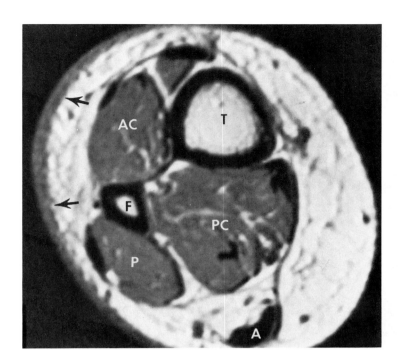

Figure 3-52   Soft Tissue Swelling. *This athlete complained of a palpable mass in the lateral aspect of the lower leg. MR scan in the axial plane at T1-weighted sequence shows diffuse thickening of the skin laterally representing soft tissue swelling. The underlying subcutaneous tissues are normal. Bones, muscles, and tendons are normal. T = tibia; F = fibula; P = peroneus muscles; AC = anterior compartment; PC = posterior compartment; A = Achilles tendon; arrows = region of soft tissue swelling.*

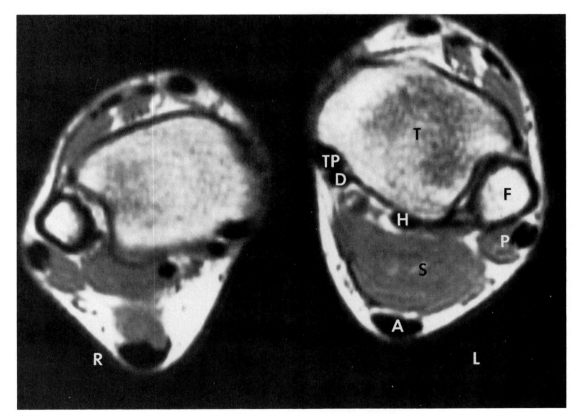

Figure 3-53   Accessory Soleus Muscle. *This young athlete had a palpable mass in the left posterior compartment. MR scan in the axial plane at T1-weighted sequence shows a large, otherwise normal-appearing left soleus muscle excluding a possible neoplasm. S = large soleus muscle; A = Achilles tendon; P = peroneus muscle and tendon; T = tibia; F = fibula; TP = tibialis posterior tendon; D = flexor digitorum longus tendon; H = flexor hallucis longus tendon.*

Subcortical and intraosseous cysts involving the ankle and tarsus may be clearly visualized on MR, CT, or TPBS (Figs. 3-54 to 3-57). Osteomyelitis (Figs. 3-58 and 3-59) and bony or soft tissue neoplasms (Figs. 3-60 and 3-61) may also occur in the athlete and cause pain with confusing clinical findings.[123–131] Osteoid osteoma can appear any-

where in the skeleton causing bone pain which may mimic a sports injury.[16] Although the plain radiograph is the initial study of choice to assess these areas, CT, MR, and TPBS may be diagnostic.[132,133] The features shown on MR are sufficiently diagnostic to separate osteomyelitis from post-traumatic arthritis.[134–139]

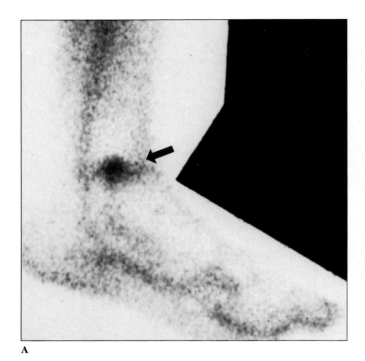

A

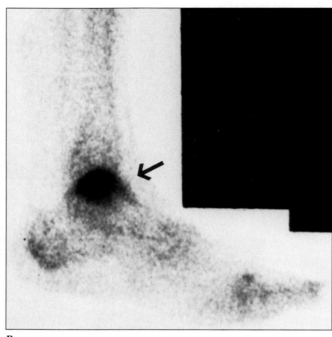

B

Figure 3-54 Subcortical Talar Cyst. *Fifty-seven-year-old male with ankle pain worsened by walking.* **A.** *Lateral blood pool image of the ankle from TPBS demonstrates mildly increased activity in the talus (arrow).* **B.** *High-resolution lateral delayed image of the ankle shows intense nuclide activity occupying most of the talar dome (arrow).* **C.** *CT scan demonstrates three well-marginated subcortical talar cysts.*

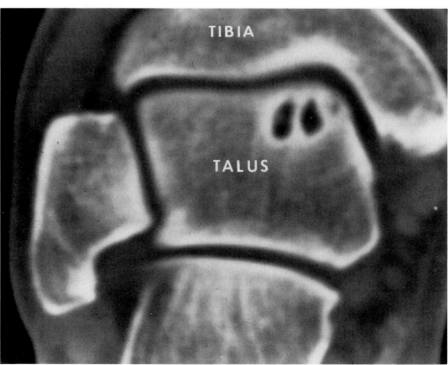

C

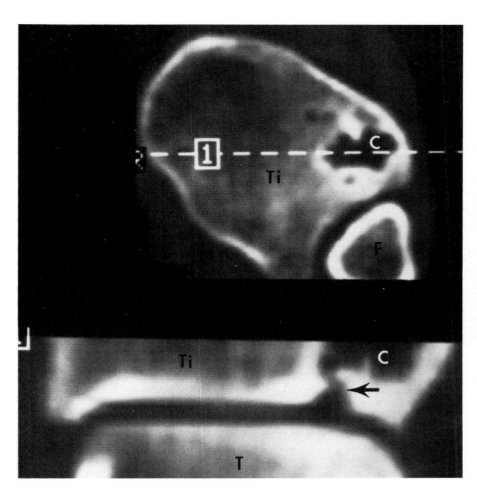

Figure 3-55 Subcortical Tibial Cyst. *CT scan (above) and reformatted coronal reconstructions (below) demonstrate a cyst within the distal portion of the tibia laterally. Reconstructions show a communicating tract from the tibiotalar joint into the cyst. Ti = tibia; C = cyst; arrow = tract; F = fibula; T = talus.*

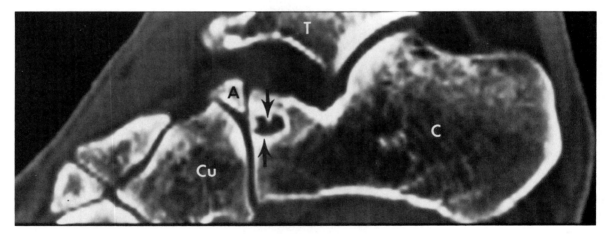

Figure 3-56 Subarticular Cysts of the Calcaneus. *CT scan reformatted in the sagittal plane through the midcalcaneus shows a subcortical cyst at the articulation of calcaneus and cuboid with an accessory ossification center adjacent to the anterior process of the calcaneus. These findings are associated with local pain accentuated by use. T = talus; C = calcaneus; CU = cuboid; A = accessory ossification center; arrows = subcortical cyst.*

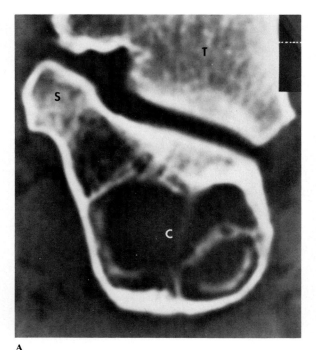

A

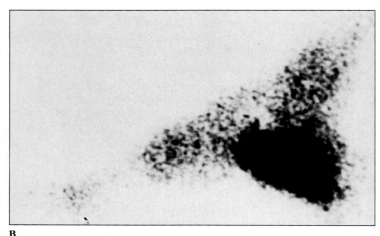

B

Figure 3-57 Calcaneal Cyst. **A.** *CT scan in the coronal plane through the anterior portion of the calcaneus at the level of the sustentaculum shows a large cyst occupying the midcalcaneus.* **B.** *De-layed image from a radionuclide bone scan shows intense nuclide activity in the calcaneus corresponding to the cyst. Bony remodeling associated with incom-plete pathologic fracture is likely present accounting for the pain that this athlete experienced. S = sustentaculum; T = talus; C = cyst.*

Figure 3-58 Metatarsal Osteomyeli-tis. *MR scan in the coronal plane at T1-weighted sequence shows loss of the nor-mal high signal from the marrow space of the 4th metatarsal. Diffuse swelling surrounding that metatarsal represents pus associated with focal osteomyelitis. At surgery, an unsuspected toothpick ab-scess was found in this jogger complain-ing of foot pain. Arrows = soft tissue abscess; metatarsals numbered 1 to 5.*

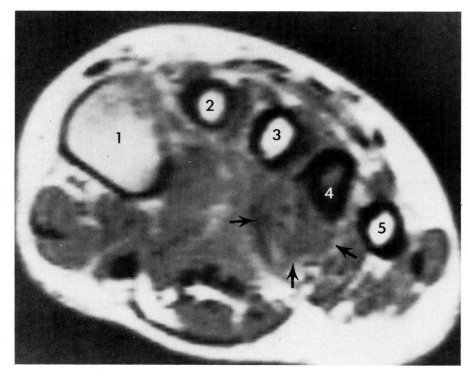

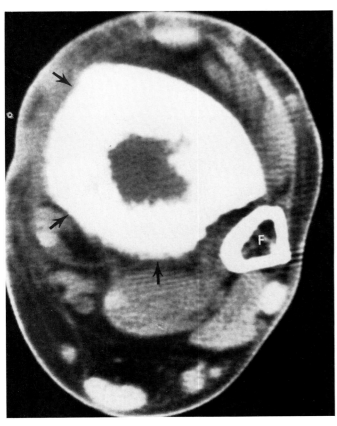

◀ **Figure 3-59** Chronic Osteomyelitis of the Tibia. *CT scan in the axial plane through the distal tibial metaphysis demonstrates chronic cortical thickening of the distal tibia with increased attenuation of its marrow space indicating chronic inflammatory reaction. The adjacent fibula is normal. Arrows = chronic cortical thickening of the tibia; F = fibula.*

Figure 3-60 Synovial Osteochondroma. **A.** *Lateral radiograph shows a calcified mass anterior to the tibiotalar joint.* **B.** *CT scan following intraarticular injection of air demonstrates a pedunculated synovial osteochondroma projecting into the tibiotalar joint space. Ti = tibia; T = talus; F = fibula; arrows = pedunculated synovial osteochondroma.*

▼

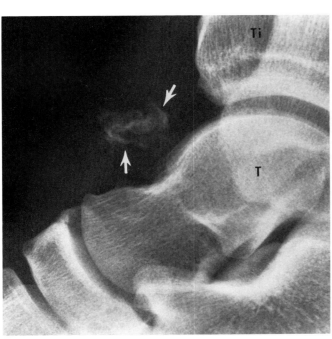

A

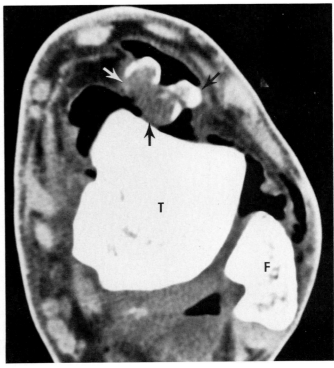

B

Any type of bony or soft tissue injury to the foot or ankle may result in reflex sympathetic dystrophy (RSD) (Fig. 3-62). TPBS is the most sensitive test for RSD.[15] Magnetic resonance has not proved useful in that diagnosis.[140] With increased interest in martial arts, it is not surprising that the first published case of TPBS confirmation of reflex sympathetic dystrophy of the ankle and foot was reported in a karate competitor.[141]

Figure 3-61 Aneurysmal Bone Cyst of a Metatarsal. *This 17-year-old runner complained of persistent severe pain following a stubbing injury to the metatarsal. Magnetic resonance image in the sagittal plane at T1-weighted sequence shows a destructive process of the distal half of the metatarsal with normal metatarsal-phalangeal joint maintenance. This lesion is characterized by an intermediate signal mass containing a lower signal fluid level (arrowheads). This represents a blood-fluid level within an aneurysmal bone cyst.*

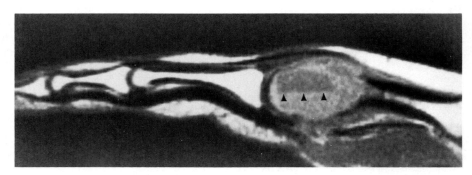

Figure 3-62 Reflex Sympathetic Dystrophy (RSD) of the Right Foot. *Right foot trauma with persistent pain, swelling, and decreased range of motion with negative radiographs was assessed with TPBS. High-resolution delayed plantar images demonstrate diffusely increased nuclide activity in the entire right ankle/foot including the tibiotalar joint, all of the tarsal joints, tarsometatarsal joints, and, to a lesser extent, the metatarsophalangeal joints. This pattern of activity in the right foot and ankle on delayed images is compatible with the diagnosis of RSD.*

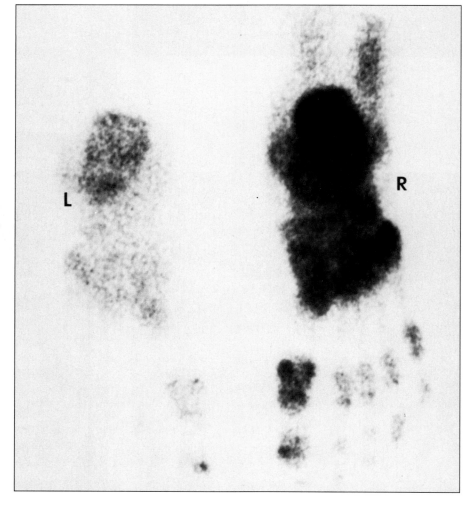

REFERENCES

1. Grahame R, Saunders AS, Maisey M: The use of scintigraphy in the diagnosis and management of traumatic foot lesions in ballet dancers. Rheumatol Rahabil 18:235–238, 1979.
2. Gray FS, Malkin L: Persistent ankle arthralgia. Complications Orthop 2:67–71, 1987.
3. Renfrew DL, El-Khoury GY: Anterior process fractures of the calcaneus. Skeletal Radiol 14:121–125, 1985.
4. Rettig AC, Shelbourne KD, Beltz HF, et al.: Radiographic evaluation of foot and ankle injuries in the athlete. Clin Sports Med 6:905–919, 1987.
5. Garrick JG, Requa RK: The epidemiology of foot and ankle injuries in sports. Clin Podiatr Med Surg 6:629–637, 1989.
6. Hamilton WG: Foot and ankle injuries in dancers. Clin Sports Med 1:143–173, 1988.
7. Hardaker WT, Margello S, Goldner JL: Foot and ankle injuries in theatrical dancers. Foot Ankle 6:59–69, 1985.
8. Sammarco HG: Dance injuries. Contemp Orthop 8(4):15–27, 1984.
9. Keyser CK, Gilula LA, Hardy DC, et al.: Soft-tissue abnormalities of the foot and ankle: CT diagnosis. AJR 150:845–850, 1988.
10. Magid D, Fishman EK: Imaging of musculoskeletal trauma in three dimensions. Radiol Clin North Am 27:945–956, 1989.
11. Stoller DW: Musculoskeletal applications of magnetic resonance imaging. Appl Radiol 11:39–48, 1988.
12. Beltran J, Noto AM, Herman LJ, et al.: Joint effusions: MR imaging. Radiology 158:133–137, 1986.
13. Holder LE: Clinical radionuclide bone imaging. Radiology 176:607–614, 1990.
14. Holder LE, Matthews LS: The nuclear physician and sports medicine, in Freeman L, Weissman H (eds): *Nuclear Medicine Annual 1984*. Raven Press, New York, 1984, pp 88–140.
15. Martire JR: The role of nuclear medicine scans in evaluating pain in athletic injuries. Clin Sports Med 6:713–737, 1987.
16. Rupani HD, Holder LE, Espinola DA, et al.: Three phase radionuclide bone imaging in sports medicine. Radiology 156:187–196, 1985.
17. Tehranzadeh J, Serafini AN, Pais MJ: *Avulsion and Stress Injuries of the Musculoskeletal System*. Karger, Basel, 1989.
18. Feldman F, Singson RD, Rosenberg ZS, et al.: Distal tibial triplane fractures: diagnosis with CT. Radiology 164:429–435, 1987.
19. Dalinka MK, Boorstein JM, Zlatkin MB: Computed tomography of musculoskeletal trauma. Radiol Clin North Am 27:933–944, 1989.
20. Mann RA: Biomechanics of running, in Mack R (ed): *The American Academy of Orthopaedic Surgery Symposium of the Foot and Leg in Running Sports*. Mosby, St. Louis, MO, 1982, pp 1–29.
21. Anderson IF, Crichton KJ, Grattan-Smith T, et al: Osteochondral fractures of the dome of the talus. J Bone Joint Surgery 71(A):1143–1152, 1989.
22. Hudson TM: Joint fluoroscopy before arthrography: detection and evaluation of loose bodies. Skeletal Radiol 12:199–203, 1984.
23. DeSmet AA, Fisher DR, Burnstein MI, et al.: Value of MR imaging in staging osteochondral lesions of the talus (osteochondritis dissecans): results in 14 patients. AJR 154:555–558, 1990.
24. Mesgarzadeh M, Sapega AA, Bonakdarpour A, et al.: Osteochondritis dissecans: analysis of mechanical stability with radiography, scintigraphy and MR imaging. Radiology 165:775–780, 1987.
25. Kaye JJ: Arthritis: roles of radiology and other imaging techniques in evaluation. Radiology 177:601–608, 1990.
26. Sims RE, Genant HK: Magnetic resonance imaging of joint disease. Radiol Clin North Am 24:179–188, 1986.
27. Naumetz VA, Schweigel JF: Osteocartilaginous lesions of the talar dome. J Trauma 20:924–927, 1980.
28. Savastano AA: Articular fractures of the dome of the talus. Phys Sports Med 10:113–119, 1982.
29. Thompson JP, Loomer RL: Osteochondral lesions of the talus in a sports medicine clinic: a new radiographic technique and surgical approach. Am J Sports Med 6:460–463, 1984.
30. Mulligan ME: Horizontal fracture of the talar head: a case report. Am J Sports Med 14:176–177, 1986.
31. Santopietro FJ: Foot and foot-related injuries in the young athlete. Clin Sports Med 3:563–589, 1988.
32. Scharling M: Osteochondritis dissecans of the talus. Acta Orthop Scand 49:89–94, 1978.
33. Mannis CI: Transchondral fracture of the dome of the talus sustained during weight training. Am J Sports Med 11:354–356, 1983.
34. Gillespy T III, Genant HK, Helms CA: Magnetic resonance imaging of osteonecrosis. Radiol Clin North Am 24:193–208, 1986.
35. Speer KP, Spritzer CE, Harrelson JM, Nunley JA: Magnetic resonance imaging of the femoral head after acute intracapsular fracture of the femoral neck. J Bone Joint Surg 72(A):98–103, 1990.
36. Vogler JB III, Murphy WA: Bone marrow imaging. Radiology 168:679–693, 1988.
37. Marymont JH, Mills GQ, Merritt WD: Fracture of the lateral cuneiform bone in the absence of severe direct trauma: diagnosis by radionuclide bone scan. Am J Sports Med 8:135–136, 1980.
38. Moss EH, Carty H: Scintigraphy in the diagnosis of occult fractures of the calcaneus. Skeletal Radiol 19:575–577, 1990.
39. Harburn TE, Ross HE: Avulsion fracture of the anterior calcaneal process. Phys Sports Med 15:73–80, 1987.
40. Davis AW, Alexander IJ: Problematic fractures and dislocations in the foot and ankle of athletes. Clin Sports Med 1:163–181, 1990.
41. Norfray JS, Rogers LF, Adams GP, et al.: Common calcaneal avulsion fracture. AJR 134:119–123, 1980.
42. Degan TJ, Morrey BF, Braun DP: Surgical excision for anterior process fractures of the calcaneus. J Bone Joint Surg 64(A):519–524, 1982.
43. Rosenberg ZS, Feldman F, Singson RD, Kane R: Ankle tendons: evaluation with CT. Radiology 166:221–226, 1988.
44. Rosenberg ZS, Cheung Y, Jahss MH, et al.: Rupture of posterior tibial tendon: CT and MR imaging with surgical correlation. Radiology 169:229–235, 1988.

45. Rosenberg ZS, Jahss MH, Noto AM, et al.: Rupture of the posterior tibial tendon: CT and surgical findings. Radiology 176:489–493, 1988.

46. Dalinka MK, Kricun ME, Zlatkin MB, Hibbard CA: Modern diagnostic imaging in joint disease. AJR 152:229–240, 1989.

47. Friedman RJ: MRI helps characterize foot, ankle abnormalities. Diagn Imaging 12(12):84–91, 1990.

48. Quinn SF, Murray WT, Clark RA, Cochran CF: Achilles tendon: MR imaging at 1.5 T. Radiology 164:767–770, 1987.

49. McBryde AM: Stress fractures in runners. Clin Sports Med 4:737–752, 1985.

50. Belkin SC: Stress fractures in athletes. Orthop Clin North Am 11:735–742, 1980.

51. Alfred RH, Bergfeld JA: Diagnosis and management of stress fractures of the foot. Phys Sports Med 15(8):83–89, 1987.

52. Hershman EB, Mailly T: Stress fractures. Clin Sports Med 1:183–214, 1990.

53. Meurman KOA: Less common stress fractures in the foot. Br J Radiol 54:1–7, 1981.

54. Shelbourne KD, Fisher DA, Rettig AC, et al.: Stress fractures of the medial malleolus. Am J Sports Med 16:60–63, 1988.

55. Lee JK, Yao L: Stress fractures: MR imaging. Radiology 169:217–220, 1988.

56. Murcia M, Brennan RE, Edeiken J: Computed tomography of stress fracture. Skeletal Radiol 8:193–195, 1982.

57. Yousem D, Magid D, Fishman EK, et al.: Computed tomography of stress fractures. J Comput Assist Tomogr 10:92–95, 1986.

58. Hunter LY: Stress fracture of the tarsal navicular. More frequent than we realize? Am J Sports Med 9:217–219, 1981.

59. Pavlov H, Torg JS, Freiberger RH: Tarsal navicular stress fractures: radiographic evaluation. Radiology 148:641–645, 1983.

60. Ting A, King W, Yocum L, et al.: Stress fractures of the tarsal navicular in long distance runners. Clin Sports Med 7:89–101, 1988.

61. Towne LC, Blazina ME, Cozen LN: Fatigue fractures of the tarsal navicular. J Bone Joint Surg 52(A):376–378, 1970.

62. Wilcox JR, Jr, Moniot AL, Green JP: Bone scanning in the evaluation of exercise-related stress injuries. Radiology 123:699–703, 1977.

63. Torg JS, Pavlov H, Cooley H, et al.: Stress fractures of the tarsal navicular. J Bone Joint Surg 64(A):700–712, 1982.

64. Prather JL, Nusynowitz ML, Snowdy HA, et al.: Scintigraphic findings in stress fractures. J Bone Joint Surg 59(A):869–874, 1977.

65. Main BJ, Jowetl RL: Injuries of the midtarsal joint. J Bone Joint Surg 57(B):89–97, 1975.

66. Goergen TG, Venn-Watson EA, Rossman DJ, et al.: Tarsal navicular stress fractures in runners. AJR 136:201–203, 1981.

67. Gordon GM, Solar J: Tarsal navicular stress fractures. J Am Podiatr Med Assoc 75:363–366, 1985.

68. Micheli LJ, Sohn BS, Solomon R: Stress fractures of the second metatarsal involving Lisfranc's joint in ballet dancers. J Bone Joint Surg 67(A):1372–1375, 1985.

69. Delee JC, Evans JP, Julian J: Stress fracture of the fifth metatarsal. Am J Sports Med 11:349–353, 1983.

70. Drez D, Young JC, Johnston RD, et al.: Metatarsal stress fractures. Am J Sports Med 8:123–125, 1980.

71. Hulkko A, Orava S, Nikula P: Stress fracture of the fifth metatarsal in athletes. Ann Chir Gynaecol 74:233–238, 1985.

72. Levy JM: Stress fractures of the first metatarsal. Am J Roentgenol 130:679–681, 1978.

73. Yokoe K, Takemoto M: Stress fracture of the proximal phalanx of the great toe: a report of three cases. Am J Sports Med 14:240–242, 1986.

74. Hulkko A, Orava S, Peltokallio P, et al.: Stress fractures of the sesamoid bones of the first metatarso-phalangeal joint in athletes. Arch Orthop Trauma Surg 104:113–117, 1985.

75. Scranton PE, Jr.: Pathologic anatomic variations in the sesamoids. Foot Ankle 1:321–326, 1981.

76. Van Hal ME, Keene JS, Lange TA, et al.: Stress fractures of the great toe sesamoids. Am J Sports Med 10:122–128, 1982.

77. Sakamoto K, Mizuta H, Okajima K, et al.: An unusual cause of metatarsal pain in a young kendo player. Am J Sports Med 17:296–298, 1989.

78. McBryde AM, Anderson RB: Sesamoid foot problems in the athlete. Clin Sports Med 1:51–61, 1988.

79. Brodsky AE, Khalil MA: Talar compression syndrome. Am J Sports Med 14:472–476, 1986.

80. Ecker ML, Ritter MA, Jacobs BS: The symptomatic os-trigonum. JAMA 204:882–884, 1967.

81. Hontas MJ, Haddad RJ, Schlesinger LC: Conditions of the talus in the runner. Am J Sports Med 14:486–490, 1986.

82. Ihle CL, Cochran RM: Fracture of the fused os trigonum. Am J Sports Med 10:47–50, 1982.

83. Hawkins RB: Arthroscopic treatment of sports-related anterior osteophytes in the ankle. Foot Ankle 9:87–90, 1988.

84. McMurray TP: Footballer's ankle. J Bone Joint Surg 32(B):68–69, 1958.

85. Parks JC, Hamilton WG, Patterson AH, et al.: The anterior impingement syndrome of the ankle. J Trauma 20:895–898, 1990.

86. Jacobs AM, Sollecito V, Oloff L, Klein N: Tarsal coalitions: an instructional review. J Foot Surg 20:214–221, 1981.

87. Wheeler R, Guevera A, Bleck EE: Tarsal coalitions: review of the literature and case report of bilateral dual calcaneonavicular and talocalcaneal coalitions. Clin Orthop 156:175–177, 1981.

88. Kaplan EG, Kaplan GS, Vaccari OA: Tarsal coalition: review and preliminary conclusions. J Foot Surg 16:136–143, 1977.

89. Elkus RA: Tarsal coalition in the young athlete. Am J Sports Med 14:477–480, 1986.

90. Conway JJ, Cowell HR: Tarsal coalition: clinical significance and roentgenographic demonstration. Radiology 92:799–811, 1969.

91. Jayakumar S, Cowell HR: Rigid flatfoot. Clin Orthop 122:77–84, 1977.

92. Kaye JJ, Ghelman B, Schneider R: Talocalcaneonavicular joint arthrography for sustentacular-talar tarsal coalitions. Radiology 115:730–731, 1975.

93. Resnick D: Radiology of the talocalcaneal articulations. Radiology 111:581–586, 1974.

94. Deutsch AL, Resnick D, Campbell G: Computed tomography and bone scintigraphy in the evaluation of tarsal coalition. Radiology 144:137–140, 1982.

95. Lee MS, Harcke HT, Kumar SJ, Bassett GS: Subtalar joint coalition in children: new observations. Radiology 172:635–639, 1989.

96. Goldman AB, Pavlov H, Schneider R: Radionuclide bone scanning in subtalar coalitions: differential considerations. AJR 138:427–432, 1982.

97. Beckly DE, Anderson PW, Pedegana LR: The radiology of the subtalar joint with special reference to talo-calcaneal coalition. Clin Radiol 26:333–341, 1975.

98. Galinski AW, Crovo RT, Ditmars JJ, Jr.: Os trigonum as a cause of tarsal coalition. J Am Podiatr Med Assoc 69:191–196, 1979.

99. Yuh WTC, Corson JD, Baraniewski HM, et al.: Osteomyelitis of the foot in diabetic patients: evaluation with plain film, ^{99m}Tc-MDP bone scintigraphy, and MR imaging. AJR 152:795–800, 1989.

100. Beltran J: MRI of the musculoskeletal system. Appl Radiol 3:23–29, 1990.

101. Brown ML, Johnson KA: Bone scintigraphy of the calcaneus. Clin Nucl Med 11:530–537, 1986.

102. Dalby RE: Stress fractures of the os calcis. JAMA 200:131–132, 1967.

103. Hopson CN, Perry DR: Stress fractures of the calcaneus in women Marine recruits. Clin Orthop 128:159–162, 1977.

104. Hullinger CW: Insufficiency fracture of the calcaneus similar to March fracture of the metatarsal. J Bone Joint Surg 26:751–757, 1944.

105. Kwong PK, Kay D, Voner RT, et al.: Plantar fasciitis: mechanics and pathomechanics treatment. Clin Sports Med 7:119–126, 1988.

106. Micheli LJ: Lower extremity overuse injuries. Acta Med Scand 711 (suppl):171–176, 1986.

107. Taunton JE, Clement DB, McNicol K: Plantar fasciitis in runners. Can J Appl Sports Sci 7:41–44, 1982.

108. Frey CC, Shereff MJ: Tendon injuries about the ankle in athletes. Clin Sports Med 7(1):103–118, 1988.

109. Heneghan MA, Wallace T: Heel pain due to retrocalcaneal bursitis (with an historical footnote on Sever's disease). Pediatr Radiol 15:119–122, 1985.

110. Jones DC, James SL: Partial calcaneal ostectomy for retrocalcaneal bursitis. Am J Sports Med 12(1):72–73, 1984.

111. Taylor PM: Osteochondritis dissecans as a cause of posterior heel pain. Phys Sports Med 10(9):53–59, 1982.

112. Schweigel JF, Knickerbocker WJ, Cooperberg P: A study of ankle instability utilizing ankle arthrography. J Trauma 17:878–881, 1977.

113. Olson RW: Arthrography of the ankle: its use in the evaluation of ankle sprains. Radiology 92:1439–1446, 1969.

114. Brostrom L, Liljedahl SO, Lindvall N: Sprained ankles. Acta Chir Scand 129:485–499, 1965.

115. Fordyce AJW, Horn CV: Arthrography in recent injuries of the ligaments of the ankle. J Bone Joint Surg 54(B):116–121, 1972.

116. Mehrez M, El Geneidy SE: Arthrography of the ankle. J Bone Joint Surg 52(B):308–312, 1970.

117. Bleichrodt RP, Kingma LM, Binnendijk B, Klein JP: Injuries of the lateral ankle ligaments: classification with tenography and arthrography. Radiology 173:347–349, 1989.

118. Beltran J, Munchow AM, Khabiri H, et al.: Ligaments of the lateral aspect of the ankle and sinus tarsi: an MR imaging study. Radiology 177:455–458, 1990.

119. Kneeland JB, Macrandar S, Middleton WD, et al.: MR imaging of the normal ankle: correlation with anatomic sections. AJR 151:117–123, 1988.

120. Noto AM, Cheung Y, Rosenberg ZS, et al: MR imaging of the ankle: normal variants. Radiology 170:121–124, 1989.

121. Erickson SJ, Smith JW, Ruiz ME, et al.: MR imaging of the lateral collateral ligament of the ankle. AJR 156:131–136, 1991.

122. Erickson SJ, Quinn SF, Kneeland JB, et al.: MR imaging of the tarsal tunnel and related spaces: normal and abnormal findings with anatomic correlation. AJR 155:323–328, 1990.

123. Baker BE, Levinsohn EM, Coren AB: Pitfalls to avoid in diagnosing pain in the athlete. Clin Sports Med 6:921–934, 1987.

124. Erlemann R, Reiser MF, Peter PE, et al.: Musculoskeletal neoplasms: static and dynamic Gd-DTPA-enhanced MR imaging. Radiology 171:767–773, 1989.

125. Feldman F, Singson RD, Staron RB: Magnetic resonance imaging of para-articular and ectopic ganglia. Skeletal Radiol 18:353–358, 1989.

126. Jelinek JS, Kransdorf MJ, Utz JA, et al.: Imaging of pigmented villonodular synovitis with emphasis on MR imaging. AJR 152:337–342, 1989.

127. Keigley BA, Haggar AM, Gaba A, et al.: Primary tumors of the foot: MR imaging. Radiology 171:755–759, 1989.

128. Lewis MM, Reilly JF: Sports tumors. Am J Sports Med 4:362–365, 1987.

129. Munk PL, Helms CA, Holt RG, et al.: MR imaging of aneurysmal bone cysts. AJR 153:99–101, 1989.

130. Sundaram M, McLeod RA: MR imaging of tumor and tumorlike lesions of bone and soft tissue. AJR 155:817–824, 1990.

131. Wetzel LH, Levine E: Soft-tissue tumors of the foot: value of MR imaging for specific diagnosis. AJR 155:1025–1030, 1990.

132. Fletcher BD, Scoles PV, Nelson AD: Osteomyelitis in children: detection by magnetic resonance. Work in Progress. Radiology 150:57–60, 1984.

133. Kuhn JP, Berger PE: Computed tomographic diagnosis of osteomyelitis. Radiology 130:503–506, 1979.

134. Beltran J, Campanini S, Knight C, McCalla M: The diabetic foot: magnetic resonance imaging evaluation. Skeletal Radiol 19:37–41, 1990.

135. Mason MD, Zlatkin MB, Esterhai JL, et al.: Chronic complicated osteomyelitis of the lower extremity: evaluation with MR imaging. Radiology 173:355–359, 1989.

136. Micheli LJ, Ireland ML: Prevention and management of calcaneal apophysitis in children: an overuse syndrome. J Pediatr Orthop 7:34–38, 1987.

137. Modic MT, Pflanze W, Feiglin DHI, Belhobek G: Magnetic resonance imaging of musculoskeletal infections. Radiol Clin North Am 24:247–258, 1986.

138. Tang JSH, Gold RH, Bassett LW, Seeger LL: Musculoskeletal infection of the extremities: evaluation with MR imaging. Radiology 166:205–209, 1988.

139. Unger E, Moldofsky P, Gatenby R, et al.: Diagnosis of osteomyelitis by MR imaging. AJR 150:605–610, 1988.

140. Koch E, Hofer HO, Sialer G, et al.: Failure of MR imaging to detect reflex sympathetic dystrophy of the extremities. AJR 156:113–115, 1991.

141. Birrer RB, Birrer CD: Martial arts injuries. Phys Sports Med 10(6):103–108, 1982.

Orthopedic overview

Traumatic injuries and overuse syndromes in the region of the pelvis, hip, and thigh are not as common as the frequently encountered knee, shoulder, and elbow problems of the active athlete. A groin pull or a pelvic stress fracture, however, can be as devastating to an athlete as an anterior cruciate ligament tear.

Keep in mind as well that the anatomy in this region is complex. The patient's history, mechanism of injury, and symptoms may not provide sufficient information with which to formulate a diagnosis. Injured structures may be deep and difficult to palpate. Anatomic variations and overlying shadows frequently make interpretation of plain radiographs difficult, especially in the area of the pelvis, sacrum, and coccyx. It is for these reasons that orthopedic surgeons often find that additional imaging techniques are not only helpful but frequently crucial in order to pinpoint the exact diagnosis prior to initiating treatment.

Acute traumatic fractures and stress fractures of the pelvis and hip may be undetectable on routine radiographs. An adolescent with hip pain and a suspected early slipped capital femoral epiphysis may have normal radiographs. A young woman aerobic dancer with pubic symphysis pain and tenderness may have normal films as well. In both these cases, a triple-phase bone scan (TBPS) is invaluable in helping to confirm or rule out the suspected diagnosis.

Injuries to the muscles and muscle attachments about the pelvis and hip are frequently quite difficult to isolate. The injured muscle may be small, deep, and well covered by more superficial layers of muscle and fat, making the physical exam less than diagnostic.

A skeletally immature gymnast may present with the sudden onset of anterolateral pelvic pain. The suspected diagnosis of an apophyseal avulsion injury may not be confirmed on plain films. A college long jumper experiences sudden thigh pain which prevents continued participation. A rectus femoris muscle disruption is suspected, but pain and swelling make the examination inconclusive. Imaging techniques which are currently available will be helpful in each of these cases. TPBS can provide information regarding increased blood flow or bone injury. CT scanning may clarify confusing radiographic findings in the situation of a bony avulsion injury. Magnetic resonance imaging may provide additional information regarding the extent and severity of muscle or tendinous disruption.

There are multiple bursas and tendons about the pelvis and hip which are subject to overuse. Trochanteric bursitis in a marathon runner or piriformis tendinitis in a ballet dancer can significantly impair function and performance. If these conditions do not respond promptly to the appropriate rest, anti-inflammatory medication, physical therapy, and perhaps steroid injection, then imaging in the form of bone scanning may be necessary to further localize and quantitate the inflammatory process.

An important issue regarding these imaging techniques centers on their clinical applicability. When and how are these diagnostic tests important to the treating physician? Certainly, not every pulled muscle warrants a bone scan or MRI. Some stress fractures can be clinically and radiographically

CHAPTER 4

PELVIS, HIP, AND THIGH

proven without a bone scan. It is imperative, however, that we not allow an athlete to return to his or her activity in the face of a potentially serious problem. Often our active athletes become quite impatient with sports medicine physicians unless we are able to quickly make a diagnosis and institute effective therapy, allowing them to continue or resume their exercises promptly. At times, it is simply not possible to arrive at a diagnosis based on clinical evidence. It is at these times that modern imaging techniques offer invaluable assistance in the care of our patients.

Working closely with our radiologic colleagues is crucial. The radiologist must know the clinical question being asked by the treating physician in order to be able to recommend the most appropriate imaging modality. Additionally, the radiologist must be provided with the essential clinical information in order to maximize the interpretation of imaging findings. With this team approach, injured athletes will derive maximal benefit from our modern imaging techniques.

MICHAEL T. SCHEERER, M.D.
Medical Director, Greater Baltimore Sports Medicine and Rehabilitation Center
Towson, Maryland

NUMEROUS SURVEYS attest to the broad spectrum of traumatic and overuse injuries in this region of the body including specific entities that are age-related for adolescents, adults, and older athletes.[1-3] The three separate anatomic areas of pelvis, hip, and thigh are combined as a unit in sports medicine primarily because of the large muscle groups that originate in the pelvis and serve the hip and thigh.[4,5]

Modern imaging plays an important role in the diagnosis of abnormalities in this region. Initial examination starts with the plain radiograph, which provides detailed images of the fine bony structure, which is crucial in the assessment of osseous injuries. Because of overlying structures in this region, computed tomography (CT) and magnetic resonance imaging (MRI) allow the anatomic separation of otherwise confusing shadows.[6,7] Triple-phase bone scanning (TPBS) is especially useful in patients with either acute injury or persistent chronic pain and with equivocal or normal radiographs.[8-12] This is best demonstrated in the hip, where failure to diagnose an occult fracture can have serious and career-threatening implications. Finally, TPBS offers the additional advantage of scanning large regions in a rapid fashion, allowing detection of unsuspected areas of pathology (Fig. 4-1). One recent study utilizing TPBS for acute hip fractures found additional significant bony pathology, other than in the hip, in 41 percent of patients.[13]

The increased utilization of MR coupled with standard CT as well as three-dimensional CT has made these modalities valuable in the evaluation of sports medicine injuries in

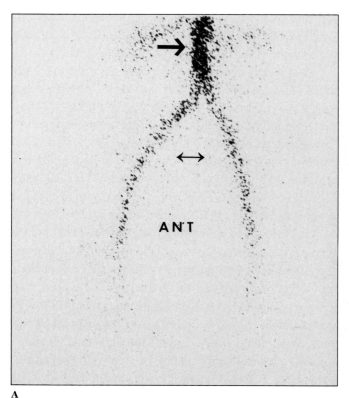

A

Figure 4-1   Normal TPBS. **A.** *Anterior view of blood flow image (first phase) showing aortoiliac arterial system. Arrow = lower abdominal aorta; double arrow = right and left common iliac arteries. (Fig. 4-1B and C continues on the opposite page.)*

this region. Additionally, CT, when combined with standard imaging techniques, fluoroscopy, or arthrography, is particularly valuable for several specific diagnostic problems. CT and fluoroscopy are each useful in helping to localize intraarticular loose bodies and periarticular calcifications. Arthrography combined with CT has been successful in helping to assess and localize osteochondral fractures, to demonstrate capsule tears caused by earlier hip dislocation, and to aid in the diagnosis of iliopsoas bursitis.[14–18]

Understanding the normal appearance of the hip dem-

onstrated on CT and MR is essential to avoid misdiagnosing the normal as disease and in recognizing early disease entities.[19] The recognition that the femoral head articulates with anterior, superior, and posterior articular surfaces of the acetabulum, forming a smooth, congruent articulating interface, is important. One must appreciate that the central area of the acetabulum contains fat and ligamentous structures which do not articulate with the femoral head in the same way that the peripheral bony articular rim does, in order to avoid possibly overcalling a centrally depressed acetabular fracture.

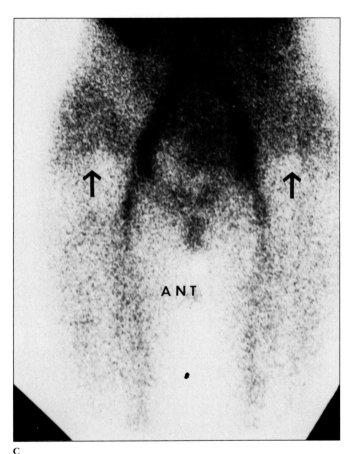

C

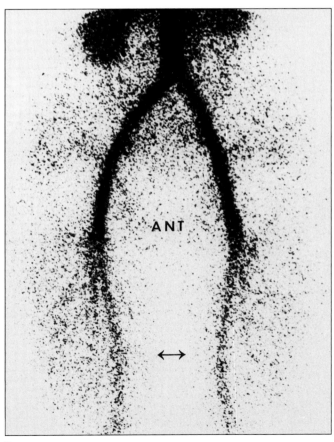

B

Figure 4-1 Normal TPBS (Continued). **B.** *Anterior view of blood flow images later into the study (approximately 20 s) demonstrates distal blood flow into the hips and thighs via the femoral arterial system. There is early distribution of isotope into the soft tissues of the pelvis, hips, and thighs. Double arrow = right and left superficial femoral arteries at the level of the mid-thighs.* **C.** *Anterior view of blood pool image (second phase) showing that most of the isotope has left the vascular system and is now accumulating in the soft tissues after 1 to 2 min. Vertical arrows = symmetric area of blood pool uptake in both hip regions. (Fig. 4-1D–F continues on next page.)*

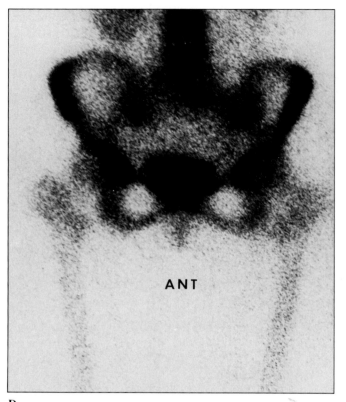

D

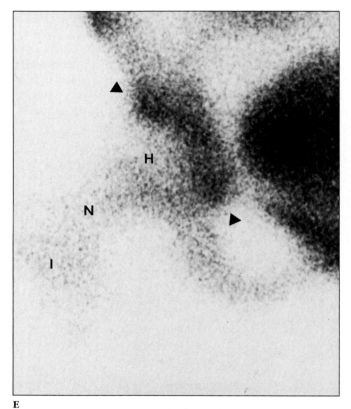

E

Figure 4-1   Normal TPBS (Continued). **D.** *Anterior view of high-resolution delayed image (third phase). Anterior view best demonstrates femoral head, acetabulum, and anterior aspects of the pelvis.* **E.** *Anterior view of high-resolution delayed images of right hip taken in magnified mode. Magnification is useful in evaluating the hip joint and in showing possible ischemic changes of the femoral head as well as subtle fractures of the neck and intertrochanteric regions. Arrowheads = superolateral and inferomedial aspects of the acetabulum, which shows a greater concentration of isotope; H = femoral head; N = femoral neck; I = intertrochanteric region of femur.* **F.** *Posterior view of high-resolution delayed image. This image best demonstrates the sacrum, sacroiliac joint, coccyx, and other posterior aspects of the pelvis.*

F

The MR appearance of the marrow about the hip undergoes evolutionary changes from early childhood through middle age and late adulthood (Fig. 4-2). The capital femoral epiphysis contains fatty marrow as early as age 2 and demonstrates a bright signal intensity on T1-weighted images throughout life.[20,21] This is in contrast to the proximal femoral metaphysis, which contains hematogenous marrow until late middle age and as such shows intermediate signal intensity on T1-weighted images until that time. Several normal areas of low-signal intensity are present, which include the bony residua of the former growth plate, the bridging trabecula within the proximal femoral metaphysis, the fovea centralis, and other anatomic features such as herniation pits of the femoral neck.[22]

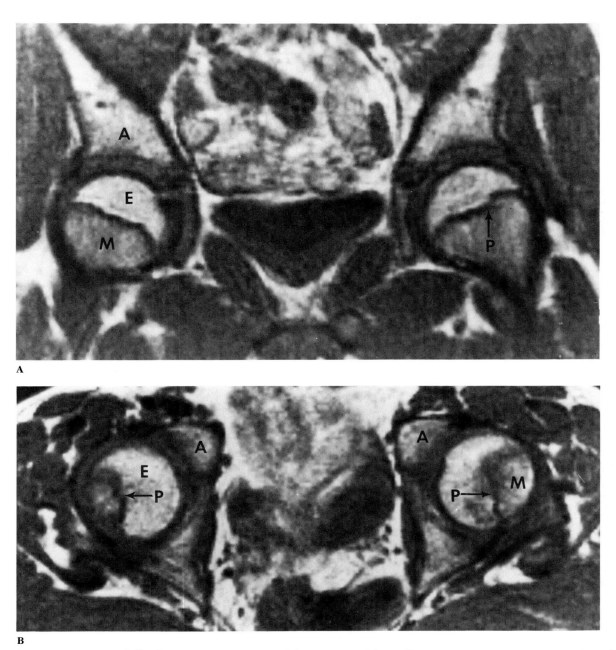

Figure 4-2 Normal Femoral Head. **A.** *Coronal scan at T1-weighted sequence through the hips of this 12-year-old male shows the femoral heads to display high signal indicating* *predominance of fatty marrow. The well-defined growth plate separates the epiphysis from the more hematogenous proximal femoral metaphysis.* **B.** *Axial scan through the same patient shows the* *normal fatty marrow centrally with the growth plate and metaphysis distally. This appearance should not be confused with focal bilateral avascular necrosis. (Fig. 4-2C–E continues on next pages.)*

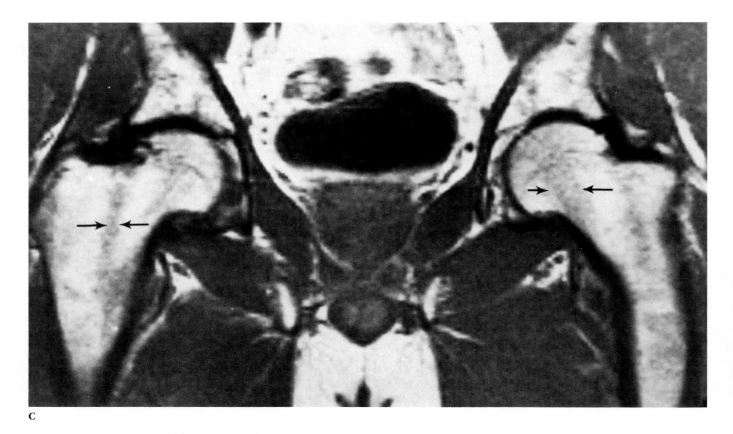

C

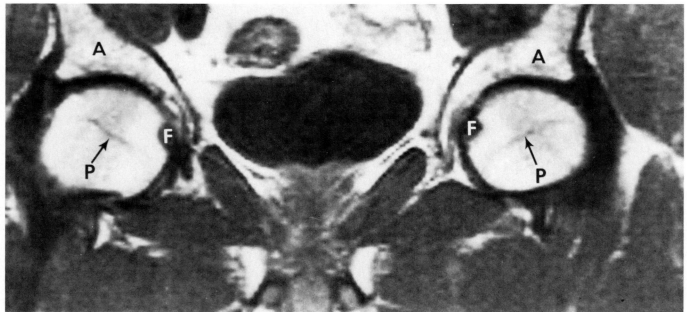

D

Figure 4-2   Normal Femoral Head (Continued). **C.** *Coronal scan at T1-weighted sequence through the midportion of the hips of this 50-year-old man shows the linear low-intensity fused growth plate still normally seen. Longitudinal regions of low signal in the proximal femoral metaphyses represent regions of trabecular prominence. The signal of the femoral metaphysis approximates that of the adjacent acetabula.* **D.** *Coronal scan of the same patient as above at a slightly more anterior level additionally demonstrates the normal low-signal indentation into the central aspect of the femoral head representing the fovea. (Fig. 4-2E continues on the opposite page.)*

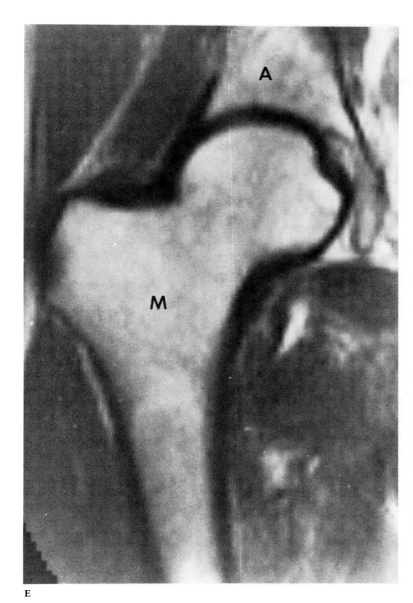

E

Figure 4-2   Normal Femoral Head (Continued). **E.** *Coronal scan at T1-weighted sequence in this osteoporotic woman shows diffuse high signal within the entire proximal femur. Much of this patient's hematogenous marrow has been replaced with fatty marrow. E = epiphysis; P = physis; M = metaphysis; F = fovea; A = acetabulum; arrows = low-signal trabecular lines.*

ACUTE PROBLEMS

Bony fracture/dislocation

Intertrochanteric hip fracture (Fig. 4-3)

Numerous studies have demonstrated the usefulness of TPBS in confirming suspected occult, acute fractures.[13,23] Despite positive physical findings, these fractures may be radiographically unapparent, especially in difficult areas such as the hip, and, therefore, TPBS is especially helpful for these patients. Early detection of hip fracture has important economic, legal, and medical implications. This is particularly true for the athlete, since failure to correctly diagnose an occult hip fracture can be catastrophic and end a career.[10,13] Intertrochanteric hip fractures have been found to have a characteristic appearance with TPBS. In patients with normal or equivocal radiographs, the sensitivity of TPBS was 97.8 percent with a negative predictive value of 99 percent. Of special interest was that other diagnoses including fractures of the pelvis, sacrum, tibia, spine, and rib were scintigraphically established in 41 percent of patients. Additionally, meticulous imaging techniques and careful scan analysis enable us to differentiate less serious, focal fractures of the greater trochanter from intertrochanteric fractures[10] (Fig. 4-3).

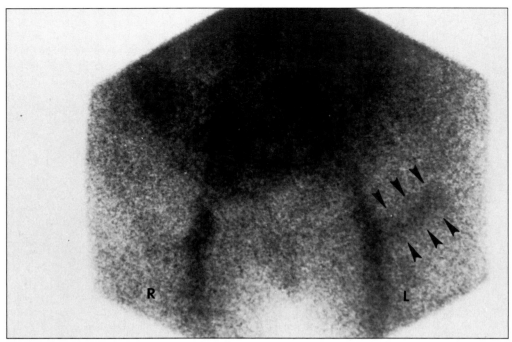

A

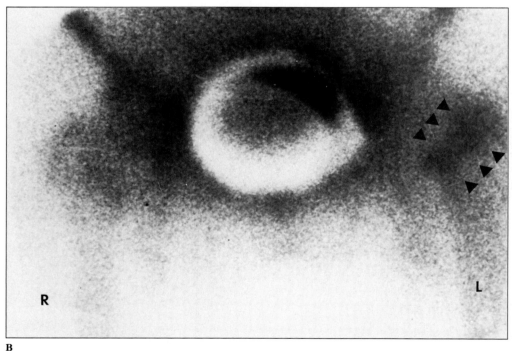

B

Figure 4-3 Intertrochanteric Fracture. **A.** *Anterior blood pool image of pelvis and hips shows asymmetry in the hip region. On the left, there is a faint, oblique area of increased nuclide activity corresponding to the intertrochanteric region of this hip not present on the opposite/right hip. This asymmetry and focal hyperemia in the left hip is an early sign on TPBS consistent with* *fracture. Black arrowheads = increased blood pool activity in left intertrochanteric region.* **B.** *Anterior high-resolution delayed image of pelvis and hip. Large white area in central portion of the film represents a lead shield placed over the bladder to decrease scatter photon activity in a patient who is unable to void (commonly seen in elderly patients or in patients with pelvic trauma).* *Asymmetry is noted on this delayed image with focal oblique area of increased nuclide activity corresponding to the intertrochanteric portion of the left hip, not seen on the opposite/right hip. The TPBS is, therefore, positive for occult fracture of the left hip not evident on radiographs. Black arrowheads = increased nuclide activity, left intertrochanteric region.*

Acetabular fracture (Figs. 4-4 and 4-5)

Although plain film radiographs are mandatory in the assessment of possible acetabular fracture, difficulty in identifying and characterizing fractures, because of overlapping bony margins, has resulted in up to one-third of nondisplaced fractures being missed on the initial plain film examination. Detailed thin-section CT images through the acetabulum provide the maximum bony information available and do so without a necessity to move the patient.[24-26] CT has virtually replaced conventional tomography for this purpose and should be performed on all patients with acetabular fracture (Figs. 4-4 and 4-5).

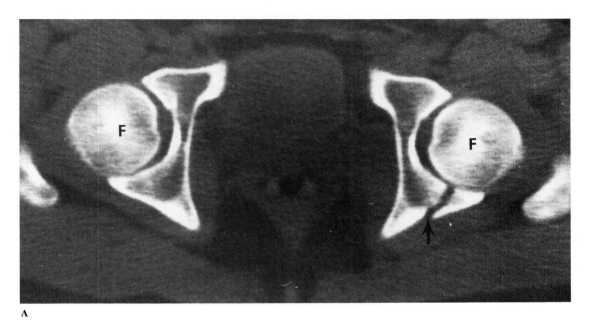

A

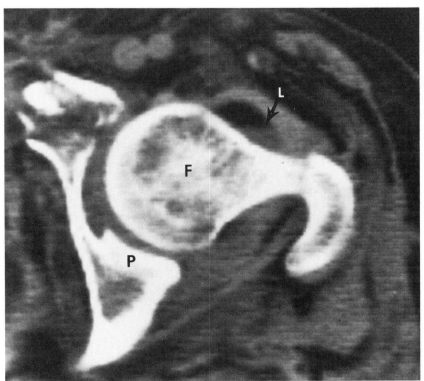

B

Figure 4-4   Acetabular Fracture. **A.** *CT scan at the midhip level shows fracture of the posterior rim of the left acetabulum with a fracture fragment making up 50 percent of the rim. The femoral head is normally seated within the acetabulum without evidence for intraarticular loose fragments.* **B.** *Axial scan at a level corresponding to the lower one-third of the femoral head shows fracture of the anterior rim of the acetabulum. The posterior articular acetabular process is seen. A fat-fluid level has developed within the joint representing marrow blood and fat having leaked through the violated cortex. Arrow = fracture; F = femoral head; P = posterior articular process; L = fat-blood level within joint capsule.*

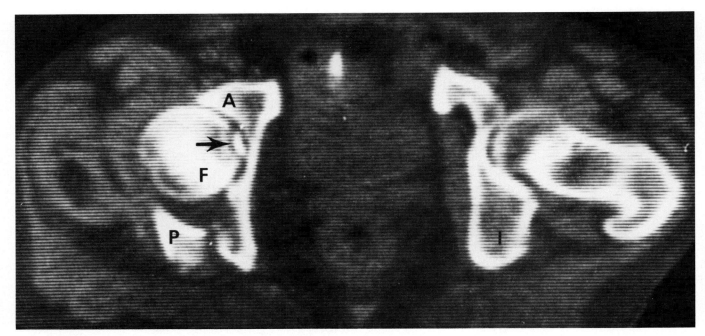

Figure 4-5 Avulsion Fracture at Attachment of Ligamentum Teres. *Axial scan through the hips following reduction of a right posterior dislocation shows a crescent-shape bony fragment within the fovea representing an avulsion fracture at the attachment of the ligamentum teres to the femoral head. The intraarticular fragment is not causing articular incongruence. A fracture of the posterior acetabular rim is also noted. A = anterior acetabular rim; P = fractured posterior acetabular rim; I = ischium; F = femoral head; arrow = avulsion fracture. [Reprinted with permission from Levinsohn EM: Computerized tomography of the extremities.* Contemporary Diagnostic Radiology *4(7):2, 1981, copyright by Williams & Wilkins.]*

Hip dislocation (Figs. 4-5 to 4-7)

CT should be considered in the postoperative reconstructed pelvis to assure removal of intraarticular loose bodies as well as restoration of articular congruence. Occasionally, a patient may present with an irreducible dislocation of the hip. This may indicate that the femoral head has buttonholed through the capsule or that the pyriformis muscle has been displaced across the acetabulum, preventing relocation.[27] Alternatively, an intraarticular loose body may be present, preventing relocation of a dislocated hip. Each of these entities may be diagnosed with CT. A major limitation of CT is its inability to visualize noncalcified cartilage. In this setting, MR or a combined CT arthrogram may be diagnostic. Although there is always concern about exposing a young patient to ionizing radiation, a well-designed CT exam may frequently provide crucial diagnostic information at an integral radiation dose not more than the plain film examination.[28,29]

Typically, three types of hip dislocation are recognized: one directed posteriorly and two varieties anteriorly. The most common is the posterior dislocation of the femoral head, which is caused by impaction of the knee or tibia into a fixed object. From 8 to 15 percent of hip dislocations are in the anterior direction and include the iliopubic type (directed anteriorly and superiorly) as well as the less common obturator type [directed anteriorly and inferiorly] (Fig. 4-6). The diagnosis of these dislocations is usually apparent from the plain film examination. In difficult circumstances, however, the CT scan is diagnostic. Previous dislocation is also frequently accompanied by avulsion of the ligamentum teres, which can be diagnosed with CT (Fig. 4-5).[32] Recurrent hip dislocation is quite infrequent, occurring in 0.3 to 1.2 percent of cases.

Dislocations may be combined with tears of the joint capsule and of the cartilaginous labrum. Anterior dislocations are associated with anterior capsule tears and posterior dislocations with posterior capsule and/or labrum tears. These entities can best be recognized with a combined CT arthrogram examination.[30,31] Contrast injected into the joint space extravasates through the capsule or labral tear into the adjacent soft tissues (Fig. 4-7). This is usually easily seen on the associated CT exam.

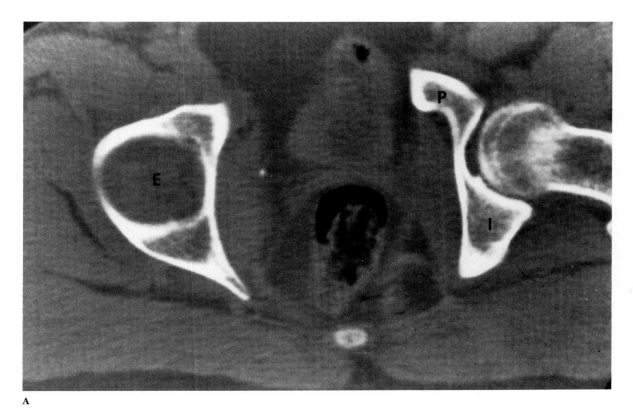

A

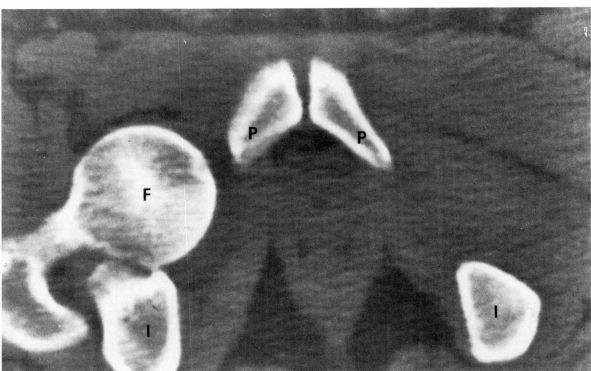

B

Figure 4-6   Hip Dislocation. **A.** *CT scan in the axial plane through the midlevel of the right acetabulum shows that acetabulum to be empty. The dislocated right femoral head is not* *visualized at this level. The left femoral head is normally contained within the left acetabulum.* **B.** *CT scan in the axial plane at the level of the obturator foramen shows inferior dislocation of the* *right femoral head. The left obturator foramen is normal. E = empty right acetabulum; P = pubic ramus; I = ischium; F = dislocated right femoral head.*

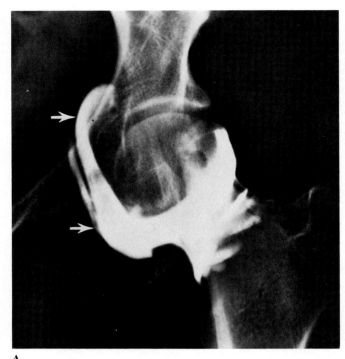

A

Figure 4-7 Capsule Tear Following Dislocation. **A.** *This patient suffered a hyperextension injury with transient anterior dislocation of the hip resulting in a capsule tear. Arthrogram shows anterior leakage of contrast through the torn capsule. (Reprinted with permission from Guyer B, Levinsohn EM: Recurrent anterior dislocation of the hip: Case report with arthrographic findings. Skeletal Radiology 10:263, 1983.)* **B.** *Arthrogram shows an inferior capsule tear resulting from posterior hip dislocation. Arrows = contrast extravasating through capsule tear.*

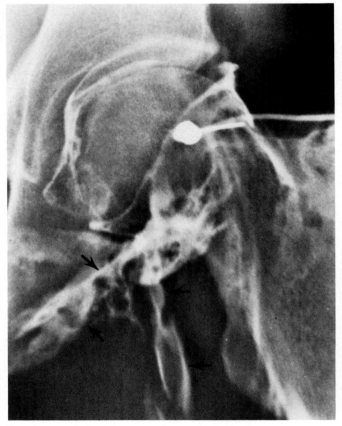

B

Fractures of the pelvis (Figs. 4-8 and 4-9)

Occult fractures of the pelvis are notoriously difficult to evaluate or confirm on plain film radiographs even when utilizing multiple oblique and lateral views. Fractures of the sacrum or coccyx as well as fracture/diastasis of the sacroiliac joint can be identified on TPBS (Figs. 4-8 and 4-9) and visualized in detail on CT exam.[9,10,33]

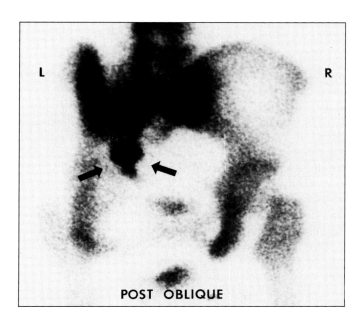

Figure 4-8   Fracture of Coccyx. *Posterior oblique view of high-resolution delayed image. In patients with suspected coccygeal fracture, oblique views are important in order to position the coccyx off the midline so that it can best be seen in oblique projection or profile. Asymmetrically intense nuclide activity is noted in the mid and lower coccygeal segments consistent with an occult fracture of the coccyx in a patient with trauma and normal radiographs. Black arrows = abnormal nuclide activity in coccyx.*

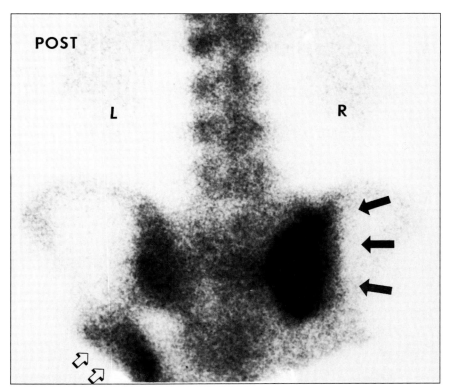

Figure 4-9   Multiple Pelvic Fractures. *Posterior view of high-resolution delayed image. Very intense nuclide activity is seen in the right sacroiliac (SI) region extending on both sides of the joint. Increased activity is also noted in the superolateral aspect of the left pubic ramus. Professional jockey suffering serious spill was noted on radiographs to have multiple rib fractures as well as fractures of the left pubic ramus. Severe right back and sacroiliac pain was noted with normal radiographs. Total body bone scan with high-resolution regional anatomic images demonstrated the known areas of fracture as well as abnormality in the right SI joint. Fractures at or adjacent to the SI joint including diastasis of this joint are difficult to visualize on radiographs, and their existence can be confirmed by bone scan. CT scans are useful in identifying the number and position of the bony fragments. Black arrows = increased activity in the right sacroiliac region; open arrows = increased nuclide activity in left pubic ramus superolaterally.*

Muscle injuries

Avulsion injuries (Figs. 4-10 and 4-11)

An apophysis is a secondary ossification center that contributes to the peripheral growth or contour of a bone but not to its longitudinal bone growth. Apophyseal avulsion injuries of the pelvis and hip in athletes are well documented in the literature.[4,5,12] Adolescents are particularly susceptible to apophyseal avulsion injuries for two reasons. First, the pelvis and hip apophyses appear and fuse later than elsewhere in the body and are, therefore, open and susceptible during adolescence, generally 13 to 17 years old. Second, apophyseal avulsion is more likely than a muscle tear in adolescents, since it is the weakest point in the ''musculotendinous unit'' (Drawing I).

The mechanism of injury is due to sudden muscle tension across an open apophysis. This occurs in one of two ways. Tension can be generated by sudden forceful concentric or eccentric contraction of a large muscle attempting to decelerate or accelerate the body. While this is the most common

way for apophyseal avulsion, it can also occur after excessive passive lengthening of a muscle, as would occur in a cheerleader performing an anteroposterior split.[5,12,34]

The displacement of the avulsed fragment is determined by the soft tissue attachments, which can prevent fragment migration as well as preserve muscle function by maintaining length. As the displacement of the fragment increases, there is more pain and muscle spasm. Avulsion fractures of the iliac crest and the anterior-inferior iliac spine are, in general, less displaced, whereas avulsions of the ischium, anterior-superior iliac spine, and lesser trochanter show more fragment displacement (Figs. 4-10 and 4-11). Treatment depends on the location of the avulsion as well as the degree of separation or attachment, and in some cases open reduction and internal fixation are necessary.[5,35] Depending on the degree of displacement and/or healing, there can be a 3- to 5-cm shortening of the musculotendinous unit.

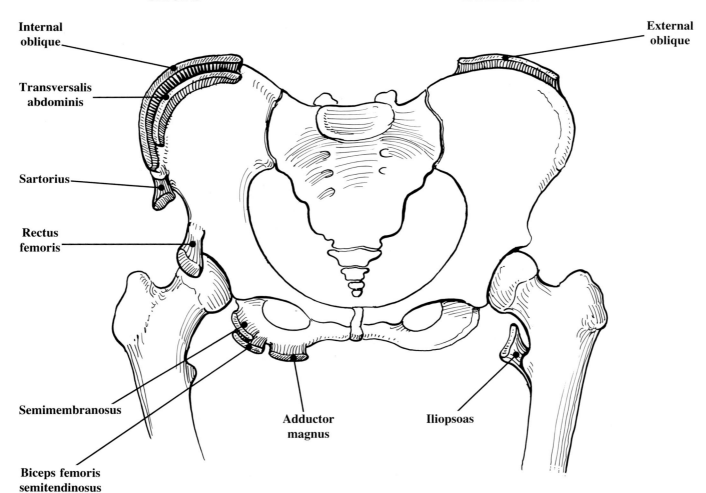

ORIGINS　　　　　　　　　　　　**INSERTIONS**

Internal oblique

Transversalis abdominis

Sartorius

Rectus femoris

Semimembranosus

Biceps femoris semitendinosus

Adductor magnus

Iliopsoas

External oblique

Drawing I Hip and Pelvic Muscle Origins and Insertions. *Avulsion injuries of the muscles of the hip are common in athletes especially during adolescence. Anatomic knowledge of the exact location of these origins and insertions is necessary for proper assessment. The right side of the pelvis demonstrates the origins of the major muscles and the left side the insertions.*

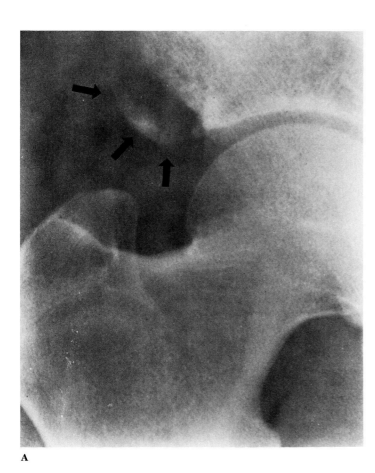

A

Figure 4-10   Avulsion Fracture of Anterior-Inferior Iliac Spine at Origin of Rectus Femoris Muscle. **A.** *Coned down anteroposterior view of right hip demonstrates avulsion fragment and/or ossification (arrows) adjacent to the right anterior-inferior iliac spine in a high school football player with acute right hip injury. The remainder of the radiographic study was normal. Clinical question existing as to whether this is a new or old avulsion fragment or whether the patient's right hip pain represents occult intertrochanteric fracture to be decided by follow-up TPBS.* **B.** *Anterior view of blood pool image of pelvis and hips (TPBS). Focal asymmetry noted with increased nuclide activity identified in superolateral aspect of right hip corresponding to abnormal area seen on radiograph. The identification of intense activity in blood pool phase is consistent with an acute injury. Black arrow = abnormal activity in superior aspect of right hip region. (Fig. 4-10C– E continues on next pages.)*

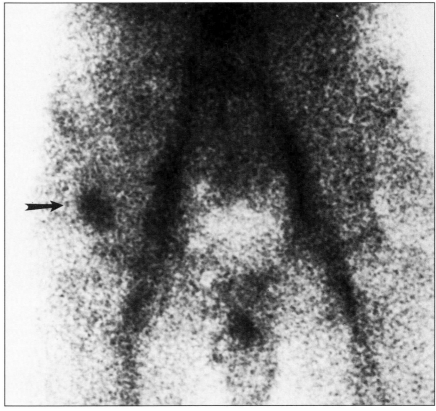

B

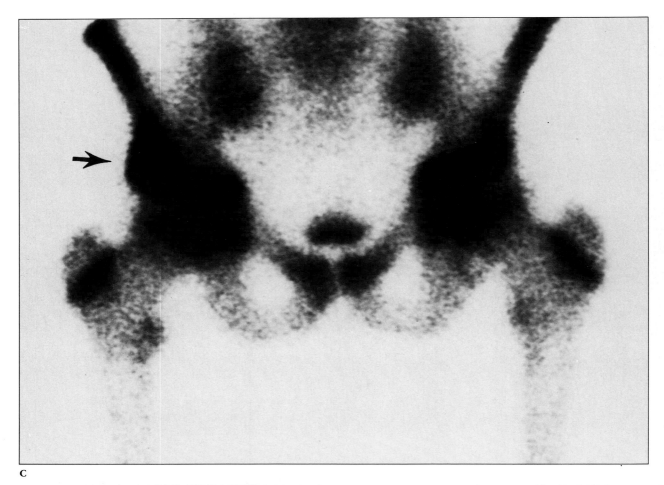

C

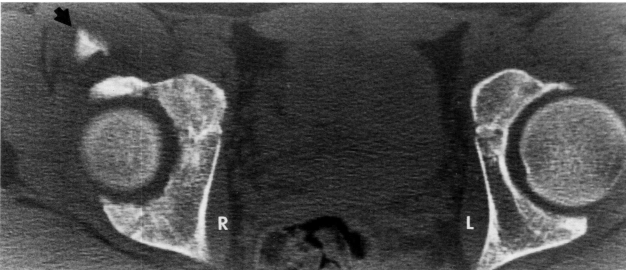

D

Figure 4-10 Avulsion Fracture of Anterior-Inferior Iliac Spine at Origin of Rectus Femoris Muscle (Continued). **C.** *Anterior view of high-resolution delayed image of pelvis and hips (TPBS). Asymmetry is noted in the right anterior-inferior iliac spine, although not as* striking as on the blood pool image. The reason for this is normal activity in the right hip region in an adolescent with increased activity in regions of epi-physeal growth plates and joints, which is normal for this age. Black arrow = asymmetrically increased activity in the region of the right anterior-inferior iliac spine. **D.** CT scan of pelvis and hip axially through the superior aspect of the hip joint. Triangular avulsion fragment (arrow) is noted on the right consistent with radiographic and TPBS findings. (Fig. 4-10E continues on the opposite page.)

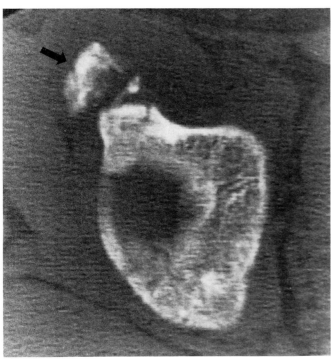

E

Figure 4-10   Avulsion Fracture of Anterior-Inferior Iliac Spine at Origin of Rectus Femoris Muscle (Continued). **E.** *Magnified coned-down CT scan with transverse cut in the right hip region at the most superior aspect of the acetabulum. This demonstrates avulsion fracture of anterior-inferior iliac spine, corresponding to the origin of the rectus femoris muscle. Black arrow = avulsion fragment (see Drawing I).*

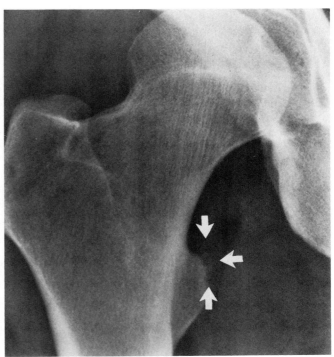

A

Figure 4-11   Avulsion Injury of Iliopsoas Insertion at the Lesser Trochanter. **A.** *Coned-down anteroposterior radiograph of right hip. There is irregularity and some fragmentation of the normally smooth cortical margin of the superior-medial aspect of the lesser trochanter. Tiny avulsion fragments are noted adjacent to the lesser trochanter. White arrows = tiny avulsion fragments adjacent to right lesser trochanter. (Fig. 4-11B continues below.)*

Figure 4-11   Avulsion Injury of Iliopsoas Insertion at the Lesser Trochanter (Continued). **B.** *Anterior view of high-resolution delayed image of pelvis and hip (TPBS) in a 30-year-old high-level female runner/athlete with acute and chronic right hip pain, suspicious radiograph, and pain on physical exam when isolating iliopsoas muscle. Nonspecific, diffuse moderate activity is noted in the right hip region in the lesser and subtrochanteric region, which is neither focal nor intense enough to represent acute fracture (earlier blood flow and blood pool images were negative). This activity did not have the typical location or appearance of a femoral neck or intertrochanteric fracture. Black arrow = increased activity in right lesser trochanter. (Fig. 4-11C continues on next page.)*

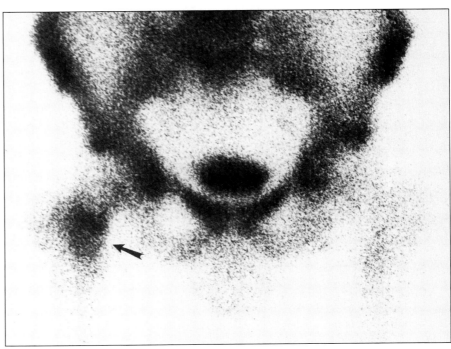

B

Figure 4-11 Avulsion Injury of Iliopsoas Insertion at the Lesser Trochanter (Continued). **C.** *Anterior high-resolution image of pelvis and hip in frog-leg projection (TPBS). Non-specific increased activity is noted in the lesser trochanter and subtrochanteric region of the right hip along the medial cortex. The diffuse nature and long length of abnormal activity seen on this study represents avulsion injury at the insertion of the right iliopsoas muscle in the lesser and subtrochanteric region of the right hip. Black arrows = increased nuclide activity, medial right trochanteric region (see Drawing I).*

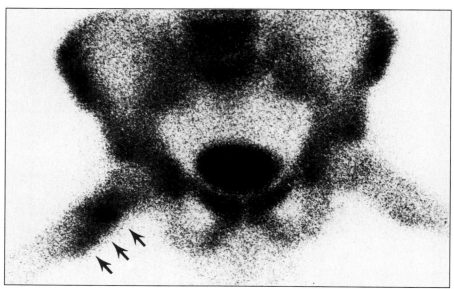

C

TABLE 4-1

Common sites of avulsion injuries of pelvis and femur

Site	Muscle	Clinical features
Iliac crest (anterior)	Transverse abdominal (O) Internal oblique Abdominal (O) External oblique Abdominal (I) Tensor fascia lata (O) Gluteus medius (O)	Running and cutting actions associated with severe or sudden abdominal muscle contractions with twisting or directional changes (runners, figure skaters, weight lifters).
Anterior-superior iliac spine	Sartorius (O)	Flexes lower leg and femur; rotates femur laterally. Less painful than inferior spine, but fragment displaces more.
Anterior-inferior iliac spine	Rectus femoris (O)	Associated with rapid or repetitive acceleration. Avulsion fragment sometimes confused with os acetabuli. Can heal with exostosis.
Ischial tuberosity	Hamstrings (O) Gracilis Biceps femoris Semimembranosus Semitendinosus	Associated with sprinting or deceleration injuries. Irregular healing may mimic tumor. Seen commonly with runners, hurdlers, jumpers, and cheerleaders. Fragment can displace several centimeters.
Greater trochanter	Gluteus medius (I)	Abducts and medially rotates femur. Point tenderness can mimic trochanteric bursitis.
Lesser trochanter	Iliopsoas (I)	Flexes femur. Avulsion fragment may displace cephalad several centimeters. Associated hematoma may calcify.

NOTE: O = origin; I = insertion.

Clinically, these injuries usually occur as the result of an "extreme effort," and the athlete will usually complain of a popping, snapping, or tearing sensation as the avulsion occurs. There is usually point tenderness and deep pain on palpation over the avulsion site. Radiographically, the injury is similar to a Salter-Harris I/II epiphyseal fracture. Each anatomic site has associated with it its own specific clinical features[5,34,36–39] (Table 4-1).

Muscle tear/hemorrhage (Fig. 4-12)

Muscle soreness accompanying or following extreme exertion is a common clinical symptom. Magnetic resonance imaging is useful in that setting, as T2-weighted sequences often show transiently increased signal within the affected muscles thought to represent muscle strain.[40] When these findings are associated with an abnormal signal more than 3 weeks after injury or with perifascial hemorrhage (Fig. 4-12), then muscle tear is the likely diagnosis.[40–41] MR is especially useful in the diagnosis and follow-up of acute muscle hematoma, since no other imaging modality is as well suited to demonstrate the size of the hematoma or to follow its resolution.

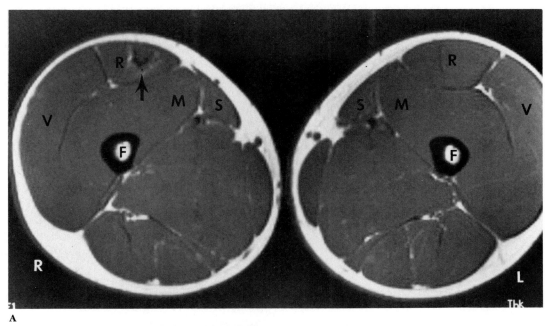

A

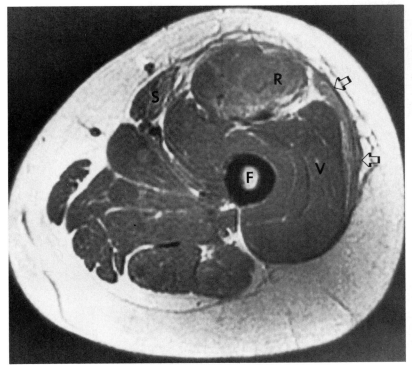

B

Figure 4-12   Muscle Tear of Rectus Femoris. **A.** *MR scan in the axial plane at T1-weighted sequence shows an abnormality in the right rectus femoris muscle. The low-signal center followed by high-signal periphery represents a region of muscle tear.* **B.** *MR scan in the axial plane at T1-weighted sequence shows abnormality of the left rectus femoris muscle. Diffuse swelling throughout the muscle with fascial thickening is noted characteristic of acute rectus femoris muscle tear. (Fig. 4-12C and D continues on next page.)*

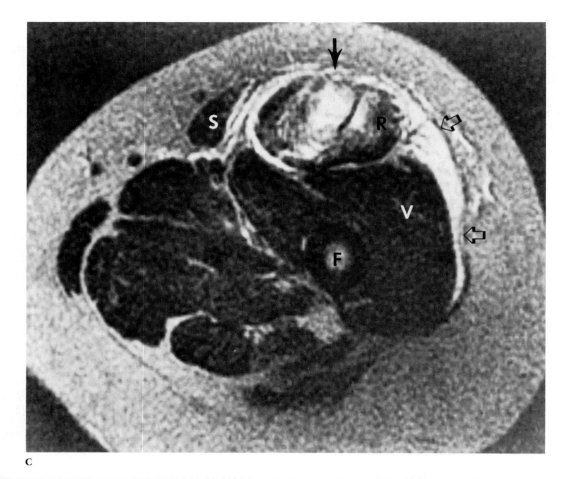

C

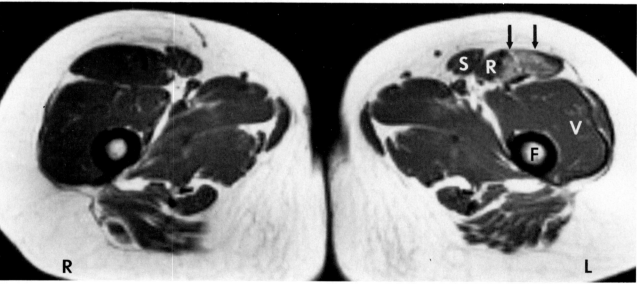

D

Figure 4-12   Muscle Tear of Rectus Femoris (Continued).   **C.** *Same patient as above at T2-weighted sequence shows regions of high signal within the rectus femoris muscle and in the adjacent planes representing areas of hemorrhage and edema from the muscle tear.*

D. *Same patient as **B** and **C**. MR scan 5 months later at T1-weighted sequence shows persisting abnormality of the rectus femoris muscle which has improved somewhat since the earliest scan. There still remain regions of altered signal intensity with persisting*

symptomatology. R = rectus femoris muscle; open arrows = hemorrhage into fascial planes; arrow = focus of muscle abnormality; M = vastus medialis muscle; S = sartorius muscle; F = femur; V = vastus lateralis muscle.

Exertional rhabdomyolysis (Fig. 4-13)

Rhabdomyolysis is a rare but sometimes catastrophic complication of severe exertional muscular trauma. Skeletal muscle injury due to exercise has been documented. There is disintegration or dissolution of muscle associated with release of muscle fiber contents into the tissue fluid space and then eventually the circulation.[42] A complication is the resulting myoglobinuria, which can lead to acute tubular necrosis and renal failure.[43]

The damaged muscle can be identified on TPBS with the mechanism of uptake similar to that seen with myocardial infarct scanning, whereby there is an influx of calcium ions into acutely necrotic muscle cells, which then bind with the phosphate from the technetium scanning agent.[44–56] The bone scanning agent shows increased uptake in areas of pain that is best visualized at 48 h after injury and virtually undetectable at 1 week (Fig. 4-13). In addition to the clinical and TPBS findings, there are also laboratory values which include increase in serum CK levels.[57]

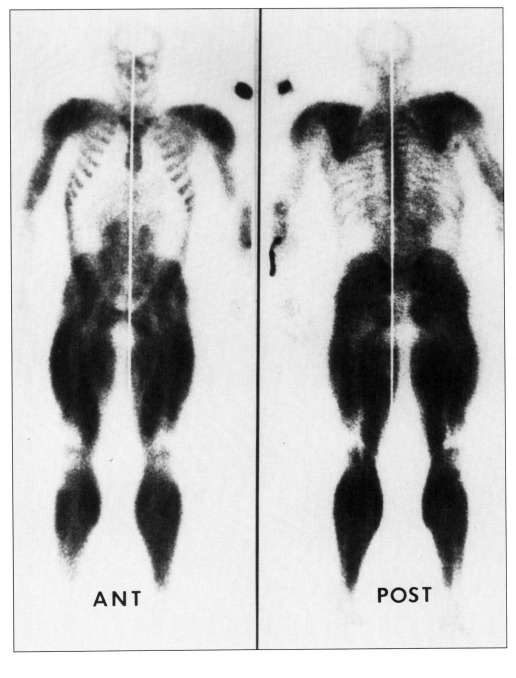

Figure 4-13 Acute Exertional Rhabdomyolysis. *Anterior and posterior total body images of TPBS demonstrate only minimal skeletal uptake but extensive deposition of the isotope in the large muscle groups of the body especially in the pelvis, hip, thigh, and lower leg which can be seen with severe exertional rhabdomyolysis.*

CHRONIC PROBLEMS

Overuse injuries (stress fractures/periostitis)

Stress fractures of the hip and pelvis are similar to those in other parts of the body. A continuum exists beginning with early bone remodeling (secondary to increased levels of stress) continuing through subclinical stress fracture and terminating in clinical stress fracture. TPBS has been shown to be exceptionally sensitive in detecting and localizing areas of overuse injury.[9–12,58] This is especially important, since studies have shown that positive radiographic findings in femoral neck stress fractures may lag behind symptoms for as long as 2 to 4 weeks. The team physician must have a high clinical index of suspicion and should pursue additional imaging tests even if plain radiographs remain normal.[59–61]

Hip and femur (Figs. 4-14 to 4-19)

In McBryde's study of 1000 consecutive fractures in runners, 14 percent were found in the femur (7 percent in the femoral neck and 7 percent in the femoral shaft).[62] Undetected femoral neck fractures have a potential for displacement with resulting serious complications such as nonunion, malunion, and in some cases eventual aseptic necrosis.[63–69] Although quite uncommon, bilateral femoral stress fractures have also been reported.[59,70] Many biomechanical studies have been performed demonstrating and measuring the large loads transmitted through the femur.[70–75] Experimental studies have shown that just walking exerts forces through the femur

equivalent to six times body weight, while running and jogging can increase these peak forces to 10 to 20 times body weight.[12,60] The highest area of strain was noted to be in the calcar area of the femur.[76,77] Additional studies have been able to identify two discrete types of femoral neck stress fractures (transverse and compression) with specific clinical features identified with each one (Table 4-2).[78]

TABLE 4-2

Femoral neck stress fractures

	Transverse type	Compression type
Location	Superior neck	Inferior neck
Age group	Older patients (except military recruits)	Younger patients
Contributing factors	Metabolic bone disease	Athletic activity
Early radiographic findings	Radiolucent cortical line	Hazy callus formation
Displacement	More common	Less common
Treatment	May require internal fixation	Conservative/non-weight-bearing

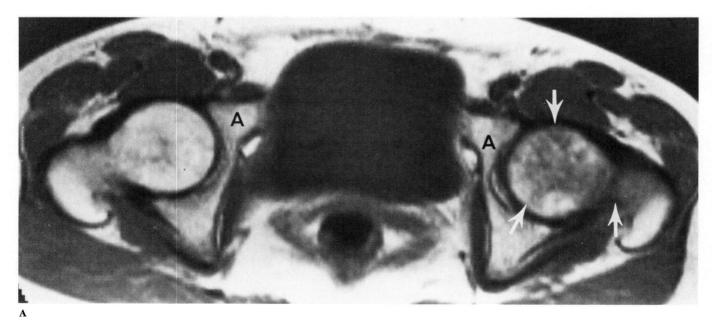

A

Figure 4-14 Stress Fracture of Femoral Neck. **A.** *MR scan at T1-weighted sequence in the axial plane at the level of the femoral heads shows diffuse low signal within the left femoral head and neck representing edematous change.* (Fig. 4-14B and C continues on the opposite page.)

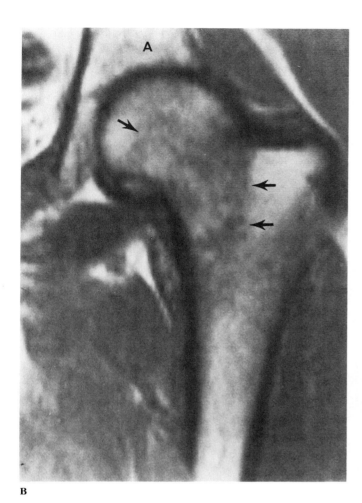

B

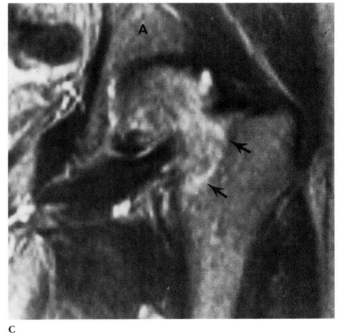

C

Figure 4-14   Stress Fracture of Femoral Neck (Continued). **B.** *MR scan at T1-weighted sequence in the coronal plane shows a focal region of diminished signal intensity in the left femoral neck representing edema and hemorrhage.* **C.** *MR scan at T2-weighted sequence in the coronal plane through the left femur of the same patient shows high signal in the femoral neck corresponding to edema and hemorrhage. These changes indicate a stress fracture at this site. Arrows = region of abnormal signal; A = acetabulum.*

As with stress fractures in other regions of the body, MR demonstrates characteristic findings. There is diminished signal in the affected portion of the bone on T1-weighted images and high signal in those same areas on T2-weighted images. These findings represent edema and/or hemorrhage into the involved bone and indicate underlying stress fracture[6,79] (Fig. 4-14). With long-standing overuse, such as in marathon runners, there may be accentuation of the trabecular pattern causing diminished signal intensity in the involved area on both T1- and T2-weighted images (Fig.

4-15). When a completed fracture occurs, the magnetic resonance scan shows a linear area of diminished signal on T1-weighted images in the area corresponding to the fracture line. Despite loss of vascularity and impending avascular necrosis, the femoral head continues to look normal for at least 48 h and likely for at least 5 days following interruption of blood supply.[80] The predominant marrow present in the femoral head is fatty in composition. From 2 to 5 days is required for necrotic changes to occur within fatty marrow.

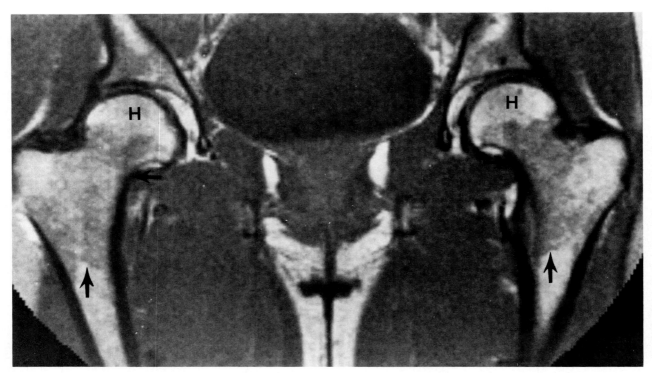

Figure 4-15 Stress Reaction of Proximal Femur. *MR scan in the coronal plane at T1-weighted sequence through the midportion of the femurs of* *this marathon runner shows large areas of diminished signal intensity in the proximal femoral metaphyses representing the changes of chronic stress* *reaction. H = femoral head; arrows = regions of diminished signal intensity representing stress reaction.*

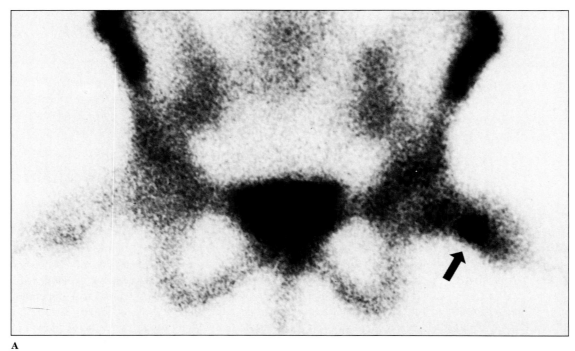

A

Figure 4-16 Stress Fracture of Femoral Neck. **A.** *Anterior view of high-resolution delayed image of the pelvis and hip in frog-leg projection (TPBS). Asymmetry is noted with increased activity in left femoral neck. Black arrow = increased left femoral neck activity.* (Fig. 4-16B and C continues on the opposite page.)

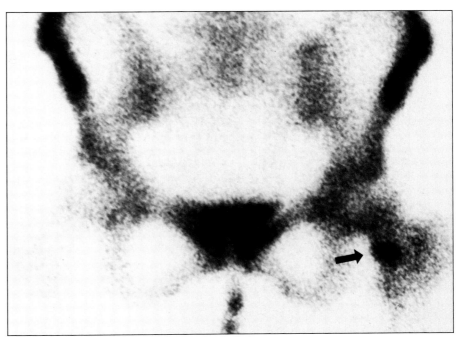

B

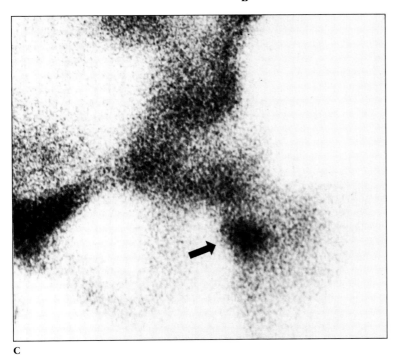

C

Figure 4-16   Stress Fracture of Femoral Neck (Continued). **B.** *Anterior view of high-resolution delayed image of pelvis and hip (TPBS). Mild to moderate asymmetry is noted with focal nuclide activity seen in the left femoral neck. Black arrow = increased activity, left femoral neck.* **C.** *Anterior view of high-resolution delayed image of left hip in magnified mode (TPBS). This view best demonstrates the abnormal nuclide activity in the left femoral neck consistent with a stress fracture. The study demonstrates the importance of multiple views in order to best visualize the abnormality including multiple projections and sometimes magnification. This 15-year-old female cross country runner and hurdler had left hip pain with negative radiographs. Black arrow = increased nuclide activity in left femoral neck.*

TPBS is the most common imaging modality to identify femoral neck stress fractures (Figs. 4-16 and 4-17). In athletes, compression-type fracture involving the concave portion of the neck is the most common type, explaining the bone scan finding of focal, intense, rounded area of activity limited to this portion of the femoral neck (i.e., the accumulation of the nuclide does not extend through the entire femoral neck but is localized to the inferior concave portion).

High-resolution delayed images are the most helpful, and very often only routine anteroposterior views are needed. However, if the suspected stress fracture is not identified on this view, then additional views, such as the frog-leg view, magnification view, computer-assisted subtraction view, or SPECT imaging, must be utilized[8,10,11] (Fig. 4-18). Additionally, serial scans can be used to follow up femoral neck stress fractures.

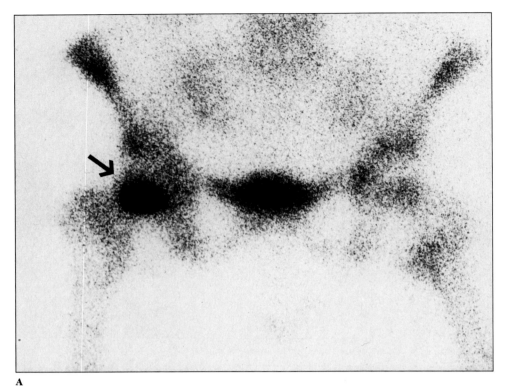

A

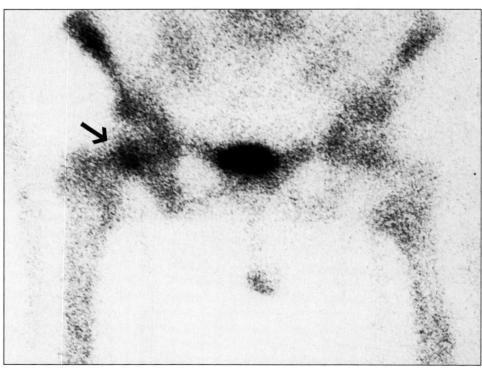

B

Figure 4-17 Stress Fracture of Femoral Neck with Follow-up. **A.** *Anterior view of high resolution delayed image of pelvis and hip (TPBS). Focal intense nuclide activity in medial aspect of right femoral neck consistent with stress fracture in a patient with right hip* *pain and negative radiographs. Black arrow = increased nuclide activity, right femoral neck.* **B.** *Anterior view of high-resolution delayed image of pelvis and hips (TPBS). This follow-up study after 2 months of non-weight-bearing demonstrates the marked improvement* *and almost complete resolution of the abnormality on bone scan. TPBS can, therefore, be used to follow up stress fractures to correlate clinical findings with scan findings. Black arrow = increased activity, right femoral neck.*

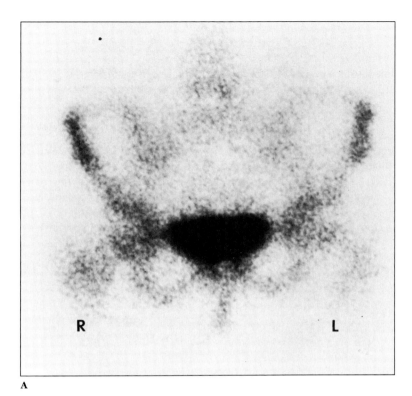

A

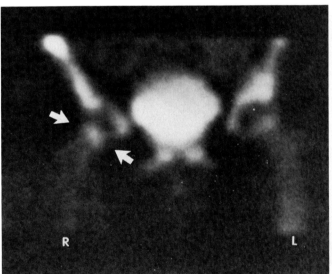

B

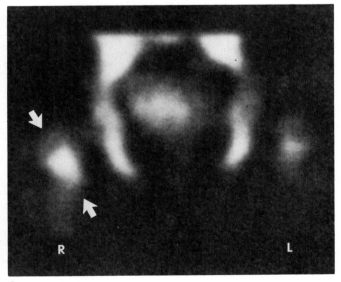

C

Figure 4-18 Stress Fracture of Femoral Neck (TPBS/SPECT). **A.** *High-resolution delayed anterior image of TPBS. Patient was a 21-year-old female college long-distance runner with right hip pain and normal radiographs. Planar image does not show any focal, intense activity in right femoral neck to suggest a stress fracture. Subtle asymmetry noted with slightly increased activity in right head and neck was inconclusive; sometimes such asymmetry is real or can be due to technical factors* including slight rotation in position of patient. Planar images were immediately followed by SPECT study. **B.** SPECT study, with computer reconstruction, of pelvis and hip in coronal plane. This cut is relatively anterior demonstrating anterior pubis and obturator foramen but barely showing femoral head or neck. Slight asymmetry is noted with increased activity in right femoral neck, when compared to left. White arrows = increased activity, right femoral neck. **C.** Additional SPECT image, with computer reconstruction, of pelvis and hip in coronal plane. This more posterior cut clearly shows asymmetry with marked nuclide uptake in right femoral neck, extending into the lesser trochanter, consistent with stress fracture. SPECT imaging can often identify in greater detail and intensity equivocal or suspicious areas noted on planar TPBS. White arrows = abnormal activity, right neck/lesser trochanter.

Many studies have placed the frequency of stress fractures of the femoral shaft in the range of 2 to 7 percent of all stress fractures occurring in athletes.[59,62,81,82] These femoral shaft stress fractures occur most commonly in the proximal third of the femur, including the subtrochanteric region (Fig. 4-19), and appear to be related to the origin of the vastus medialis muscle and the insertion of the adductor brevis muscle. As with other stress fracture sites, the increased traction or tensile force exerted on the bone by these muscles is ultimately responsible for the resulting appearance on radiographs and TPBS. Delayed bone scan images show a focal "hot spot" oriented along the medial femoral cortex. Delayed radiographic findings in the proximal third of the femoral shaft may include periosteal thickening or a radiolucent linear/oblique fracture line.[60,81] Fractures of the proximal and midshaft invariably heal without complications or displacement. Several studies have shown that when occurring in athletes and/or military recruits, distal femoral stress fractures have an increased incidence of displacement that may require internal fixation.[83,84]

Pelvis (Figs. 4-20 and 4-21)

Overuse injuries or syndromes in the pelvis include osteitis and stress fractures. *Osteitis pubis* and *pubic symphysitis* are two general terms that describe a symptom complex commonly used to represent pelvic changes secondary to a wide variety of causes. Inflammatory response of the symphysis pubis secondary to stress, trauma, childbirth, genitourinary infection, and surgery (prostate or bladder) is reported. When used in a sports medicine context, it represents an overuse syndrome, perhaps better named *pubic stress symphysitis,* which is separated from other pelvic and pubic problems because it is nonseptic and nonavulsive in nature. Osteitis pubis in the athlete represents an osteitis associated with overuse at the origin of the large adductor muscles. The major offending muscles include the adductor longus, which has its origin at the front of the pubis near the crest and symphysis, and the adductor brevis, which has its origin at the body and inferior ramus of the pubis. In athletes, this presents as groin pain radiating either to the peroneal region

Figure 4-19 Stress Fracture, Subtrochanteric Femur. *Anterior view of high-resolution delayed image of TPBS. Focal activity demonstrated in subtrochanteric region at the junction of the proximal and middle thirds of the femur on the medial aspect of the bone. This is a typical position and appearance of subtrochanteric stress fracture of the femur in a long-distance runner. Back arrow = increased activity, right proximal femur.*

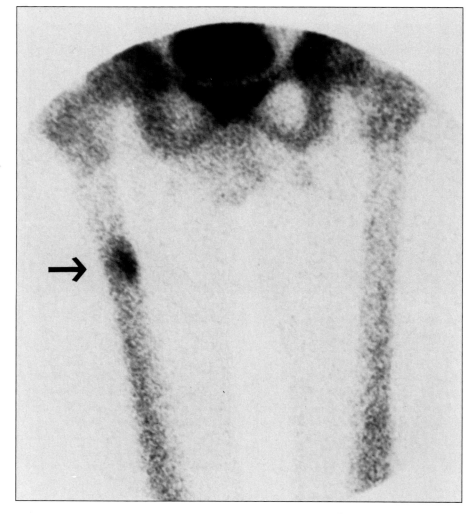

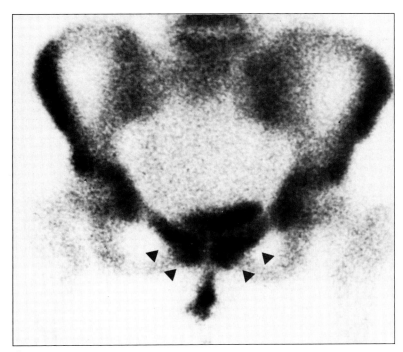

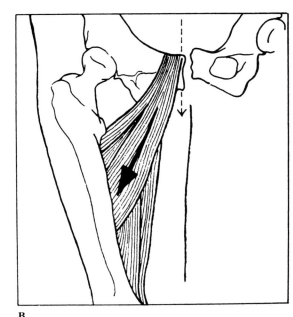

A   **B**

Figure 4-20 Overuse/Stress Osteitis Pubis. **A.** *Anterior view of high-resolution delayed image of the pelvis and hips (TPBS) symmetrically. Increased nuclide activity is noted on both sides of the symphysis pubis extending superolaterally to both the right and left pubic rami in this female athlete. This diffuse activity in the midline of the symphysis pubis in a patient with groin pain is most consistent with stress or overuse osteitis pubis. (Horizontal activity seen above the symphysis pubis represents residual isotope in the bladder. Additionally, vertical, poorly defined activity seen below the symphysis pubis represents leakage of isotope or contamination on the gown probably after voiding). Arrowheads = increased activity in the midline on both sides of the symphysis pubis.* **B.** *Anatomic drawing shows the muscular attachments of the larger adductor muscles, which are responsible for the osteitis pubis syndrome. The adductor longus arises from the front of the pubis near the crest and symphysis, and the adductor brevis arises from the body and inferior ramus of the pubis. Overuse of these large muscles causes tearing or microavulsions from their origins at or adjacent to the symphysis pubis accounting for the abnormality seen on the bone scan above. Arrow = powerful thrust of the adductor muscles tearing away from their insertion at or adjacent to the symphysis pubis). (From Martire JR: The role of nuclear medicine scans in evaluating pain in athletic injuries.* Clinics in Sports Medicine *6:713–737. Reproduced with permission.)*

or along the course of the adductor muscles to the thigh. TPBS findings include diffuse, nonspecific uptake in the region of the symphysis pubis (more commonly bilateral than unilateral), corresponding to the attachment or origin of the large adductor muscles. Later radiographic changes may include asymmetry or widening of the symphysis and one or more of the following: cortical loss, erosion, sclerosis, hypertrophic change, or periosteal reaction [85–91] (Fig. 4-20). Usually the treatment is conservative and symptomatic in nature and includes limitation of exercise until symptoms subside or completely resolve. However, in recurrent or more severe cases, wedge resection of the symphysis pubis is a treatment option.[87]

Pelvic stress fractures have been reported to range from 1 to 6 percent of all stress fractures in athletes.[62,92] Studies have shown a disproportionately high number of pelvic stress fractures in females and in long-distance or marathon runners. There are several additional unique features of pubic stress fractures that are worth mentioning. First, they always occur with increased training or during marathon running and are rarely seen in new runners or during a low level of training. Therefore, these stress fractures are thought to be due to increased or excessive repetition of muscular contraction rather than a change in muscular force. They appear to be a response to tensile as opposed to compressive forces. Second, certain biomechanical differences may account for a "fatigue mechanism" in females making them more susceptible to pubic stress fractures. Compared to the male, the female skeleton is more slender, the pubic symphysis shallower, the margins of the ischiopubic ramus less inverted, and the obturator foramen more triangular. This creates a situation with a greater female reliance on hip extension whereby strong tensile forces create muscular stress on the pubic ramus and ischium as the hip is repeatedly extended.

In summary, pubic stress fractures are mechanical disruptions of the bones of the pelvis from excessive, repetitive muscular activity or stress at the ischiopubic ramus, which is the origin of external hip rotators and adductors of the hip joint. Similarly, this type of injury has also been reported in soldiers.[12,92–95]

In a study by Noakes et al.,[93] there is a clinical triad seen in marathon or long-distance runners with pelvic stress fractures: (1) severe groin pain preventing any running activity, (2) positive standing sign (inability to stand solely on the affected foot/leg due to the pain), (3) severe, exquisite pain on deep palpation of the inferior pubic ramus. Radiographs are only infrequently positive in pelvic stress fracture, whereas the TPBS is invariably diagnostic.[9,11,93] When the radiographs are positive, they will reveal a nondisplaced fracture of the inferior pubic ramus. TPBS reveals a single or focal "hot spot" in the same area, which is characteristic for a stress fracture. This is in contrast to traumatic or overuse osteitis pubis, which shows diffuse nonspecific bi-lateral uptake. This very specific and unique pelvic/pubic stress fracture commonly seen in female long-distance and marathon runners occurs at the origin of the gracilis muscle and has been termed the *gracilis syndrome*[95,96] (Fig. 4-21).

Another pelvic overuse problem is the *pyriformis syndrome,* involving spasm and pain along the course of this muscle which has the sciatic nerve running along its lower border and occasionally within the muscle itself. This muscle, which is an external hip rotator and thigh abductor, has its origin from the anterior surface of the sacrum, the anterior capsule of the sacroiliac joint, and the gluteal surface of the ilium. It exits the pelvis through the greater sciatic foramen and inserts on the superior border of the greater trochanter. This syndrome is thought to result from overuse, with a history of trauma identified in only 50 percent of the cases. Patients present with buttock or low back pain and normal radiographs. The bone scan shows a linear band of increased activity along the entire course of the muscle.[97–99]

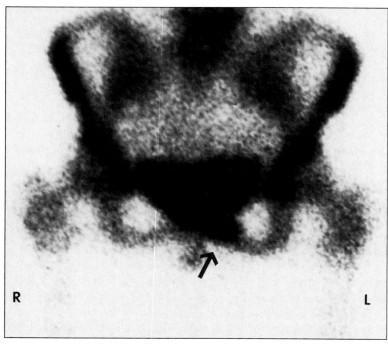

A

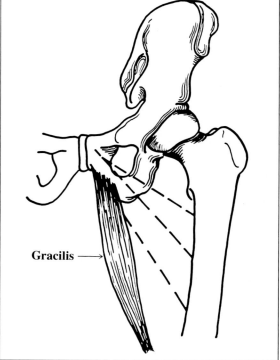

Gracilis →

B

Figure 4-21 Gracilis Syndrome/Pubic Stress Fracture. **A.** *Anterior view of high-resolution delayed image of pelvis and hips (TPBS). Focally increased activity is noted at the most medial aspect of the left ischial ramus, somewhat obscured by overlying activity within the bladder. Black arrow = focally increased nuclide activity at* the origin of the left gracilis muscle. **B.** *Anatomic drawing demonstrates origin and course of left gracilis muscle which arises from the lower half of the body of the pubis and the entire inferior pubic ramus and adjoining parts of the ischial ramus. Overuse activity is responsible for tearing or microavulsions at the origin of the gracilis causing an* osteitis noted on the above scan as a focally abnormal area of increased activity. (From Martire JR: The role of nuclear medicine scans in evaluating pain in athletic injuries. Clinics in Sports Medicine 6:713–737. Reproduced with permission.)

Thigh (Figs. 4-22 to 4-24)

In the midthigh, there is an unusual and unique overuse syndrome associated with periostitis at the insertion of the adductor muscles. *Thigh splints, or adductor insertion avulsion syndrome,* is to the thigh what shin splints is to the tibia. Primarily reported in female military recruits, it appears to be associated with continued forced overstriding and the resulting periostitis and characteristic TPBS appearance[100] (Table 4-3, Figs. 4-22 to 4-24, Drawing II).

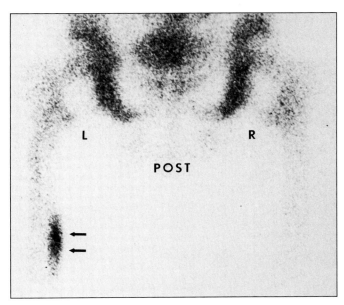

Figure 4-22 Unilateral Thigh Splints. *Posterior view of high-resolution delayed image of pelvis and hips (TPBS). Linear/vertical activity is noted along the medial femoral cortex in a female runner with left thigh pain. This moderately long segment of activity is consistent with periostitis from overuse injury with tearing at the insertion of the large adductor muscles along the proximal and middle thirds of the femur. This periostitis of the femur (thigh splints) has a similar mechanism to shin splints in the lower leg (see Drawing II). Black arrows = increased activity, middle third of left femoral shaft medially.*

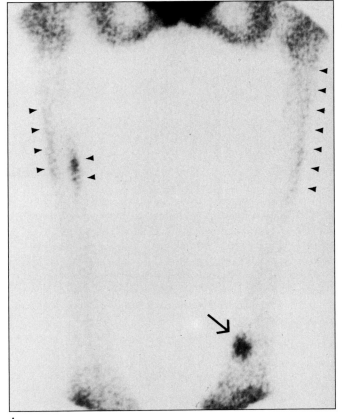

A

Figure 4-23 Bilateral Thigh Splints. **A.** *Anterior view of high-resolution delayed images of both femoral shafts (TPBS) in 16-year-old female basketball player with bilateral thigh pain. Mildly increased activity is seen in the middle third of both femoral shafts consistent with thigh splints. Additional focal area of increased activity is seen in the left distal femur. Black arrowheads = increased femoral shaft activity; black arrow = increased activity, left femur distally. (Fig. 4-23B continues on next page.)*

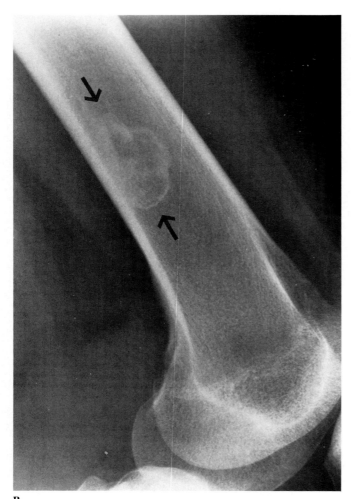

B

Figure 4-23   Bilateral Thigh Splints (Continued).
B. *Coned-down lateral radiograph of left femur demonstrates rather well circumscribed fibrous cortical defect, which accounts for the abnormal focus of activity noted on bone scan. This activity on bone scan shows that the benign defect is still metabolically active. This case illustrates that all focal "hot spots" in long bones do not represent fractures. Arrows = superior and inferior margins of fibrous cortical defect in distal left femur.*

TABLE 4-3
Clinical features of thigh splints

Also called *adductor insertion avulsion syndrome*.
Predominantly females of short stature.
Most commonly reported in military recruits.
Overuse of one or more adductor muscles associated with forced striding or overstriding (long marching step).
Periostitis of femur similar to pathophysiology of shin splints in tibia.
Severe pain on active resistance to hip adduction and external rotation.
Increased adductor tone and tenderness.
Radiographs may show periosteal reaction/thickening.
Positive TPBS shows linear/vertical activity in medial upper and mid-third of femur corresponding to adductor insertion; activity midlateral represents gluteus maximus insertion periostitis.
Usually bilateral.

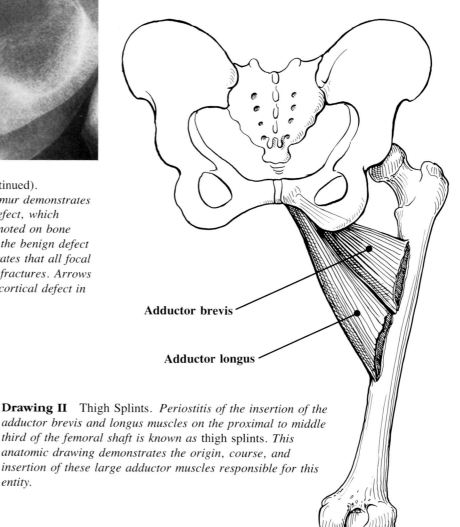

Adductor brevis

Adductor longus

Drawing II   Thigh Splints. *Periostitis of the insertion of the adductor brevis and longus muscles on the proximal to middle third of the femoral shaft is known as* thigh splints. *This anatomic drawing demonstrates the origin, course, and insertion of these large adductor muscles responsible for this entity.*

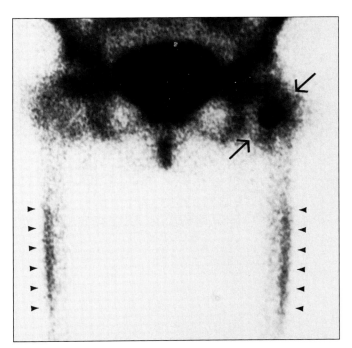

Figure 4-24   Bilateral Thigh Splints and Left Femoral Neck Stress Fracture. *Anterior view of high-resolution delayed image of hips and femurs in 37-year-old female involved with aerobics. Increased activity in the middle thirds of both right and left femoral shafts consistent with thigh splints. This activity is somewhat more prominent laterally than medially. This could be a combination not only of increased uptake in the insertion of the adductor muscles (medially) but also in the gluteus maximus (laterally). The patient also complained of left hip pain. Despite normal radiographs of the left hip and femur, TPBS revealed unsuspected left femoral neck stress fracture. Arrowheads = increased activity in the middle third of both femurs; black arrows = left femoral neck stress fracture.*

Bursitis (Figs. 4-25 and 4-26)

Bursitis is often a diagnosis made by exclusion. Radiographs are normal, and TPBS, CT, or MR imaging is performed to identify the chronic cause for hip or groin pain in order to exclude a more serious entity such as a stress fracture.

Trochanteric bursitis has a very subtle but typical TPBS pattern of increased curvilinear uptake either at or adjacent to the greater trochanter on blood pool and delayed images (Fig. 4-25). This entity can be seen in athletes of all ages and shows a pattern which is clearly distinct from femoral neck stress fracture, intertrochanteric fracture, greater trochanter fracture, or degenerative arthritis of the hip.[2,101]

The iliopsoas bursa is a normally occurring structure which, when enlarged, may present as a painful groin mass. Enlargement is often associated with preexisting joint abnormality. Diagnosis may be suspected on CT or MR examination and confirmed with a combined CT arthrogram.[102–105] The iliopsoas bursa lies posterior to the iliopsoas tendon and lateral to the femoral vessels and overlies the hip joint capsule between the pubocapsular and iliocapsular ligaments.[106,107] Communication of the iliopsoas bursa with the hip joint occurs in 9 to 15 percent of patients[108] (Fig. 4-26).

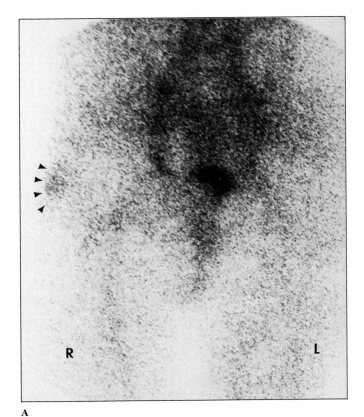

A

Figure 4-25   Trochanteric Bursitis. **A.** *Anterior blood pool image of pelvis and hips (TPBS) demonstrates a small focal area of increased activity at the lateral aspect of the right hip. Middle-aged patient complaining of chronic and recurrent right hip pain.* (Fig. 4-25B continues on next page.)

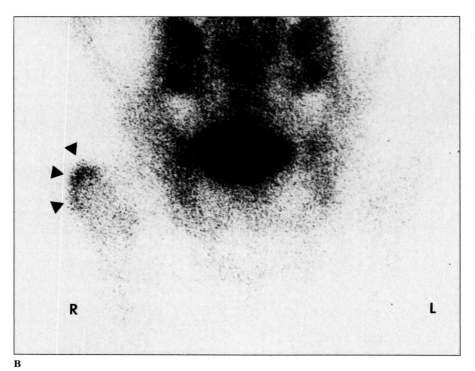

B

Figure 4-25   Trochanteric Bursitis (Continued). **B.** *Anterior view of high-resolution delayed image of pelvis and hips (TPBS) shows curvilinear, focal activity at or adjacent to the right greater trochanter. This type of appearance is most consistent with trochanteric bursitis due to inflammation in the bursa adjacent to the greater trochanter. Arrowheads = increased activity in right trochanteric bursa.*

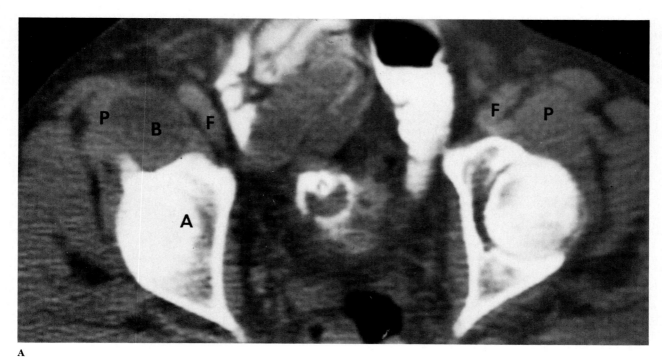

A

Figure 4-26   Iliopsoas Bursitis. **A.** *CT scan in the axial plane through the acetabulum demonstrates a region of diminished attenuation anterior to the right acetabulum displacing the iliopsoas muscle anteriorly and femoral vessels medially.* (Fig. 4-26B continues on the opposite page.)

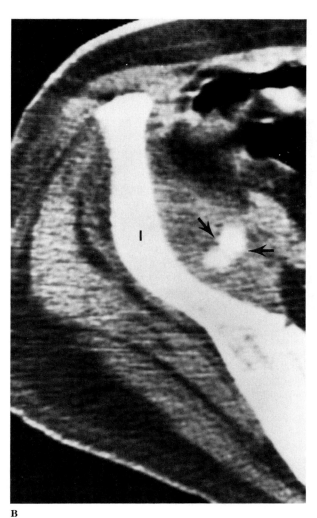

B

Figure 4-26 Iliopsoas Bursitis (Continued). **B.** *CT scan in the axial plane following a right hip arthrogram shows contrast tracking anterior to the right iliacus muscle representing an extension of the iliopsoas bursa. A = right acetabulum; F = femoral vessels; P = iliopsoas muscle; B = distended iliopsoas bursa; I = right iliac bone; arrows = contrast within right iliopsoas bursa.*

Avascular necrosis (Fig. 4-27)

CT, MR, and nuclear bone scans have each been used to provide important diagnostic information concerning avascular necrosis. A number of studies report a high level of diagnostic accuracy provided by these modalities.[109–114] Recent reports suggest that MR is the most sensitive and accurate modality in the early diagnosis of avascular necrosis of the femoral head with an accuracy in the range of 94 percent.[112,114–120] Since prognosis may be related to early treatment, the diagnosis of avascular necrosis before radiographic findings occur may be beneficial.[121] Ficat[122] devised a commonly used staging system for avascular necrosis (Table 4-4). In the earliest stage 0 disease, patients are asymptomatic with normal radiographs and normal nuclear bone scans but with a positive MR scan. At that stage, there is some evidence to suggest that early treatment may prevent progression of the disease.

Typically, avascular necrosis presents with a variety of magnetic resonance imaging patterns.[65,123–126] Commonly, a linear area of diminished density or a ring of diminished density at T1-weighted sequences is seen. With T2 weight-

ing, an inner border of high-signal intensity may be seen in up to 80 percent of cases.[127–128] Edema within the bone marrow may be an early feature.[129] This is nonspecific and may also be seen with transient osteoporosis, early stress fracture, occult fracture, and osteomyelitis. Joint effusion causing distention of the joint capsule is a nearly constant finding[128,130] (Fig. 4-27).

TABLE 4-4

Stages of avascular necrosis of the femoral head

Stage	Clinical symptoms	Radiographic findings	Nuclear bone scan	MR
0	−	−	−	+
1	−	−	+	+
2	+	+	+	+
3	+	+	+	+

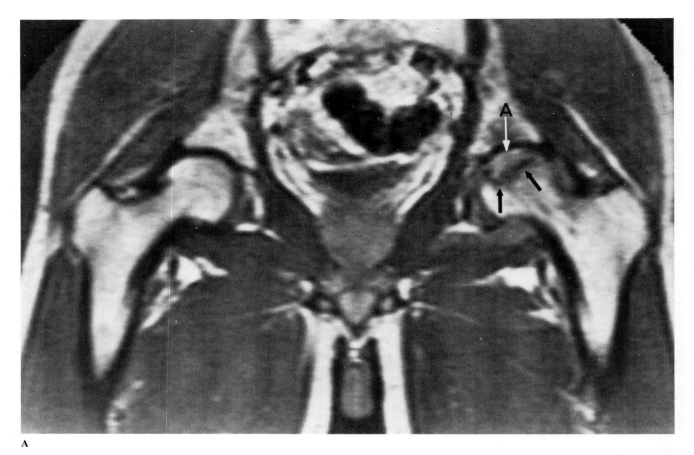

A

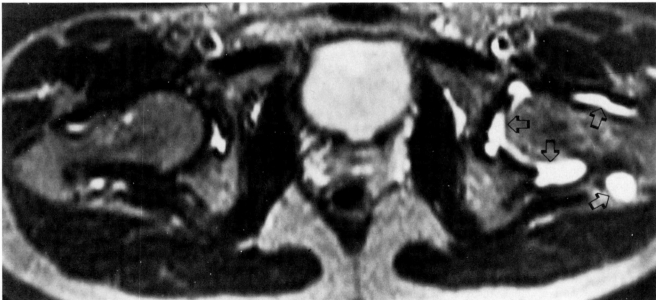

B

Figure 4-27   Avascular Necrosis of Femoral Head. **A.** *MR scan at T1-weighted sequence in the coronal plane shows a ring of low-signal intensity in the left femoral head surrounding a focus of intermediate signal intensity. These changes are characteristic for* *avascular necrosis of the left femoral head.* **B.** *MR scan at T2-weighted sequence in the axial plane shows distended joint capsule from left hip effusion. The high signal within the joint space indicates joint fluid. Tiny areas of increased signal in the right hip indicate* *a normal volume of synovial fluid on the right side. Arrows = low-signal margin to the region of avascular necrosis of the left femoral head; A = avascular necrotic focus; open arrows = left joint effusion.*

In advanced cases of avascular necrosis, magnetic resonance and computed tomography both show femoral head flattening with subcortical compression fracture.[131,132] Numerous studies have compared the relative accuracy of nuclear bone scanning, MR, and bone marrow pressure measurement in the diagnosis of avascular necrosis of the femoral head[112,114,116] (Table 4-5).

DIAGNOSTIC PROBLEMS

Infection (Figs. 4-28 to 4-30)

Septic arthritis and osteomyelitis are urgent medical/surgical problems that can often mimic athletic injuries. A combination of TPBS, CT, and/or MRI can be utilized[133–138] (Figs. 4-28 to 4-30) to secure the diagnosis.

TABLE 4-5

Comparative results in the diagnosis of avascular necrosis of the femoral head

	Nuclear bone scan, %	MR, %	Bone marrow pressure, %
Sensitivity	78–86[112,116]	89–100[112,114,116]	92[116]
Specificity	75–100[112,116]	71–100[112,114,116]	57[116]
Accuracy	76[116]	94[116]	80[116]

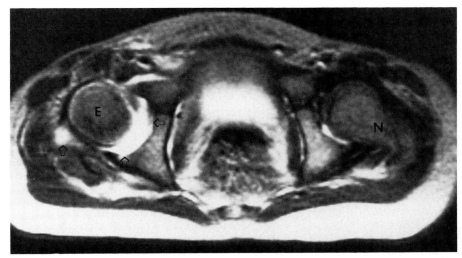

A

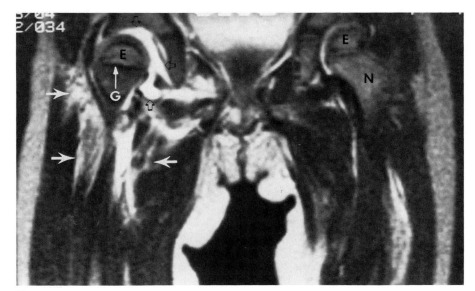

B

Figure 4-28   Septic Arthritis of the Hip. **A.** *MR scan in the axial plane at T2-weighted sequence shows right hip effusion.* **B.** *MR scan in the coronal plate at T2-weighted sequence through the hips demonstrates high-signal collection surrounding the right femoral head as well as increased signal permeating the periarticular muscles. These findings indicate an inflammatory right hip effusion with edema in the periarticular soft tissues. E = proximal femoral epiphysis; N = femoral neck; G = growth plane; arrows = region of edematous change within muscles; open arrows = joint effusion.*

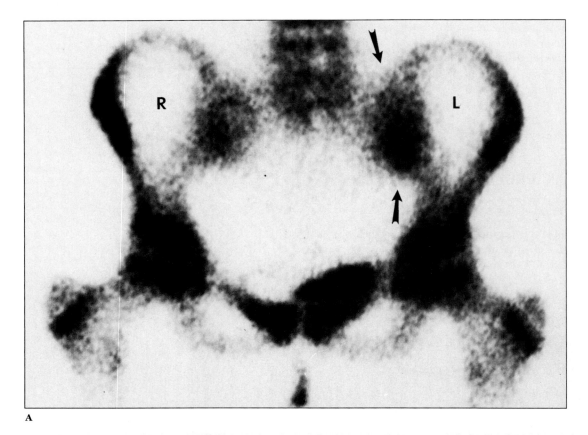

A

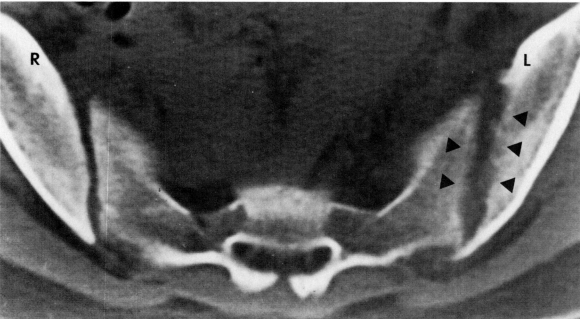

B

Figure 4-29   Septic Arthritis of Sacro-iliac Joint. **A.** *Anterior view of high-resolution delayed image of pelvis and hip. The patient is a 15-year-old female basketball player with left sacroiliac (SI) joint pain. Asymmetry is noted with increased activity in the left SI joint* *when compared with the right. Arrows = increased activity in left SI joint.* **B.** *On the basis of this suspicious bone scan, follow-up CT scan of the pelvis was performed. Axial scan at the level of the SI joint demonstrates widening of the left SI joint with bony destruction* *suggestive of septic arthritis. Further tests revealed pyogenic septic arthritis of left SI joint. Sacroiliac and back pain was, therefore, due to septic arthritis rather than athletic overuse injury. Black arrowheads = abnormal left SI joint with widening and bony destruction.*

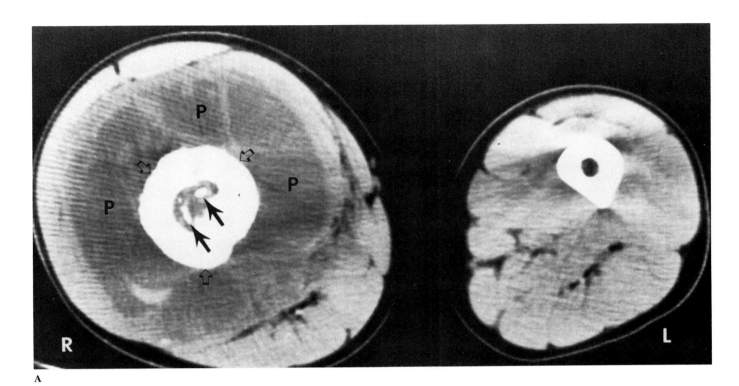

A

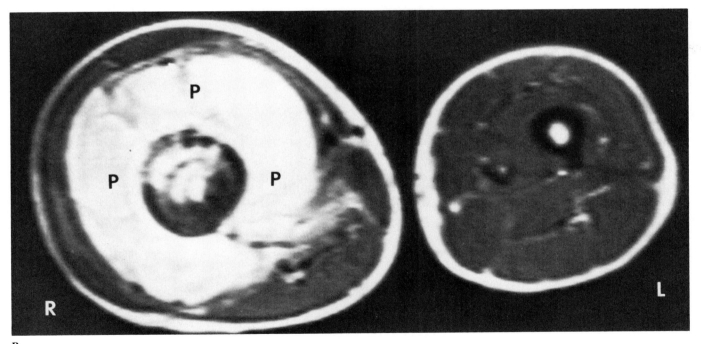

B

Figure 4-30   Osteomyelitis of Femur. **A.** *CT scan in the axial plane shows marked swelling of the right thigh with soft tissue collection between overlying muscles and thickened cortex. Bony fragments within the medullary canal represent the sequestra associated with osteomyelitis.* **B.** *MR scan at T2-weighted sequence shows a large area of high signal representing subperiosteal pus. CT optimally displays the bony abnormality. Magnetic resonance is most effective in showing soft tissue abnormality. Arrows = bony sequestrum; open arrows = involucrum of chronic periosteal apposition; P = subperiosteal collection of pus.*

Vascular (Figs. 4-31 and 4-32)

Arterial and venous problems of the pelvis and thigh associated with pain and swelling can present diagnostic difficulty in athletes. Until the last 5 years, contrast venography was the imaging tool of choice in diagnosing thrombophlebitis, but Doppler sonography has now replaced this as the test of choice, and in some circumstances CT can also identify the defect[139–143] (Fig. 4-31). The blood flow phase of TPBS is primarily intended to identify athletic injuries that are acute and relatively hyperemic in nature. Occasionally and incidentally, arterial/venous abnormalities and malformations are noted and then pursued in greater detail by MRI or angiography (Fig. 4-32).

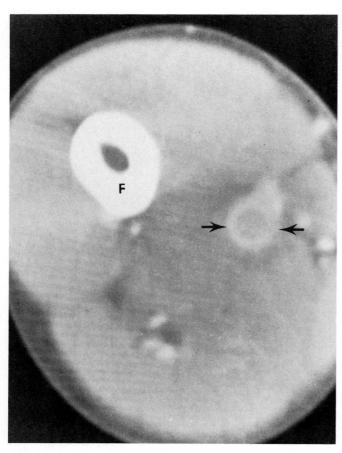

Figure 4-31   Thrombophlebitis of Deep Femoral Vein. *CT scan through the midthigh in the axial plane following intravenous contrast injection shows a ring of increased density surrounding a lucency. This corresponds to a focus of thrombophlebitis involving the deep femoral vein. F = femur; arrows = hyperintense venous wall indicating thrombophlebitis.*

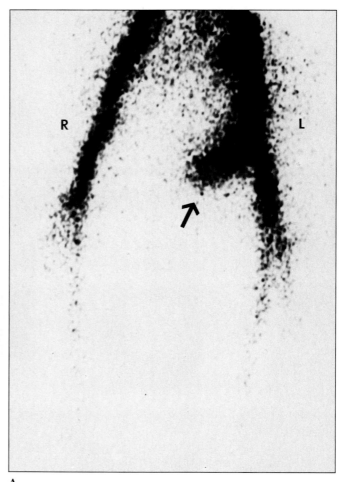

A

Figure 4-32   Arteriovenous Malformation (AVM) of Internal Iliac Artery. **A.** *Anterior view of blood pool phase of pelvis and hips (TPBS). Middle-aged male complaining of left hip and groin pain with physical activity. Flow portion of the scan demonstrates nuclide activity in the left internal iliac region representing either an AVM or a large vascular, pelvic mass. Blood pool and delayed portions of TPBS were normal. Arrow = abnormal blood vessel in region of left internal iliac artery. (Fig. 4-32B and C continues on the opposite page.)*

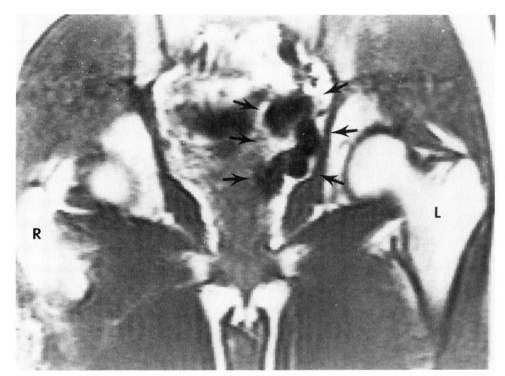

B

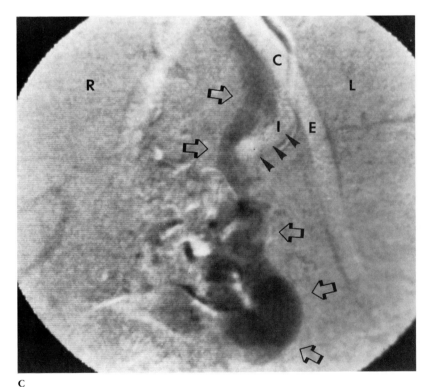

C

Figure 4-32 Arteriovenous Malformation (AVM) of Internal Iliac Artery (Continued). **B.** *MRI of pelvis and hip demonstrates large, abnormal, serpentine vascular structure in left hemipelvis corresponding to the AVM seen on the flow portion of the TPBS.*

Black arrows = large left arteriovenous malformation of left internal iliac artery. **C.** *Anterior view of digital subtraction angiogram of pelvis. Study demonstrates large arteriovenous malformation of the left internal iliac artery. C = left common iliac artery; E*

= left external iliac artery; I = left internal iliac artery; black arrowheads = contrast in proximal portion of left internal iliac artery just before AVM; open arrows = contrast entering venous portion of large AVM coursing inferiorly and then cranially.

Bone tumor (Figs. 4-33 and 4-34)

Benign or malignant bone lesions can mimic athletic injuries and have been, therefore, termed as *sports tumors* in the literature [144,145] (Figs. 4-33 and 4-34).

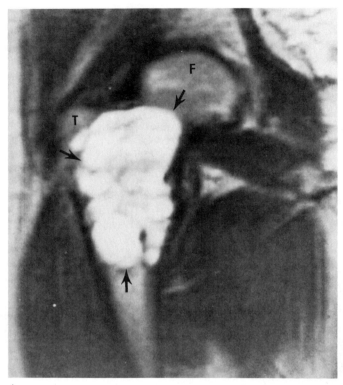

A

Figure 4-33 Bone Cyst of Femur. **A.** *MR scan at T2-weighted sequence through the proximal metaphysis of the femur shows a large area of bubbly appearing high signal indicating a bone cyst.* **B.** *MR scan at T1-weighted sequence shows this same area to demonstrate intermediate signal intensity. This signal pattern, although not specific, is consistent with bone cyst. F = femoral head; T = greater trochanter; arrows = cystic abnormality.*

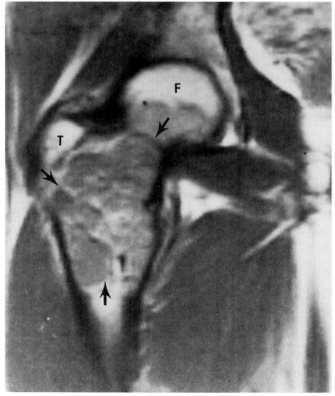

B

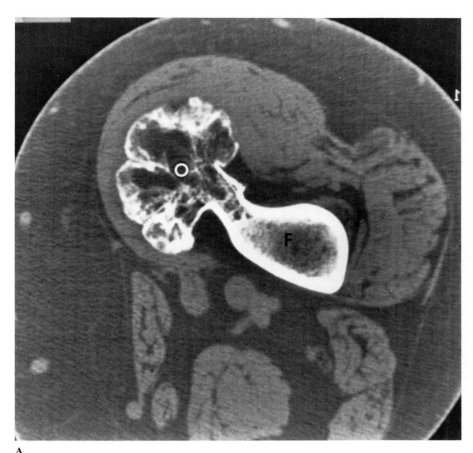

A

Figure 4-34   Osteochondroma of the Femur. **A.** *CT scan in the axial plane through the distal thigh demonstrates a cauliflowerlike projection directed medially off the distal metaphysis of the femur displacing overlying muscles. The medullary space of the femur is contiguous with that of this benign bony proliferation. The appearance is characteristic for osteochondroma.* **B.** *Three-dimensional reconstruction derived from the axial scan demonstrates the appearance of this benign neoplasm from the posterior perspective.* **C.** *Three-dimensional reconstruction from the superior perspective shows the extent of this benign neoplasm. F = normal femoral metaphysis; O = osteochondroma; P = patella; M = medial femoral condyle; I = intercondylar notch; L = lateral femoral condyle; Ma = marrow space.*

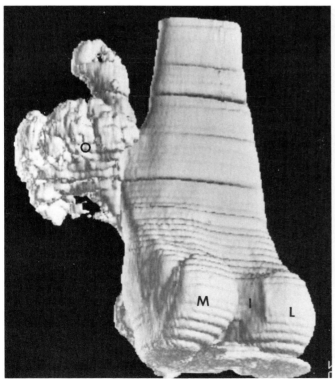

B

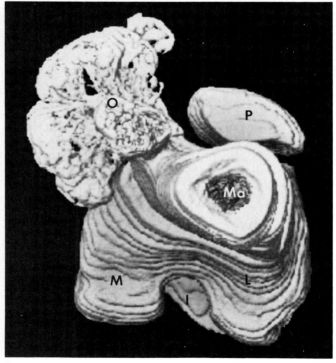

C

Slipped femoral capital epiphysis (SFCE)
(Fig. 4-35)

This entity occurs in the 9 to 17-year-old age group, with the problem representing a shift or movement of the femoral head on the shaft. Although the exact cause is not known, it is thought to be nontraumatic in nature. The resulting pain, often referred to the thigh or knee, is the most frequent clinical complaint and often associated with a limp. On radiographs, there is widening of the radiolucent growth plate on the affected side, and the epiphysis of the involved femoral head is slightly displaced dorsally and/or medially. The TPBS pattern is quite specific, reflecting the response to abnormal movement of the growth plate on the affected side appearing as increased activity in this area on both blood pool and high-resolution delayed images. When compared with the normal or opposite side, the affected side shows nonspecific increased activity through the growth plate (Fig. 4-35). Early diagnosis is essential, since early intervention with surgical pinning prevents further slippage as well as potential complications of aseptic necrosis and/or osteoarthritis.[9]

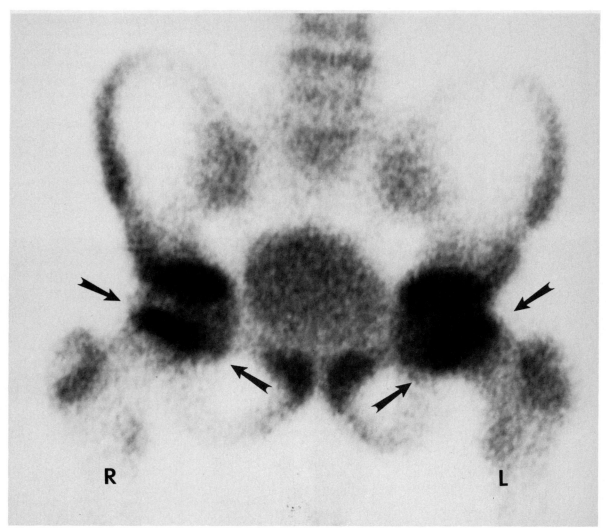

Figure 4-35 Slipped Femoral Capital Epiphysis. *Anterior view of delayed high-resolution image of TPBS in 13-year-old with left hip pain for 1 month exacerbated with any type of athletic activity. Radiographs were equivocal for left slipped femoral capital epiphysis (SFCE). This study demonstrates asymmetry of the hip epiphysis which is open and quite active in this adolescent patient. On the right, or asymptomatic, side, the physis is seen as a sharply delineated band of activity of normal size and shape. On the left, the physis activity is poorly marginated and widened compatible with a diagnosis of SFCE representing movement of the femoral head on the shaft. Arrows = nuclide activity in physes.*

REFERENCES

1. Lloyd-Smith R, Clement DB, McKenzie DC, et al.: A survey of overuse and traumatic hip and pelvic injuries in athletes, Phys Sports Med 10:131–142, 1985.
2. Nicholas JA, Friedman MJ: Orthopedic problems in middle-aged athletes. Phys Sports Med 7(12):53–64, 1979.
3. Waters PM, Millis MB: Hip and pelvic injuries in the young athlete. Clin Sports Med 7:513–525, 1988.
4. Fernbach SK, Wilkinson RH: Avulsion injuries of the pubis and proximal femur. AJR 137:581–584, 1981.
5. Metzmaker JN, Pappas AM: Avulsion fractures of the pelvis. Am J Sports Med 13:349–358, 1985.
6. Crues JV, Lynch TCP: MR effective in detecting traumatic bone injuries. Diagn Imaging 38:118–121, 1990.
7. Dalinka MK, Boorstein JM, Zlatkin MB: Computed tomography of musculoskeletal trauma. Radiol Clin North Am 27:933–944, 1989.
8. Holder LE: Clinical radionuclide bone imaging. Radiology 176:607–614, 1990.
9. Holder LE, Matthews LS: The nuclear physician and sports medicine, in Freeman L, Weissman H (eds): *Nuclear Medicine Annual 1984*. Raven Press, New York, 1984, pp 88–140.
10. Martire JR: The role of nuclear medicine scans in evaluating pain in athletic injuries. Clin Sports Med 6:713–737, 1987.
11. Rupani HD, Holder LE, Espinola DA, et al.: Three phase radionuclide bone imaging in sports medicine. Radiology 156:187–196, 1985.
12. Tehranzadeh J, Serafini AN, Pais MJ: *Avulsion and Stress Injuries of the Musculoskeletal System.* Karger, Basel, 1989.
13. Holder LH, Schwarz C, Wernicke PG, et al.: Radionuclide bone imaging in the early detection of fractures of the proximal femur (hip): multifactorial analysis. Radiology 174:509–515, 1990.
14. Bressler EL, Marn CS, Gore RM, et al.: Evaluation of ectopic bone by CT. AJR 148:931–935, 1987.
15. Hudson TM: Joint fluoroscopy before arthrography: detection and evaluation of loose bodies. Skeletal Radiol 12:199–203, 1984.
16. Magid D, Fishman EK: Imaging of musculoskeletal trauma in three dimensions: an integrated two-dimensional/three dimensional approach with computed tomography. Radiol Clin North Am 27:945–956, 1989.
17. Mesgarzadeh M, Sapega AA, Bonakdarpour A, et al.: Osteochondritis dissecans: analysis of mechanical stability with radiography, scintigraphy and MR imaging. Radiology 165:775–780, 1987.
18. Ozonoff MB: Controlled arthrography of the hip: a technique of fluoroscopic monitoring and recording. Clin Orthop 93:260–264, 1973.
19. Weinreb JC, Cohen JM, Maravilla KR: Iliopsoas muscles: MR study of normal anatomy and disease. Radiology 156:435–440, 1985.
20. Littrup PJ, Aisen AM, Braunstein EM, et al.: Magnetic resonance imaging of femoral head development in roentgenographically normal patients. Skeletal Radiol 14:159–163, 1985.
21. Mitchell DG, Rao VM, Dalinka M, et al.: Hematopoietic and fatty bone marrow distribution in the normal and ischemic hip: new observations with 1.5-T MR imaging. Radiology 161:199–202, 1986.
22. Nokes SR, Vogler JB, Spritzer CE, et al.: Herniation pits of the femoral neck: appearance at MR imaging. Radiology 172:231–234, 1989.
23. Matin PM: Appearance of bone scans following fractures including immediate and long term studies. J Nucl Med 20:1227–1231, 1979.
24. Lasda NA, Levinsohn EM, Yuan HA, et al.: Computerized tomography in disorders of the hip. J Bone Joint Surg 60(A):1099–1102, 1978.
25. Sauser DD, Billimoria PE, Rouse GA, et al.: CT evaluation of hip trauma. AJR 135:269–274, 1980.
26. Shirkhoda A, Braschear HR, Staab EV: Computed tomography of acetabular fractures. Radiology 134:683–688, 1980.
27. Canale ST, Manugian AH: Irreducible traumatic dislocations of the hip. J Bone Joint Surg 61(A):7–14, 1979.
28. Guyer B, Smith DS, Cady RB, et al.: Dosimetry of computerized tomography in the evaluation of hip dysplasia. Skeletal Radiol 12:123–127, 1984.
29. Peterson HA, Klassen RA, McLeod RA, et al.: The use of computerized tomography in dislocation of hip and femoral neck anteversion in children. J Bone Joint Surg 63(B):198–208, 1981.
30. Guyer B, Levinsohn EM: Recurrent anterior dislocation of the hip: case report with arthrographic findings. Skeletal Radiol 10:262–264, 1983.
31. Klein A, Sumner TE, Volberg FM, et al.: Combined CT-arthrography in recurrent traumatic hip dislocation. AJR 138:963–964, 1982.
32. Glynn TP Jr, Kreipke DL, DeRosa GP: Computed tomography arthrography in traumatic hip dislocation: intra-articular and capsular findings. Skeletal Radiol 18:29–31, 1989.
33. Schneider R, Yacovone J, Ghelman B: Unsuspected sacral fractures: detection by radionuclide bone scanning. Am J Roentgenol 144:337–341, 1985.
34. Clancy WG, Foltz AS: Iliac apophysitis in stress fractures in adolescent runners. Am J Sports Med 4:214–218, 1976.
35. Wootton JR, Cross MJ, Holt KW: Avulsion of the ischial apophysis: the case for open reduction and internal fixation. J Bone Joint Surg 72(B):625–627, 1990.
36. Mozes M, Papa MZ, Zweig A, et al.: Iliopsoas injury in soccer players. Br J Sports Med 19(3):168–170, 1985.
37. Rockett JF: Three-phase radionuclide bone imaging in stress injury of the anterior iliac crest. J Nucl Med 31:1554–1556, 1990.
38. Schneider R, Kaye J, Ghelman B: Adductor avulsive injuries near the symphysis pubis. Radiology 120:567–569, 1976.
39. Tehranzadeh J, Kurth L, Elyaderani MK, et al.: Combined pelvic stress fracture and avulsion of the adductor longus in a middle-distance runner, a case report. Am J Sports Med 10:108–111, 1982.
40. Fleckenstein JL, Weatherall PT, Parkey RW, et al.: Sports-related muscle injuries: evaluation with MR imaging. Radiol 172:793–798, 1989.
41. Zagoria RJ, Karstaedt N, Koubek TD: MR imaging of rhabdomyolysis. J Comput Assist Tomogr 10:268–270, 1986.
42. Hagerman FC, Hikida RS, Staron RS, et al.: Muscle damage in marathon runners. Phys Sports Med 11:39–46, 1984.

43. Demos MA, Gitin EL, Kagen LJ: Exercise myoglobinemia and acute exertional rhabdomyolysis. Arch Intern Med 134:669–673, 1974.

44. Boyd JF: Fatal rhabdomyolysis in marathon runner. Lancet 1(8541):1089, 1987.

45. Frymoyer PA, Giammarco R, Farrar FM, et al.: Technetium-99m-medronate bone scanning in rhabdomyolysis. Arch Intern Med 45:1991–1995, 1985.

46. Hamilton RW, Gardner LB, Penn AS: Acute tubular necrosis caused by exercise-induced myoglobinuria. Ann Intern Med 77:77–82, 1972.

47. Lentle BC, Percy JS, Rigal WM, et al.: Localization of Tc-99m pyrophosphate in muscle after exercise. J Nucl Med 19:223–224, 1978.

48. Olerud JE, Homer LD, Carroll HW: Incidence of acute exertional rhabdomyolysis. Arch Intern Med 136:692–697, 1976.

49. Schiff HB, MacSearraigh ET, Kallmeyer JC: Myoglobinuria, rhabdomyolysis and marathon running. Q J Med 188:463–472, 1978.

50. Siegel AJ, Warhal MJ, Evans WJ, et al.: Focal myofibrillar necrosis in skeletal muscle of trained marathon runners after competition. Med Sci Sports Exerc 15:164, 1983.

51. Siegel BA, Engel WR, Derrer EC: Localization of technetium-99m diphosphonate in acutely injured muscle: relationship to calcium deposition. Neurology 27:230–238, 1977.

52. Stewart PJ, Rosen GA: Case report: acute renal failure following a marathon. Phys Sports Med 8(4):61–63, 1980.

53. Thomas BD, Motley CP: Myoglobinemia and endurance exercise: a study of twenty-five participants in a triathelon competition. Am J Sports Med 12:113–119, 1984.

54. Tiidus PM, Ianuzzo CD: Effects of intensity and duration of muscular exercise on delayed soreness and serum enzyme activities. Med Sci Sports Exerc 15:461–465, 1983.

55. Valk P: Muscle localization of Tc-99m MDP after exertion. Clin Nucl Med 9:493–494, 1984.

56. Ziskind A, Huang P: Jet-ski rhabdomyolysis. JAMA 255:1879–1880, 1986.

57. Matin P, Lang G, Garetta R, et al.: Scintigraphic evaluation of muscle damage following extreme exercise. J Nucl Med 24:308–311, 1983.

58. El-Khoury GY, Wehbe MA, Bonfiglio M, et al.: Stress fracture of the femoral neck: a scintigraphic sign for early diagnosis. Skeletal Radiol 6:271–273, 1981.

59. Devas MB: Stress fractures of the femoral neck. J Bone Joint Surg 47(B):728–738, 1984.

60. Lombardo SJ, Benson SL: Stress fractures of the femur in runners. Am J Sports Med 10:219–227, 1982.

61. Mogle DD, Bowden RW: Fracture of the human femoral bone. J Biomech 17:203–213, 1984.

62. McBryde AM: Stress fractures in runners. Clin Sports Med 4:737–752, 1985.

63. Blatz DJ: Bilateral femoral and tibial shaft stress fractures in a runner. Am J Sports Med 9:322–325, 1981.

64. Blickenstaff MD, Morris JM: Fatigue fracture of the femoral neck. J Bone Joint Surg 45(A):1031–1047, 1966.

65. Bluemm RG, Falke THM, Ziedses des Plantes Jr. BG, et al.: Early Legg-Perthes disease (ischemic necrosis of the femoral head) demonstrated by magnetic resonance imaging. Skeletal Radiol 14:95–98, 1985.

66. Cady GW, White ES, Lapointe JN: Displaced fatigue fracture of the femoral neck. J Bone Joint Surg 57(A):1022–1027, 1975.

67. Erne P, Burkhardt A: Femoral neck fatigue fracture. Arch Orthop Trauma Surg 97:213–220, 1980.

68. Hershman EB, Mailly T: Stress fractures. Clin Sports Med 1:183–214, 1990.

69. Kaltsas D: Stress fractures of the femoral neck in young adults. J Bone Joint Surg 63(B):33–37, 1981.

70. Hajek MR, Noble HB: Stress fractures of the femoral neck in joggers. Am J Sports Med 10:112–116, 1982.

71. Oh I, Harris WH: Proximal strain distribution in the loaded femur. J Bone Joint Surg 60(A):75–85, 1978.

72. Reilly DT, Burstein AH: The mechanical properties of cortical bone. J Bone Joint Surg 56(A):1001–1020, 1974.

73. Rybicki EF, Simonen FA, Webb BB: On the mathematical analysis of stress in the human femur. J Biomech 5:203–215, 1972.

74. Skinner HB, Cook SD: Fatigue failure stress of the femoral neck: a case report. Am J Sports Med 7:89–101, 1988.

75. Woo SL, Kuei SC, Amiel D, et al.: The effect of prolonged physical training on the properties of the long bone: a study of Wolff's law. J Bone Joint Surg 63(A):780–787, 1981.

76. Toridis TG: Stress analysis of the femur. J Biomech 2:163–174, 1969.

77. Viano DC, Stalknaker RL: Mechanisms of femoral fracture. J Biomech 13:701–715, 1980.

78. Bargren JH, Tilson DH, Brideford OE: Prevention of displaced fatigue fractures of the femur. J Bone Joint Surg 53(A):1115–1117, 1971.

79. Lynch TCP, Crues JV, Morgan FW, et al.: Bone abnormalities of the knee: prevalence and significance at MR imaging. Radiology 171:761–766, 1989.

80. Speer KP, Spritzer CE, Harrelson JM, et al.: Magnetic resonance imaging of the femoral head after acute intracapsular fracture of the femoral neck. J Bone Joint Surg 72(A):98–103, 1990.

81. Butler JE, Brown SL, McConnell BG: Subtrochanteric stress fractures in runners. Am J Sports Med 10:228–232, 1982.

82. Hershman EB, Lombardo J, Bergfeld JA: Femoral shaft stress fractures in athletes. Clin Sports Med 1:111–119, 1990.

83. Hulkko A, Orava S: Stress fractures of the femur in runners. Am J Sports Med 10:219–227, 1982.

84. Provost RA, Morris JM: Fatigue fracture of the femoral shaft. J Bone Joint Surg 51(A):487–498, 1969.

85. Cochrane GM: Osteitis pubis in athletes. Br J Sports Med 5:233–235, 1971.

86. Coventry MB, Mitchell WC: Osteitis pubis: observations based on a study of 45 patients. JAMA 178:898–905, 1961.

87. Grace JN, Sim FH, Shives TC, et al.: Wedge resection of the symphysis pubis for the treatment of the osteitis pubis. J Bone Joint Surg 71(A):358–364, 1989.

88. Hanson PG, Angevine M, Juhl JH: Osteitis pubis in sports activities. Phys Sports Med 6:111–114, 1978.

89. Koch RA, Jackson DW: Pubic symphysitis in runners. A report of two cases. Am J Sports Med 9:62–63, 1981.

90. Pearson RL: Osteitis pubis in a basketball player. Phys Sports Med 16(7):69–72, 1988.

91. Rold JF, Rold BA: Pubic stress symphysitis in a female distance runner. Phys Sports Med 14:61–65, 1986.

92. Latshaw RF, Kantner TR, Kalenak A, et al.: A pelvic stress fracture in a female jogger. Am J Sports Med 9:54–56, 1981.

93. Noakes TD, Smith JA, Lindenberg G, et al.: Pelvic stress fractures in long distance runners. Am J Sports Med 13:120–123, 1985.

94. Pavlov H, Nelson TL, Warren, RF, et al.: Stress fractures of the pubic ramus. J Bone Joint Surg 64(A):1020–1025, 1982.

95. Meurman KOA: Stress fracture of the pubic arch in military recruits. Br J Radiol 53:521–524, 1980.

96. Wiley JJ: Traumatic osteitis pubis—the gracilis syndrome. Am J Sports Med 11:360–363, 1983.

97. Karl RD, Yedinak MA, Hartshorne MF, et al.: Scintigraphic appearance of the piriformis muscle syndrome. Clin Nucl Med 10(5):361–363, 1985.

98. Pace J, Nagle D: Piriformis syndrome. West J Med 124:435–439, 1976.

99. Retzloff E, Berry A, Haight A, et al.: The piriformis muscle syndrome. J Am Osteopath Assoc 73:799, 1974.

100. Charkes MD, Siddhivarn N, Schneck CD: Bone scanning in the adductor insertion avulsion syndrome ("thigh splints"). J Nucl Med 28:1835–1838, 1987.

101. Christensen SB, Arnoldi CC: Distribution of ^{99m}Tc-phosphate compounds in osteoarthritic femoral heads. J Bone Joint Surg 62(A):90–96, 1980.

102. Binek R, Levinsohn EM: Enlarged iliopsoas bursa. Clin Orthop 221:158–163, 1987.

103. Penkava RR: Iliopsoas bursitis demonstrated by computed tomography. AJR 135:175–176, 1980.

104. Sartoris DJ, Danzig L, Gilula L, et al.: Synovial cysts of the hip joint and iliopsoas bursitis: a spectrum of imaging abnormalities. Skeletal Radiol 14:85–94, 1985.

105. Steinbach LS, Schneider R, Goldman AB, et al.: Bursae and abscess cavities communicating with the hip: diagnosis using arthrography and CT. Radiology 156:303–307, 1985.

106. Armstrong P, Saxton H: Ilio-psoas bursa. Br J Radiol 45:493–495, 1972.

107. Chandler SB: The iliopsoas bursa in man. Anat Rec 58:235–240, 1933.

108. Staple TW: Arthrographic demonstration of iliopsoas bursa extension of the hip joint. Radiology 102:515–516, 1972.

109. Bensahel H, Bok B, Cavailles F, et al.: Bone scintigraphy in Perthes' disease. J Pediatr Orthop 3:302–305, 1983.

110. Danigelis JA, Fisher RL, Osonoff MB, et al.: ^{99m}Tc polyphosphate bone imaging in Legg-Perthes disease. Radiology 115:407–413, 1975.

111. Majid M, Frankel RS: Radionuclide imaging in skeletal inflammatory and ischemic disease in childhood. AJR 126:832–841, 1976.

112. Markisz JA, Knowles RJR, Altchek DW, et al.: Segmental patterns of avascular necrosis of the femoral heads: early detection with MR imaging. Radiology 162:717–720, 1987.

113. Ponseti IV, Maynard JA, Weinstein SL, et al.: Legg-Calve-Perthes Disease. J Bone Joint Surg 65(A):797–807, 1983.

114. Thickman D, Axel L, Kressel HY, et al.: Magnetic resonance imaging of avascular necrosis of the femoral head. Skeletal Radiol 15:133–140, 1986.

115. Baker LL, Blanco JAP, Young SW: MRI of avascular necrosis of the hip: state of the art and review. Radiol Report 2:222–230, 1990.

116. Beltran J, Herman LJ, Burke JM, et al.: Femoral head avascular necrosis: MR imaging with clinical-pathologic and radionuclide correlation. Radiology 166:215–220, 1988.

117. Gillespy T III, Genant HK, Helms CA: Magnetic resonance imaging of osteonecrosis. Radiol Clin North Am 24:193–208, 1986.

118. Glickstein MF, Burk DL Jr, Schiebler ML, et al.: Avascular necrosis versus other diseases of the hip: sensitivity of MR imaging. Radiology 169:213–215, 1988.

119. Mitchel MD, Kundel HL, Steinberg ME, et al.: Avascular necrosis of the hip: comparison of MR, CT and scintigraphy. AJR 147:67–71, 1986.

120. Patten RM, Shuman WP: MRI of osteonecrosis. MRI Decisions 4:2–13, 1990.

121. Robinson HJ, Hartleben PD, Lund G, et al.: Evaluation of magnetic resonance imaging in the diagnosis of osteonecrosis of the femoral head. J Bone Joint Surg 71(A):650–663, 1989.

122. Ficat RP: Idiopathic bone necrosis of the femoral head: early diagnosis and treatment. J Bone Joint Surg 67(B):3–9, 1985.

123. Hauzeur JP, Pasteels JL, Schoutens A, et al.: The diagnostic value of magnetic resonance imaging in non-traumatic osteonecrosis of the femoral head. J Bone Joint Surg 71(A):641–649, 1989.

124. Lang P, Jergensen HA, Moseley ME, et al.: Avascular necrosis of the femoral head: high-field strength MR imaging with histologic correlation. Radiology 169:517–524, 1988.

125. Mitchel DG, Joseph PM, Fallon M, et al.: Chemical-shift MR imaging of the femoral head: an in vitro study of normal hips and hips with avascular necrosis. AJR 148:1159–1164, 1987.

126. Totty WG, Murphy WA, Ganz WI, et al.: Magnetic resonance imaging of the normal and ischemic femoral head. AJR 143:1273–1280, 1984.

127. Mitchell DG, Rao VM, Dalinka MK, et al.: Femoral head avascular necrosis: correlation of MR imaging, radiographic staging, radionuclide imaging and clinical findings. Radiology 162:709–715, 1987.

128. Mitchell DG, Steinberg ME, Dalinka MK, et al.: Magnetic resonance imaging of the ischemic hip. Clin Orthop 244:60–77, 1989.

129. Turner DA, Templeton AC, Selzer PM, et al.: Femoral capital osteonecrosis: MR finding of diffuse marrow abnormalities without focal lesions. Radiology 171:135–140, 1989.

130. Shuman WP, Castagno AA, Baron RL, et al.: MR imaging of avascular necrosis of the femoral head: value of small field-of-view sagittal surface-coil images. AJR 150:1073–1078, 1988.

131. Magid D, Fishman EK, Scott WW Jr, et al.: Femoral head avascular necrosis: CT assessment with multiplanar reconstruction. Radiology 157:751–756, 1985.

132. Mitchell DG, Kressel HY, Arger PH, et al.: Avascular necrosis of the femoral head: morphologic assessment by MR imaging with CT correlation. Radiology 161:739–742, 1986.

133. Fletcher BD, Scoles PV, Nelson AD: Osteomyelitis in children: detection by magnetic resonance. Radiology 150:57–60, 1984.

134. Kaye JJ: Arthritis: roles of radiography and other imaging techniques in evaluation. Radiology 177:601–608, 1990.

135. Kuhn JP, Berger PE: Computed tomographic diagnosis of osteomyelitis. Radiology 130:503–506, 1979.

136. Mason MD, Zlatkin MB, Esterhai JL, et al.: Chronic complicated osteomyelitis of the lower extremity: evaluation with MR imaging. Radiology 173:355–359, 1989.

137. Modic MT, Pflanze W, Feiglin DHI, et al.: Magnetic resonance imaging of musculoskeletal infections. Radiol Clin North Am 24:247–258, 1986.

138. Unger E, Moldofsky P, Gatenby R, et al.: Diagnosis of osteomyelitis by MR imaging. AJR 150:605–610, 1988.

139. Aitken AG, Godden DJ: Real-time ultrasound diagnosis of deep vein thrombosis: a comparison with venography. Clin Radiol 38:309–313, 1987.

140. Aronen HJ, Pamilo M, Suoranta ST, et al.: Sonography in differential diagnosis of deep venous thrombosis of lower leg. Acta Radiol 28:457–459, 1987.

141. Cronan JJ, Dorfman GS, Grusmark J: Lower extremity deep venous thrombosis: further experience with and refinements of ultrasound assessment. Radiology 168:101–107, 1988.

142. Mackey JW, Webster JA: Deep vein thrombosis in marathon runners. Phys Sports Med 9(5):91–98, 1981.

143. Sidler GJ, Bugaieski SM, Sunderlin J, et al.: Case report: difficulty in diagnosing and treating deep vein thrombosis in a competitive basketball player. Phys Sports Med 13(7):113–118, 1985.

144. Baker BE, Levinsohn EM, Coren AB: Pitfalls to avoid in diagnosing pain in the athlete. Clin Sports Med 6:921–934, 1987.

145. Lewis MM, Reilly JF: Sports tumors. Am J Sports Med 4:362–365, 1987.

Orthopedic overview

Until approximately 1983, the physician's ability to provide a patient with an accurate diagnosis of shoulder joint pathology was limited. Imaging techniques available at that time included plain radiography, sonography, arthrography, and triple-phase bone scanning (TPBS). In the highly competitive athlete, we simply were unable to provide adequately accurate information required in decision making for playability and treatment. Arthrography in pitchers undergoing rotator cuff surgery was frequently found to be false-negative, and sonography was inconsistent and unreliable.

The development of arthroscopic techniques for visualizing intraarticular anatomy and pathology allowed orthopedic surgeons to visualize the glenoid labrum, biceps tendon attachment, and glenohumeral ligaments in a manner that previously could only be appreciated in the anatomy laboratory. Coincident with the emergence of arthroscopy has been the development of combined CT arthrography and magnetic resonance imaging (MRI), allowing us to combine the imaging diagnosis with the arthroscopic findings. Thus, an appreciation for a new subset of pathologic entities has become possible. Additionally, anatomic studies and additional views of the acromion, such as the supraspinatus outlet view, have given us tools to predict impending impingement pathology as well as a method to determine the sufficiency of decompression following anterior acromioplasty.

MRI allows us the luxury of detecting soft tissue and nonossified pathologic tissue under the acromion as well as within the acromioclavicular joint, which cannot be appreciated on any other study. It enables us to study the effects of continuous exercise of the musculotendinous units about the shoulder and to image overuse tendinitis. Partial rotator cuff tears, invisible on arthrography, are now routinely diagnosed. Recognition of atrophy or fatty degeneration of the muscles inserting on the rotator cuff, allows the orthopedic surgeon to prognosticate the likely outcome of open cuff repair before undertaking such a procedure.

CT arthrography allows us to image the labrum in a manner far superior to any other imaging method. The results obtained with CT arthrography correlate closely with those of arthroscopy. In evaluating the throwing or racket sport athlete, however, our inability to image the shoulder in the abducted and externally rotated position is a limiting factor. One wonders how many more defects in the labra might be detected with provocative stress. Those experienced in looking at CT arthrograms of the shoulder have occasionally noticed the appearance of heterotopic calcification or ossification in the region of the posterior capsular attachment to the glenoid. When this is seen, TPBS is indicated in helping to determine the age (metabolic activity) of this reactive new bone formation. One wonders whether the ossification seen on CT corresponds to what we have previously referred to as the *Bennett lesion* identified on radiographs of professional pitchers.

Those experienced with glenohumeral joint pathology have long recognized that labral and rotator cuff disease, which is seen in patients who are less than 35 years of age, differs substantially from that seen in patients

CHAPTER 5

SHOULDER AND HUMERUS

who are over 45 years of age. In the younger athlete, one frequently sees glenohumeral instability resulting from stretching of the glenohumeral ligaments. This leads to labral abrasion, causing cleavage and partial tears. This is entirely different from the labral detachment associated with acute glenohumeral dislocation. Rotator cuff tears occur secondary to change in the resting length of the musculotendinous units, aggravated by friction between the rotator cuff and the coracoacromial artication. In the older patient, rotator cuff tears most often occur in the lateral critical zone of the rotator cuff (within a centimeter of the greater tuberosity). Macrotears of the cuff usually occur following an acute injury. It is important for the clinician to convey his clinical considerations to the radiologist in order to optimize the imaging plan.

The use of MRI for detecting physeal injuries of the sternoclavicular joint in the preadolescent and adolescent can help the orthopedic surgeon to avoid unnecessary and risky surgery. The identification of growth plate fracture is an important diagnosis now possible with magnetic resonance scanning. Posterior dislocations remain important diagnostic entities which require urgent open reduction if morbidity is to be minimized.

TPBS is the imaging gold standard in the detection of stress fractures. I have found it particularly helpful in the diagnosis of early stress fractures of the coracoid process and in humeral shaft stress fractures which are reported in javelin throwers. The early diagnosis of an incomplete stress fracture is important, since that condition is far easier to treat than the completed fracture identified later as the result of an acute event. Obviously, unexplained bone pain or muscle pain in a patient with normal radiographs requires further evaluation. TPBS has been extremely helpful in this situation. The use of sonography to evaluate rotator cuff tears has been reported and shows promise. Unfortunately, this modality is exceedingly operator-dependent and the results are not always reliable. Sonography has been helpful in assessing the biceps tendon, and real time sonography allows us to watch tendons as they move.

These new imaging tools enable us to accurately diagnose a number of athletic injuries and conditions. Careful clinical examination and routine radiographs should be obtained first in all cases of athletic injury in the shoulder and humerus. Neoplasms, Hill-Sachs lesions, osteophytes, loose bodies, and even avascular necrosis can frequently be readily diagnosed on the plain radiograph in a reliable and economic way.

CHARLES E. SILBERSTEIN, M.D., M.SC.
Medical Director, The Bennett Institute for Sports Medicine and Fitness, The Children's Hospital and Center for Reconstructive Surgery, Baltimore, Maryland
Orthopedic Surgeon, Baltimore Orioles Professional Baseball Team, and The Johns Hopkins University Intercollegiate Athletic Teams
Clinical Assistant Professor of Orthopedic Surgery
The Johns Hopkins University School of Medicine
Baltimore, Maryland

HOULDER PAIN in the athlete is a common clinical problem often caused by lesions of the rotator cuff, glenohumeral capsule, glenoid labrum, and acromioclavicular and sternoclavicular joints. The spectrum of disorders also includes bicipital tendon abnormality, osteochondral loose bodies, avascular necrosis, and calcific tendinitis. The high degree of mobility allowed by the glenohumeral articulation and the stresses applied to the glenoid labrum, rotator cuff, and sternoclavicular and acromioclavicular joints subject these areas to specific injuries and pathologic alteration.[1]

An effective arsenal of imaging tests has been devised to assist in the diagnosis of pathologic abnormalities about the shoulder. Routine radiographs are generally the first imaging tools used and are helpful in assessing fracture, including the Hill-Sachs compression fracture of the humeral head and Bankart fracture of the glenoid. These fractures result from previous shoulder dislocation. Plain radiographs additionally are useful in demonstrating calcific peritendinitis, bicipital groove abnormality, and tuberosity injury as well as some cartilage and soft tissue abnormalities. Triple-phase bone scanning (TPBS) has proved effective in helping to show occult and stress fractures about the shoulder. Tears of the rotator cuff are effectively visualized with either single or double contrast shoulder arthrography, magnetic resonance (MR) imaging, and, in some hands, shoulder sonography.[2–4] Tears of the glenoid labra from previous dislocation are nicely shown with either arthrography of the shoulder combined with CT[5] or with magnetic resonance imaging. The accuracy of these modalities in the assessment of the rotator cuff is indicated in Table 5-1 and of the glenoid labrum in Table 5-2.

TABLE 5-1

Reported comparative accuracy of diagnosis for rotator cuff lesions

	Arthrography, %			CT arthrography, %			Sonography, %			MR, %		
	Sensitivity	Specificity	Accuracy	Sensitivity	Specificity	Accuracy	Sensitivity	Specificity	Accuracy	Sensitivity	Specificity	Accuracy
Complete tear	92[48] 71[41]	100[48] 71[41]	94[48] 98–99[46] 75[3]	50[5]	100[5]	96[5]	63[48] 91[4]	91[4]	60[48] 97[3]	100[40] 97[39] 92[48] 91[41] 80[51]	95[40] 94[39] 100[48] 88[41] 94[51]	91[50] 95[39] 94[48] 100[41] 89[51]
Partial tear			71[3]	NR[a]	NR	NR	NR	NR	NR	89[39] 69[51]	84[39] 94[51]	84[39] 84[51] 91[41]
Tendinitis			NR	NR	NR	NR	NR	NR	NR	93[40]	87[40]	

[a] NR = not reported.

TABLE 5-2

Reported accuracy of diagnosis for glenoid and bicipital tendon abnormalities

	CT Arthrography, %			Sonography, %			MR, %		
	Sensitivity	Specificity	Accuracy	Sensitivity	Specificity	Accuracy	Sensitivity	Specificity	Accuracy
Glenoid tear (all tears)	86[67] 95[56] 100[60]	93[40] 97[69]	88[40] 100[69]	NR[a]	NR	NR	88[40]	93[40]	92–95[59]
Anterior labrum	83[5]	86[59]	92[59]						
Posterior labrum	100[5]	97[59]	77[59]						
Fracture	69[13] 93[5]								
Capsule tear	100[60]			NR	NR	NR			NR
Biceps tendon abnormality	96[5]			Claimed superior to arthrogram[4]					NR
Loose bodies	100[5]			NR	NR	NR			NR

[a] NR = not reported.

In the broad spectrum of overuse and inflammatory entities of the shoulder, TPBS demonstrates generalized but nonspecific uptake. There is a wide variety of acute, subacute, and chronic entities where TPBS is helpful in narrowing the differential diagnosis and/in localizing both the area and etiology of symptoms.[6-10] These include occult fracture, posttraumatic arthritis, synovitis, heterotopic bone formation, postsurgical ossification, infection, stress fracture, and periostitis.[9,11] Although MR has been most useful in diagnosing lesions of the rotator cuff and labrum, it has also been helpful in assessing bicipital tendon pathology, intraarticular loose bodies, and synovial disease.[12]

NORMAL ANATOMY OF THE SHOULDER

The mobility of the shoulder depends on the large humeral head articulating within a shallow glenoid fossa. A redundant glenohumeral capsule allows a wide range of motion. Stability is achieved by both the osseous and soft tissue structures. The soft tissues which enhance stability include the scapular muscles, rotator cuff, fibrous capsule, glenohumeral ligaments, and glenoid labrum. The rotator cuff is derived from the tendons of the supraspinatous, infraspinatous, teres minor, and subscapularis muscles. The supra- and infraspinatous muscles are inserted onto the superior aspect of the greater tuberosity of the humerus. The teres minor inserts posteriorly onto the greater tuberosity, and the subscapularis inserts onto the lesser tuberosity.

Three anterior glenohumeral ligaments—the superior, middle, and inferior—which strengthen the capsule anteriorly, are present.[13] Openings exist between the superior and middle glenohumeral ligaments and between the middle and inferior glenohumeral ligaments in most people.[14] The superior glenohumeral ligament thickens and becomes intracapsular, inserting near the attachment of the biceps tendon.[13] With flexion of the humerus, the biceps tendon glides within the bicipital tendon groove. In approximately 12 percent of people, flattening of the bicipital groove is present, which predisposes the tendon to medial dislocation (Fig. 5-1). Lateral dislocation of the biceps tendon does not occur.

The shallow bony glenoid is deepened into a glenoid fossa by the circumferential fibrous labrum. The labrum is larger anteriorly than posteriorly and is pliable with its shape depending on the position of the humeral head.[15] With internal rotation of the humerus, the anterior joint space becomes more capacious and the anterior labrum assumes a triangular shape. The posterior capsule inserts into the posterior labrum, which is normally slightly rounded.[16] With CT arthrography the anterior labrum and capsule are best seen with the humerus in either internal rotation or in the neutral position.[5,13] By adding additional imaging with the shoulder in external rotation, sensitivity is increased an additional 10 percent.[17]

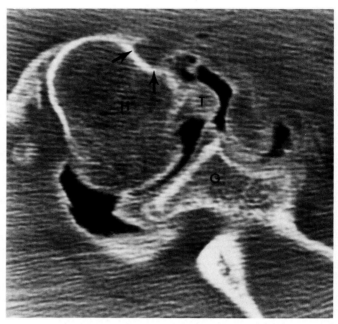

Figure 5-1   Dislocated Biceps Tendon. *Axial CT scan following double-contrast shoulder arthrogram shows medial dislocation of the biceps tendon. Flattening of the bicipital tendon groove is a predisposing condition. T = medially dislocated biceps tendon; arrows = flat bicipital groove; H = humerus; G = bony glenoid.*

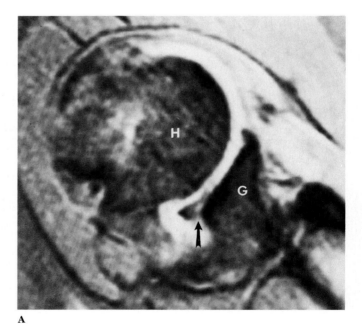

A

Figure 5-2   Glenoid Fracture. **A.** *Axial scan at short TR gradient echo (FISP, 20°) sequence shows fracture of the posterior glenoid rim following posterior shoulder dislocation.* (Fig. 5-2B continues on the opposite page.)

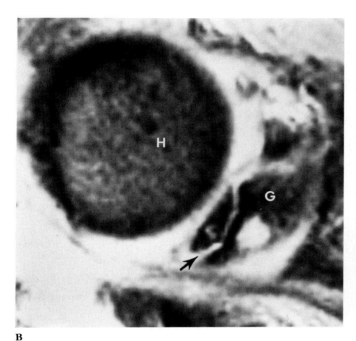

B

Figure 5-2 Glenoid Fracture (Continued). **B.** *Axial scan at short TR gradient echo (FISP, 20°) sequence shows fracture of the superior margin of the bony glenoid from anterior dislocation. Arrow = fracture line; H = humerus; G = bony glenoid.*

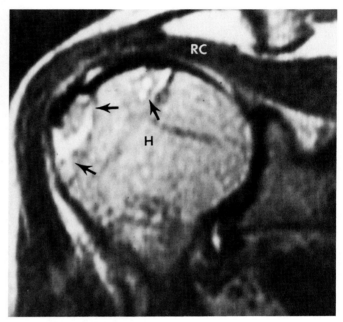

Figure 5-3 Greater Tuberosity Fracture. *MR scan in the coronal oblique plane at T1-weighted sequence shows a focus of high signal between greater tuberosity fragments and the humeral head representing acute fracture. The rotator cuff appears intact. Arrows = fractures; RC = rotator cuff; H = humerus.*

ACUTE PROBLEMS

Fractures of the scapula, clavicle, and humerus (Figs. 5-2 to 5-6)

Fractures involving the scapula, clavicle, and humerus are often effectively seen on plain radiographs, which in most cases provide an adequate imaging examination for diagnosis. The axillary view may be necessary to visualize fracture of the anterior or posterior rim of the bony glenoid, and the bicipital groove view may be needed to demonstrate subtle fractures of the greater and lesser tuberosities of the humerus. These fractures may be clearly seen on either CT or MR. In problem cases, CT is indicated for a more detailed evaluation (Figs. 5-2 to 5-5). Occasionally, occult fracture may not be detected adequately with plain radiographs, and in that situation TPBS is useful. TPBS is helpful in identifying the metabolic activity (and age) of avulsion injuries in or around the shoulder.[18] Fracture of the coracoid may be difficult to visualize on plain radiographs, and TPBS may suggest its presence (Fig. 5-6). Coracoid fracture may occur as an isolated entity or may be associated with acromioclavicular joint injury.[19–27]

Figure 5-4   Humerus Fracture. *MR* ▶
scan in the coronal plane at T1-weighted
sequence shows a linear band of low-
signal crossing the humeral neck in this
elderly recreational athlete. Normal
signal within the marrow space excludes
pathologic fracture. H = humeral head;
arrows = acute fracture.

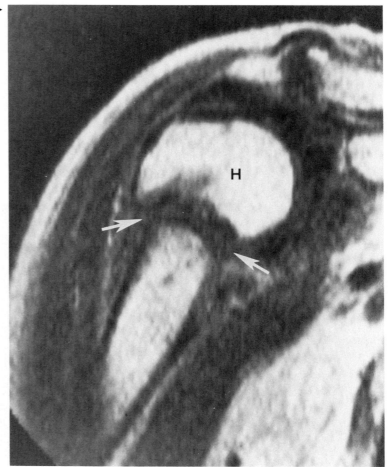

Figure 5-5   Distal Clavicular
Nonunion. *This athlete complained of a*
chronic snapping sensation in his
shoulder following previous injury. CT
scan through the distal clavicle
demonstrates nonunion of a distal shaft
fracture. C = clavicle proximal to
nonunion; arrows = nonunion site;
D = clavicular fragment distal to
nonunion site.
▼

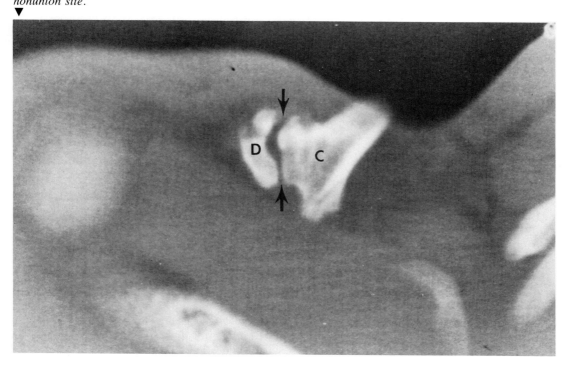

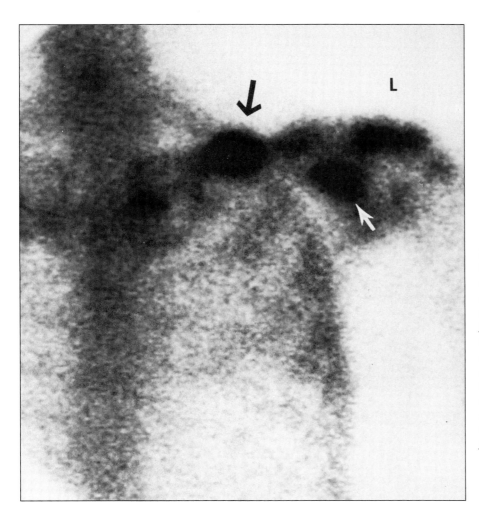

Figure 5-6 Occult Fracture of the Left Coracoid Process. *Female athlete with a known fracture of left midclavicle as well as A/C separation. Focal pain in the region of coracoid persisted for 1-month following injury despite normal radiographs. TPBS shows an intense area of increased nuclide activity in the left midclavicle consistent with fracture (black arrow). Increased activity is seen across the left A/C joint. Focally increased nuclide activity is present in the coracoid representing an occult fracture (white arrow).*

Sternoclavicular and acromioclavicular joints (Figs. 5-7 to 5-16)

Injuries about the sternoclavicular joint may lead to either fracture or dislocation of the proximal portion of the clavicle. The normal articular anatomy of this joint is shown in Fig. 5-7. Anatomically, less than one-half of the articular surface of the proximal portion of clavicle articulates with the sternum. Stability depends largely on the rhomboid ligament, intraarticular fibrocartilagenous disk, interclavicular ligament, and sternoclavicular joint capsule.[28] Dislocations involving the sternoclavicular joint account for only 2.5 percent of all shoulder dislocations.[13,28] Although most sternoclavicular dislocations are secondary to motor vehicle accidents, athletic injuries are the second leading cause. Dislocations may be either anterosuperior or posterior. The anterosuperior dislocations are more frequent.[28] Since the proximal clavicular physis does not fuse until approximately 21 years of age, an apparent dislocation before that age may instead represent a growth plate fracture (Salter fracture) of the proximal clavicle. Posterior dislocation or fracture-dislocation of the proximal portion of the clavicle at the sternoclavicular joint may compress the retrosternal great vessels and trachea (Fig. 5-8). Clinical suspicion of posterior dislocation of the sternoclavicular joint is best confirmed by obtaining 5-mm-thick CT scans in the axial plane through that joint.[29] Anterosuperior dislocation may require coronal reconstructions derived from 1- to 2-mm-thick contiguous axial scans through the sternoclavicular joint to demonstrate the presence and direction of dislocation (Fig. 5-9). Magnetic resonance imaging of a suspected clavicular dislocation at the sternoclavicular joint may provide the diagnosis of a growth plate fracture of the proximal clavicle by demonstrating disruption of the proximal clavicular physis. In that situation, surgical treatment is indicated if symptomatic retrosternal compression of vital structures develops. If great vessel or airway compression is not present, with conservative management one should expect healing and remodeling to occur with maintenance of sternoclavicular stability.

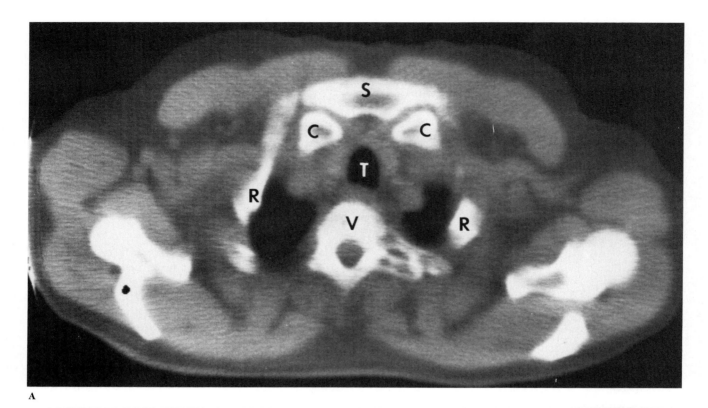

A

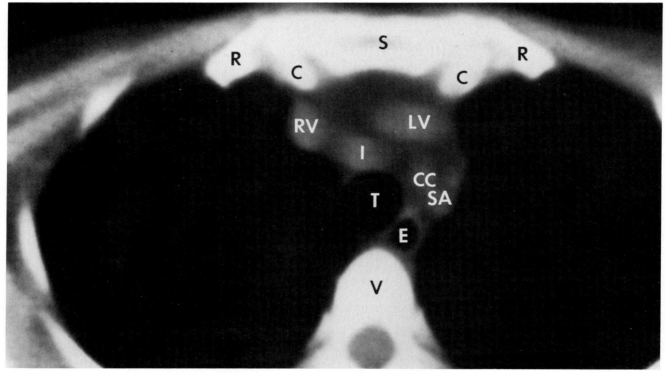

B

Figure 5-7 Normal Sternoclavicular Joint. **A.** *Axial CT scan through the sternoclavicular joint demonstrates the normal articulation of the proximal portion of clavicle with the posterolateral aspect of the sternum. The normal ar-* *ticulation of the first rib with the sternum is seen.* **B.** *Axial CT scan caudal to that shown in* **A** *shows the articulation of the first rib with the sternum. The retrosternal great vessels, trachea, and esophagus are noted. S = sternum;* *C = clavicle; R = first rib; T = trachea; E = esophagus; V = vertebral body; SA = left subclavian artery; CC = left common carotid artery; LV = left subclavian vein; I = innominate artery; RV = right subclavian vein.*

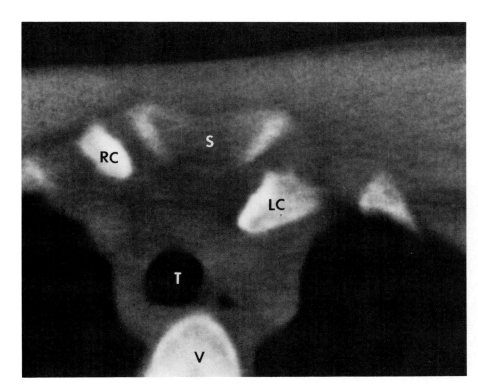

Figure 5-8 Posterior Dislocation of the Clavicle at the Sternoclavicular Joint. *Axial CT scan at the level of the sternoclavicular joints shows the proximal portion of the left clavicle to be displaced posteriorly causing clavicular impingement on the upper mediastinum. The right sternoclavicular joint is normal. S = sternum; LC = displaced left clavicle; RC = right clavicle; V = vertebral body; T = trachea.*

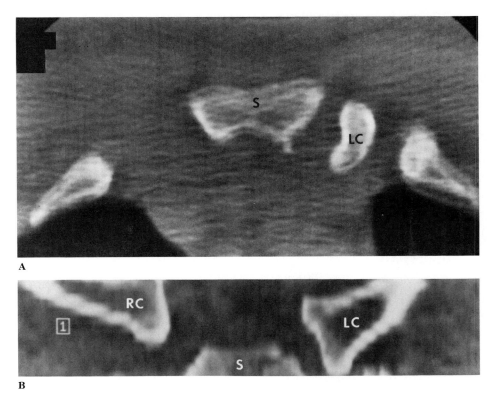

A

B

Figure 5-9 Superior Dislocation of the Clavicle at the Sternoclavicular Joint. **A.** *Axial CT scan shows a normal left sternoclavicular joint. The right clavicle* *has been displaced superiorly and is not imaged at this level.* **B.** *Image reformatted in the coronal plane shows upward displacement of the right* *clavicle. S = sternum; RC = right clavicle; LC = left clavicle.*

Injuries to the acromioclavicular and sternoclavicular joints may cause persistent pain despite normal radiographs. CT may be helpful in directing attention to the traumatized joint, which may be the site of fracture (Fig. 5-10), dislocation,[30] or arthritis (Fig. 5-11). Fracture with displacement of the costochondral junction of either the first or second rib can mimic sternoclavicular dislocation (Fig. 5-12). CT or MR may be necessary to diagnose this entity accurately. Normal anatomic landmarks (Fig. 5-13) as well as the post-traumatic changes of arthritis and synovitis can be suggested by TPBS[1,9,31] (Figs. 5-14 and 5-15). Occasionally, occult rib or sternal fracture, not visible on routine radiographs, may be suspected based on focally increased nuclide activity following a TPBS (Fig. 5-16).

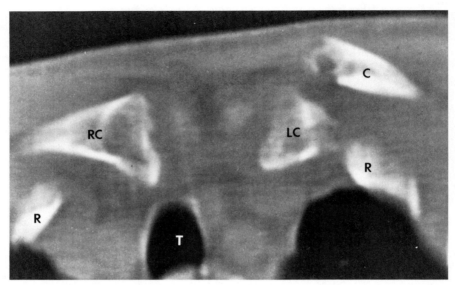

Figure 5-10 Left Clavicular Fracture. *Axial CT scan through the upper portion of the sternoclavicular joints shows normally articulating proximal clavicles. A fracture of the left clavicle has occurred with anterior displacement of its shaft. RC = right clavicle; LC = normal left sternoclavicular articulation; C = anteriorly displaced left clavicular shaft; T = trachea; R = first rib.*

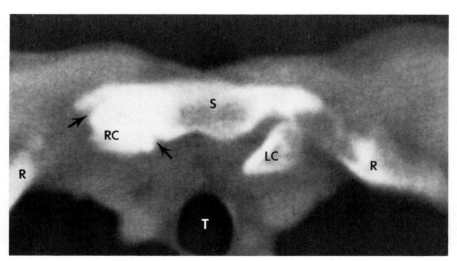

Figure 5-11 Degenerative Arthritis of the Sternoclavicular Joint. *Axial CT scan at the level of the sternoclavicular joints shows joint space loss with periarticular bony sclerosis (arrows). These features are typical for degenerative arthritis. The left sternoclavicular joint is normal. S = sternum; LC = left clavicle; RC = right clavicle; R = first rib; T = trachea.*

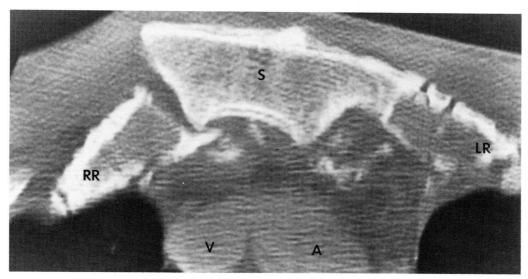

Figure 5-12 Fracture with Displacement of the Costochondral Junction. *Axial CT scan through the junction of the first rib with the sternum shows posterior displacement of the right costochondral junction. S = sternum; LR = left first rib; RR = right first rib; A = aortic arch; V = superior vena cava.*

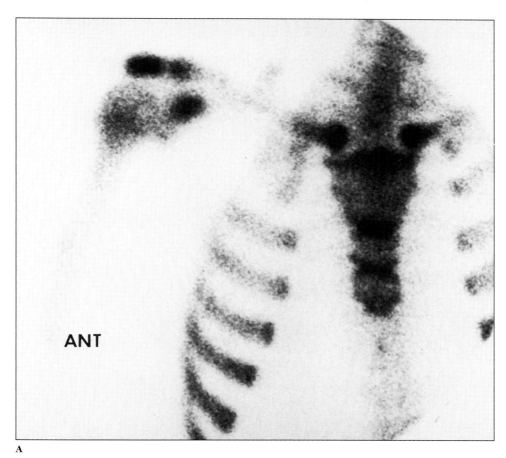

Figure 5-13 High-Resolution Delayed Images from TPBS of the Normal Shoulder and Thorax. **A.** *Anterior view defines the acromioclavicular (A/C) and sternoclavicular (S/C) joints. In addition, the humeral head, glenoid, coracoid process, and sternum are well seen.* (Fig. 5-13B and C continues on next page.)

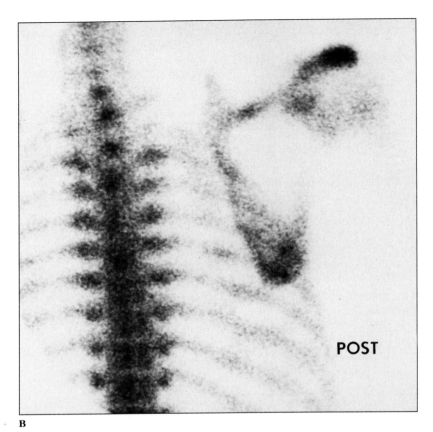

B

Figure 5-13   High-Resolution Delayed Images from TPBS of the Normal Shoulder and Thorax (Continued). **B.** *Posterior view shows the entire scapula, posterior ribs, and uncovertebral junctions.* **C.** *Posterior oblique views demonstrate ribs, scapula, and glenohumeral joint.*

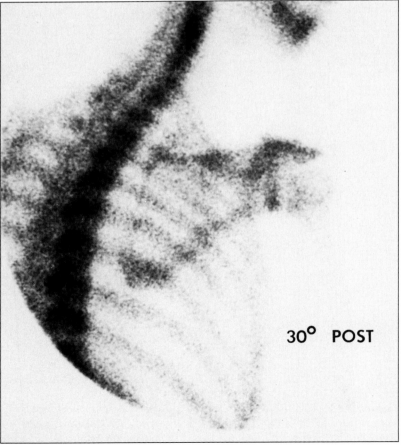

C

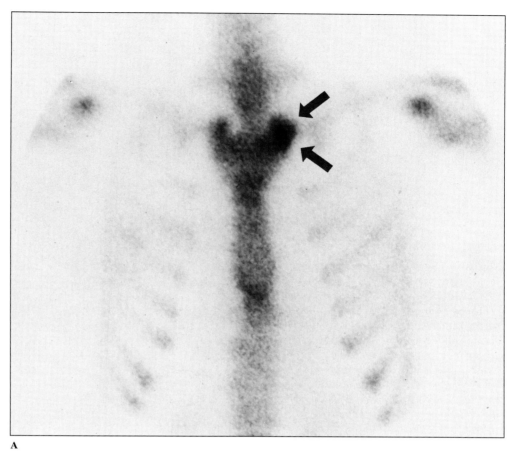

A

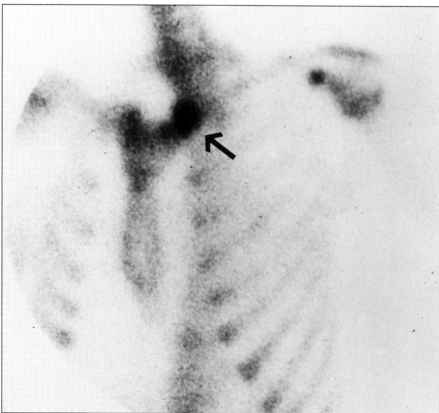

B

Figure 5-14 Posttraumatic Sternoclavicular Joint Arthritis/ Synovitis. *Male rugby player with persistent pain and normal radiographs.* **A.** *High-resolution anterior delayed images from a TPBS show focally increased activity in the left sternoclavicular joints (arrows).* **B.** *Oblique view delineates increased activity in the left sternoclavicular joint consistent with the clinical diagnosis of posttraumatic arthritis/synovitis.*

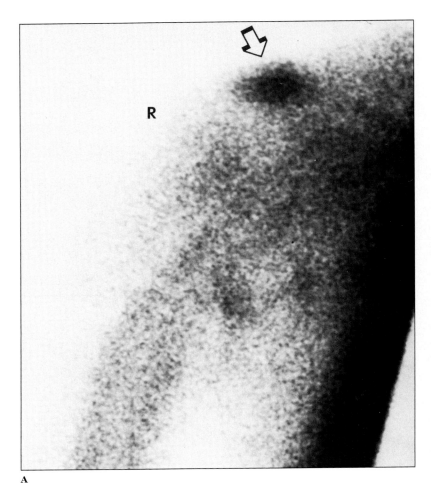

Figure 5-15 Posttraumatic Acromioclavicular Joint Arthritis/Synovitis. *Male racquetball player with a history of right A/C joint injury has persistent pain and normal radiographs.* **A.** *Anterior blood pool images from a TPBS of the right shoulder show early increased nuclide uptake in the right acromioclavicular joint area (open arrow) consistent with hyperemia and/or inflammation.* **B.** *High-resolution magnified anterior image of the right shoulder shows markedly increased activity in the right acromioclavicular joint (black arrows).* H = humerus; C = coracoid. (Fig. 5-15C continues on the opposite page.)

A

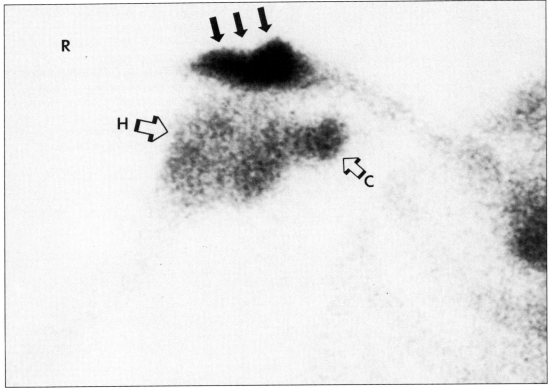

B

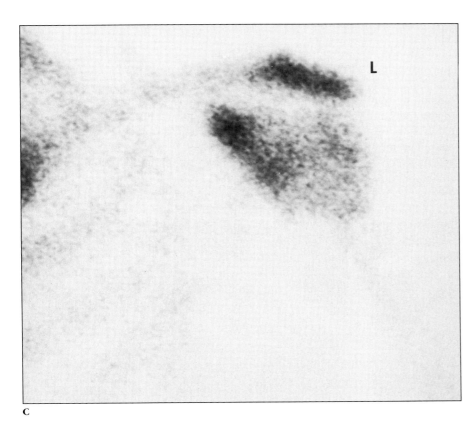

Figure 5-15   Posttraumatic Acromioclavicular Joint Arthritis/Synovitis (Continued). **C.** *Normal left shoulder.*

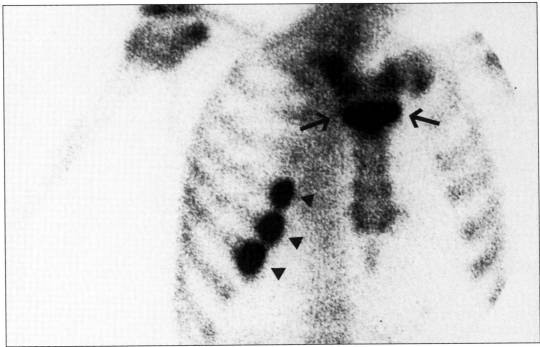

Figure 5-16   Fractured Sternum and Ribs. *Male rugby player with posttraumatic thoracic pain and normal radiographs. TPBS shows abnormal areas of increased nuclide activity which were not appreciated on the radiographic examination. Fractures of the anterior aspects of the right 4th, 5th, and 6th ribs (arrowheads) and of the sternum (arrows) are present.*

Impingement syndrome and rotator cuff pathology (Figs. 5-17 to 5-27)

Tendons of the supraspinatous, infraspinatous, subscapularis, and teres minor muscles coalesce to form the rotator cuff, which inserts onto the greater tuberosity of the humerus. The tendinous tissue that makes up the distal 1 to 2 cm of the rotator cuff is relatively hypovascular.[32] It is in this critical area that rotator cuff tears usually occur. The musculotendinous junction is located superiorly and medially to the humeral head. Parallel and superior to the supraspinatous tendon is a fat plane which borders the subacromial-subdeltoid bursa (Fig. 5-17). There is general agreement that degeneration and tear within the rotator cuff is preceded by chronic impingement into the rotator cuff by hypertrophic capsule and bony spurs extending down from the acromioclavicular joint.[15,33,34] This impinging tissue obliterates the

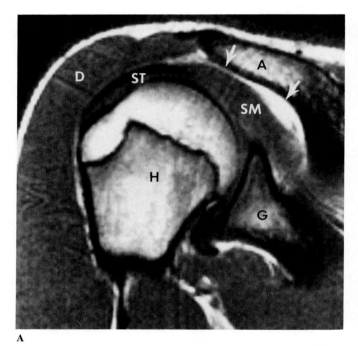

A

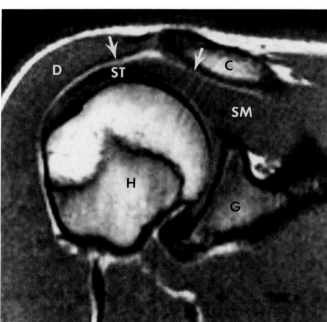

B

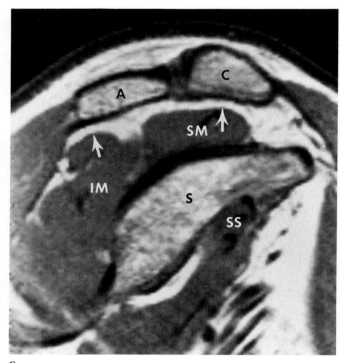

C

Figure 5-17 Normal Rotator Cuff. **A.** *Coronal oblique image (parallel to the axis of scapula) at T1-weighted sequence shows continuity of the supraspinatus muscle and tendon. A normal fat plane is present beneath the clavicle and deltoid muscle. Uniformly low signal is present within the normal rotator cuff.* **B.** *Coronal oblique image at T1-weighted sequence at a slightly more anterior level to the above shows direct continuity of the supraspinatus muscle and tendon without any increase in intratendinous signal. Normal subclavicular and subacromial fat planes are present.* **C.** *Sagittal oblique image (perpendicular to the axis of the scapula) at T1-weighted sequence shows the normal relationship of the supraspinatus muscle to the acromioclavicular joint. (Fig. 5-17D continues on the opposite page.)*

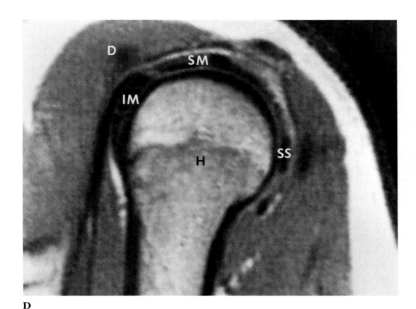

D

Figure 5-17 Normal Rotator Cuff (Continued).
D. *Sagittal oblique image at T1-weighted sequence peripherally shows the normal rotator cuff beneath the deltoid muscle. SM = supraspinatus muscle; ST = supraspinatus tendon; IM = infraspinatus muscle; SS = subscapularis muscle; D = deltoid muscle; C = clavicle; A = acromion; S = scapula; H = humerus; G = glenoid; arrows = normal subacromial fat.*

Figure 5-18 Rotator Cuff Impingement. *Coronal oblique image at T1-weighted sequence shows a hypertrophic acromioclavicular capsule impinging upon the upper aspect of the supraspinatus tendon. Focal areas of increased signal within that tendon indicate tendinitis. Obliteration of the subacromial fat has occurred. C = clavicle; A = acromion; H = humerus; S = supraspinatus muscle; open arrows = region of supraspinatus tendinitis; HC = hypertrophic AC capsule.)*

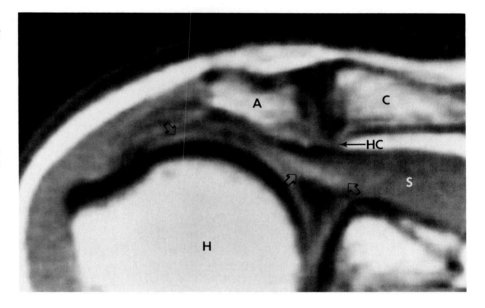

subacromial fat plane leading to tendinitis of the supraspinatous tendon.[35,36] The coronal-oblique plane (parallel to the axis of the scapula and supraspinatous tendon) is optimal for assessing the rotator cuff and subacromial space on the magnetic resonance scan.[32,37] The earliest changes of impingement involve the development either of osteophytes or of capular hypertrophy at the acromioclavicular joint (Figs. 5-18 and 5-19). This hypertrophic tissue impinges on the fat planes surrounding the subacromial-subdeltoid bursa, obliterating or displacing that plane from beneath the acromioclavicular joint and acromion process.[38,39] Early changes of tendinitis within the supraspinatous tendon cause focal areas of increased signal to develop within the substance of the supraspinatous tendon.[35,40,41] Histologically, edema and hemorrhage within the rotator cuff is found. Later, fibrosis within this region develops. Most patients with edema, hemorrhage, and fibrosis will respond to conservative management.[40,42] With the progressive development of rotator cuff tear, however, discontinuity of the supraspinatous tendon occurs. Fluid within the glenohumeral joint enters the tear and fills the subacromial-subdeltoid bursa (Figs. 5-20 and 5-21). Occasionally, fluid may additionally fill the acromioclavicular joint (Fig. 5-22). The presence of rotator cuff discontinuity with fluid present within the rotator cuff and subacromial bursa is diagnostic for rotator cuff tear.[35,37,40] Later, tendinous retraction and muscle atrophy supervene.[40]

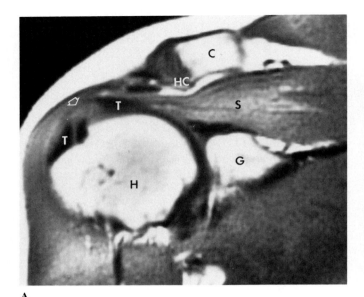

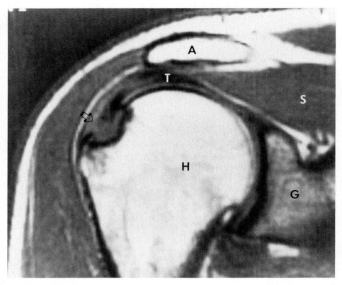

Figure 5-20 Rotator Cuff Tear. *Coronal oblique image at T1-weighted sequence shows increased signal within a disrupted supraspinatus tendon representing a rotator cuff tear. S = supraspinatus muscle; T = supraspinatus tendon; H = humerus; A = acromion process; G = glenoid; open arrow = rotator cuff tear.*

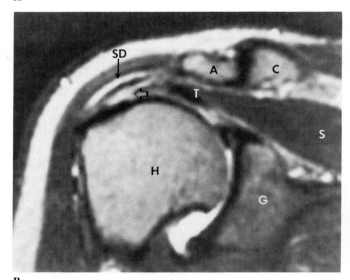

Figure 5-19 Rotator Cuff Tear. **A.** *Coronal oblique image at T1-weighted sequence shows impingement of the supraspinatus muscle by hypertrophic changes involving the acromioclavicular (AC) joint. A region of increased signal occupies the supraspinatus tendon just proximal to its insertion into the greater tuberosity.* **B.** *Coronal oblique image at T2-weighted sequence shows high signal within the joint space, supraspinatus tendon and subdeltoid bursa representing joint effusion and fluid filling a tendinous gap. These are diagnostic findings for rotator cuff tear. S = supraspinatus muscle; HC = hypertrophied AC joint capsule; T = supraspinatus tendon; H = humerus; G = glenoid; C = clavicle; A = acromion; SD = fluid in subdeltoid bursa, open arrow = rotator cuff tear.*

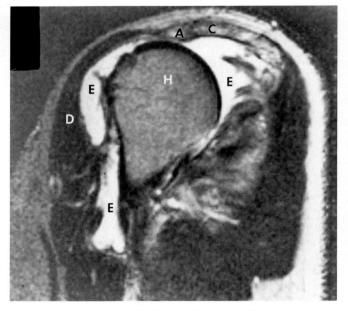

Figure 5-21 Rotator Cuff Tear. *Sagittal oblique image at T2-weighted sequence shows excess fluid to be present. This is nearly always seen when rotator cuff tear is present. E = effusion; D = deltoid; H = humeral head; C = clavicle; A = acromion process.*

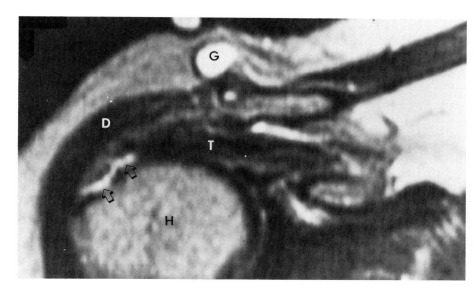

Figure 5-22 Rotator Cuff Tear with AC Joint Ganglion. *Coronal oblique image at T2-weighted sequence shows high signal at the site of attachment of the rotator cuff to the greater tuberosity indicating a rotator cuff tear. A globular focus of high signal present directly above the AC joint represents a ganglion. Open arrows = rotator cuff tear; G = ganglion; S = supraspinatous tendon; D = deltoid muscle; H = humeral head.*

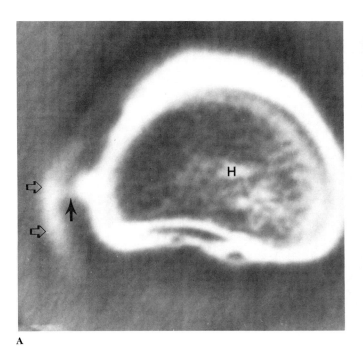

A

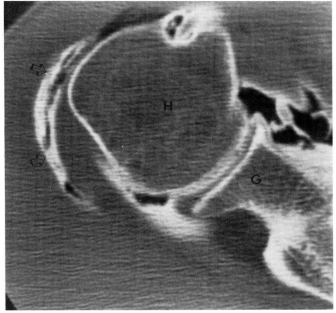

B

Figure 5-23 Rotator Cuff Tear.
A. *Axial CT scan at the level of the apex of the humeral head following a double contrast arthrogram demonstrates the* *site of rotator cuff tear (arrow).*
B. *Axial CT scan at the midglenoid level shows contrast in the subdeltoid bursa. Arrow = rotator cuff tear; open* *arrows = contrast with the subdeltoid bursa; H = humeral head; G = bony glenoid.*

Rotator cuff tear can accurately be diagnosed with shoulder arthrography (Fig. 5-23). Some debate exists as to the relative value of double-contrast shoulder arthrography compared with single-contrast examination in confirming this diagnosis.[43–45] Both examinations, however, have been shown to be highly accurate in the detection of complete rotator cuff tear.[41,46–50] Magnetic resonance is more accurate than shoulder arthrography in visualizing partial tears of the rotator cuff.[38,39,41,51] This is particularly true for those tears which originate from the superior aspect of the rotator cuff, which without MR would require subacromial bursography to identify.[43]

Since the shoulder is eccentrically located anatomically and its important structures are small, the availability of "off-centered" detailed imaging is necessary to adequately demonstrate the rotator cuff and the fibrous glenoid labrum.[37]

The advent of MR arthrography holds a promise of enhancing the sensitivity and accuracy of diagnosis of rotator cuff abnormality.[52,53] This requires the injection of a dilute solution of paramagnetic fluid into the glenohumeral joint.

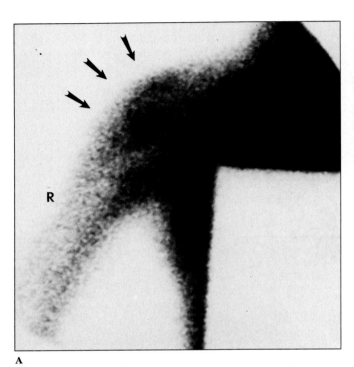

A

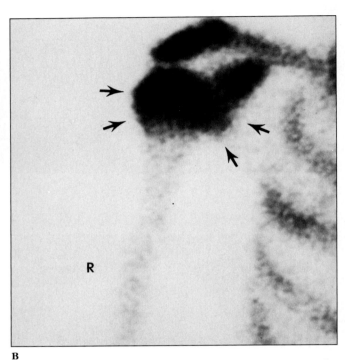

B

Figure 5-24 Adhesive Capsulitis. *Female tennis player with persistent right shoulder pain and normal radiographs.* **A.** *Anterior blood pool image of right shoulder from TPBS demonstrates mildly increased nuclide activity over the right humeral head and shoulder joint (arrows).* **B.** *High-resolution anterior delayed image demonstrates increased nuclide activity (arrows) in the right humeral head, shoulder joint, A/C joint, and acromion process.* **C.** *Shoulder arthrogram demonstrates reduced joint capacity with scalloping of the lateral capsular margin (arrows). There is a smaller than normal axillary recess with spillage of contrast from the recess. These features indicate adhesive capsulitis.*

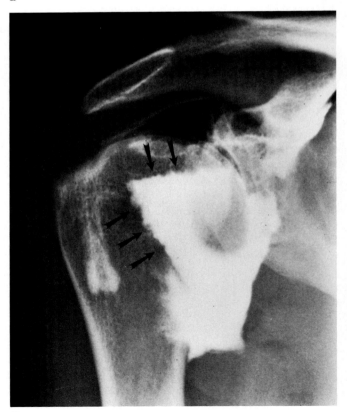

C

Injected fluid coats the rotator cuff, filling otherwise imperceptible cuff tears. Routine MR depends on the presence of native joint fluid to demonstrate rotator cuff pathology and seems less accurate and sensitive than is either routine arthrography or MR arthrography.

In patients with impingement or with chronic or recurrent pain without a history of acute injury, TPBS is not especially helpful. Such entities as frozen shoulder (Fig. 5-24), tendinitis, capsulitis (Figs. 5-25 and 5-26), capsule tear (Fig. 5-27), rotator cuff tear, and insertional injuries all produce bone scans that appear similar and have nonspecifically increased nuclide uptake overlying the humeral head and shoulder joint. These scans are helpful in ruling out other coexisting pathology but are not helpful in narrowing the differential diagnosis from the broad spectrum listed above.

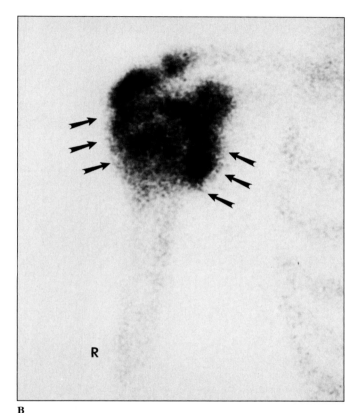

B

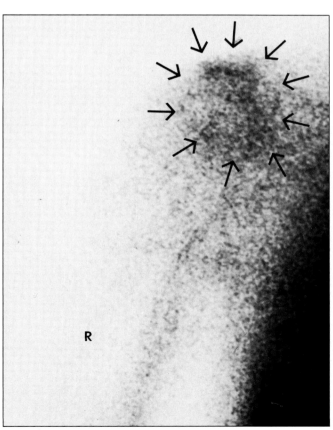

A

Figure 5-25 "Frozen Shoulder"/Rotator Cuff Tear. *Male athlete with right shoulder pain, decreased motion and normal radiographs.* **A.** *Anterior blood pool image of right shoulder from TPBS shows increased nuclide uptake around the shoulder joint especially superiorly and medially (arrows).* **B.** *High-resolution delayed anterior image of right shoulder demonstrates increased uptake (arrows) over the right humeral head, shoulder joint, A/C joint, and coracoid process.* (Fig. 5-25C continues on next page.)

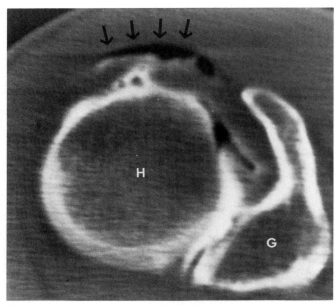

C

Figure 5-25 ''Frozen Shoulder''/
Rotator Cuff Tear (Continued). **C.** *CT
scan following shoulder arthrogram
shows extravasation of air and contrast
anteriorly (arrows) diagnostic of rotator
cuff tear. H = humerus; G = glenoid.*

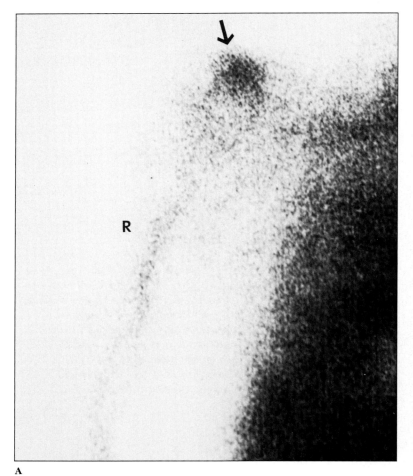

A

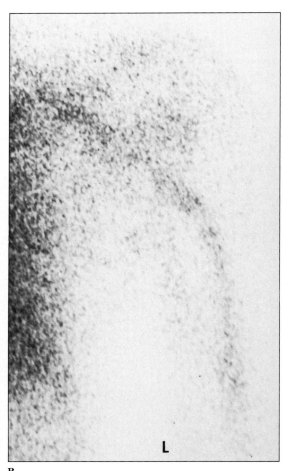

B

Figure 5-26 ''Frozen Shoulder''/
Capsulitis. *Male athlete with persistent
right shoulder pain and normal
radiographs.* **A.** *Anterior blood pool*
*image of the right shoulder from TPBS.
Increased nuclide activity (arrows) is
present in the superomedial aspect of
right should joint.* **B.** *Comparison blood*
*pool of the opposite left shoulder is
normal.* (Fig. 5-26C and D continues on
the opposite page.)

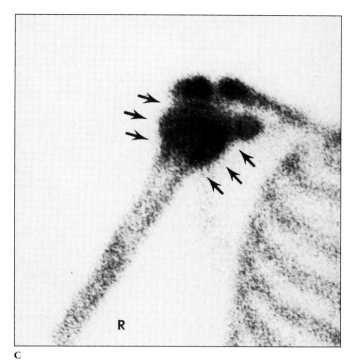

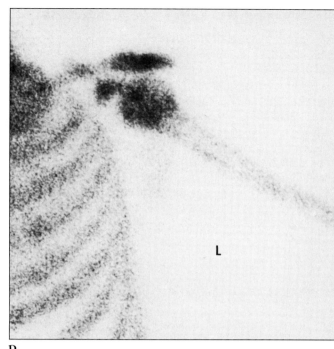

C

D

Figure 5-26 ''Frozen Shoulder''/ Capsulitis (Continued). **C.** *High-resolution delayed anterior image of right shoulder shows increased nuclide* *activity involving the entire right humeral head and right shoulder joint (arrows). Increased activity is also seen in the right A/C joint and coracoid* *process.* **D.** *Comparison delayed view of left shoulder shows normal activity.*

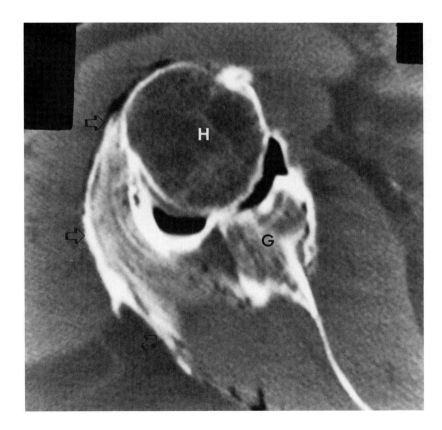

Figure 5-27 Capsule Tear. *Axial CT scan at the midglenoid level following double-contrast arthrogram shows contrast extravasating posteriorly through a defect in the joint capsule. This appearance may mimic rotator cuff tear. H = humeral head; G = glenoid; open arrows = contrast leakage through posterior capsule tear.*

Glenohumeral instability (Figs. 5-28 to 5-38)

The anatomy of the shoulder provides for maximal articular motion at the risk of potential instability predisposing the shoulder joint to subluxation and dislocations. Approximately 95 percent of shoulder dislocations are in the anterior direction. The anterior inclination of the bony glenoid favors posterior stability.[54] Remaining dislocations are posterior (2 to 4 percent), inferior (1 percent), and superior (1 percent). The primary lesion associated with anterior dislocation seems to be stretching of the inferior glenohumeral ligament, which normally reinforces the anterior aspect of the capsule.[55] Anterior instability is often associated with tear of the anterior-inferior aspect of the glenoid labrum or detachment of the labrum from the joint capsule[56] (Figs. 5-28 and 5-29). Pos-

terior instability is associated with a combined tear of the posterior labrum and capsule[56] (Fig. 5-30). In patients with recurrent anterior dislocation, 70 to 96 percent show tear of the labrum and 78 to 85 percent demonstrate capsular redundancy.[57] Three types of capsule insertions are recognized. Type I and type II insertions allow for close approximation of the articular capsule to the anterior labrum. Type III insertion exists when the joint capsule inserts directly onto the body of the scapula, which provides a region of redundancy to develop between the labrum and capsule. The likelihood of anterior instability is markedly increased if type III insertion is present.[58]

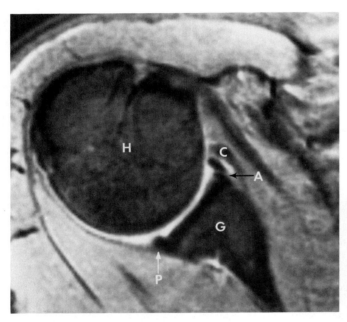

Figure 5-28   Anterior Glenoid Labrum Tear. *MR scan at T2-weighted sequence through the midglenoid shows deformity of the anterior labrum with tear of the capsular insertion. A = torn anterior labrum; C = abnormal anterior capsule; P = normal posterior labrum; G = bony glenoid; H = humeral head.*

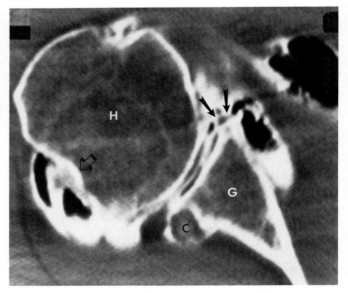

Figure 5-29   Anterior Glenoid Labrum Tear, Posterior Bony Cyst. *Axial CT scan through the level of the midglenoid following double-contrast arthrogram shows extensive tear of the anterior labrum. Lucency of the posterior bony glenoid represents a degenerative cyst. A Hill-Sachs deformity is present. Arrows = anterior labral tear; C = posterior cyst; open arrow = Hill-Sachs defect; H = humeral head; G = glenoid.*

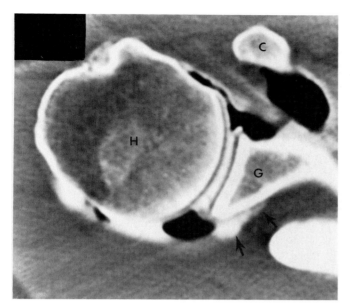

Figure 5-30   Posterior Glenoid Labrum Tear. *Axial CT scan following double-contrast arthrogram shows blunting of the posterior glenoid labrum with leakage of contrast along the posterior surface of the glenoid. These changes follow posterior glenohumeral dislocation. Arrows = abnormal posterior leakage of contrast; G = bony glenoid; H = humerus; C = coracoid process.*

Figure 5-31   Normal Glenoid Labrum. *A–F are from a thin-section axial CT examination which followed a double contrast shoulder arthrogram. The scans progress from superior to inferior and show the normal glenohumeral joint. The posterior glenoid labrum is a smooth triangular structure firmly adherent to the posterior rim of the bony glenoid. The anterior glenoid labrum may be slightly blunted, as in this case. The joint capsule is smooth and intact. Superior middle and inferior glenohumeral ligaments are present anteriorly. The bicipital tendon lies within the bicipital groove. H = humeral head; G = bony glenoid; C = coracoid process; P = posterior glenoid labrum; A = anterior glenoid labrum; GL = glenohumeral ligaments; B = bicipital tendon; S = bicipital tendon sheath. (Fig. 5-31C–F continues on next page.)*

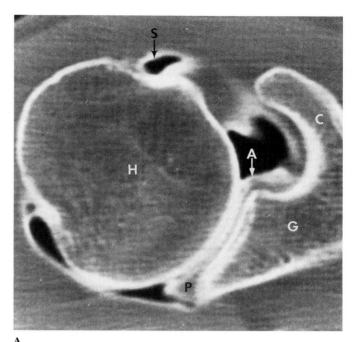

A

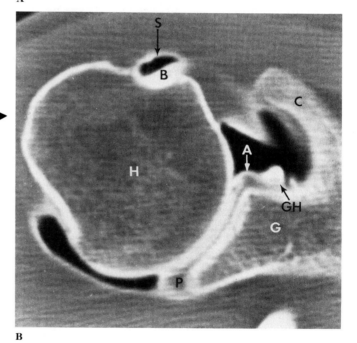

B

Although magnetic resonance provides good visualization of the glenoid labrum,[59] the combined CT arthrogram is an extremely accurate and sensitive tool for visualization of the labrum and the adjacent capsule and is the preferred examination for assessing instability.[57,60,61] The normal anatomic appearance of the glenoid labrum demonstrated with CT arthrography (Fig. 5-31) and with MR (Fig. 5-32) are shown. In addition to the capsular and labral features described, avulsion fractures of the glenoid and compression fractures of the humeral head caused from previous dislocation can be identified with CT arthrogram[62,63] (Figs. 5-33 to 5-37). Although this examination requires the intraarticular injection of a small amount of contrast, air, and epinephrine prior to thin-section CT scanning, rendering this a minimally invasive procedure, the morbidity is extremely low.[2,64,65] CT arthrography is equally accurate when compared to arthrotomography but is easier to perform and requires less radiation.[63,66–68]

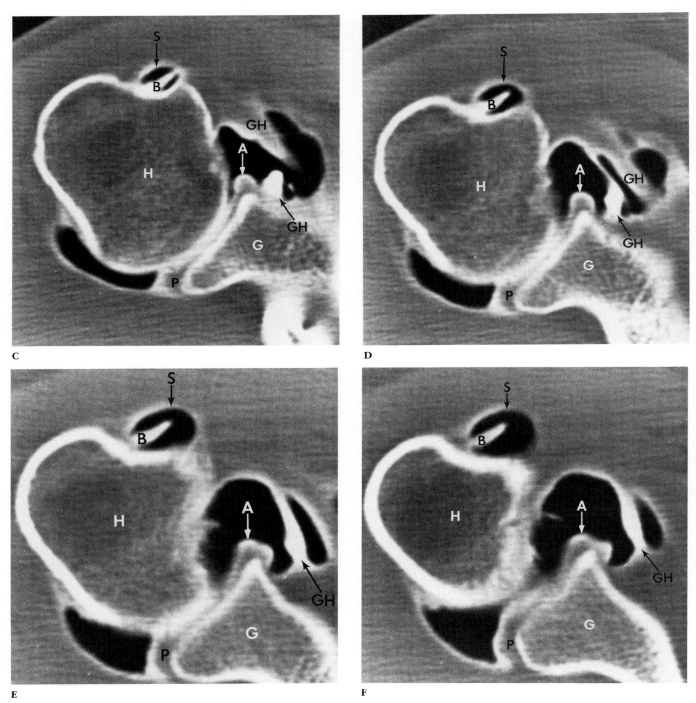

Figure 5-31   Normal Glenoid Labrum. **A–F** (Continued). *See previous page for description.*

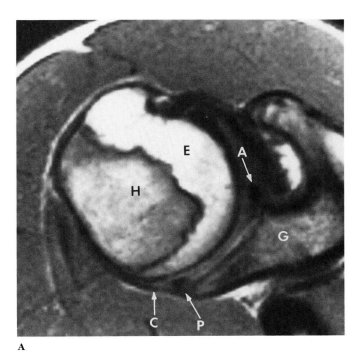

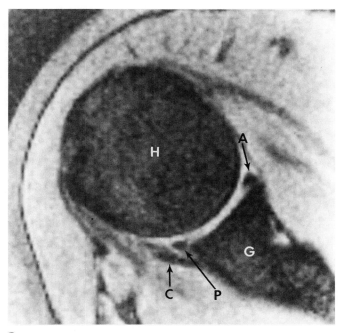

A

B

Figure 5-32   Normal Glenoid Labrum. **A.** *Axial image at T1-weighted sequence shows the normal, triangular-shape anterior and posterior glenoid labra.* **B.** *Axial image at short TR gradient echo sequence shows intact anterior and posterior labra and joint capsule. H = humeral head; E =* *proximal humeral epiphysis; P = posterior cartilaginous labrum; A = anterior cartilaginous labrum; C = joint capsule; G = bony glenoid.*

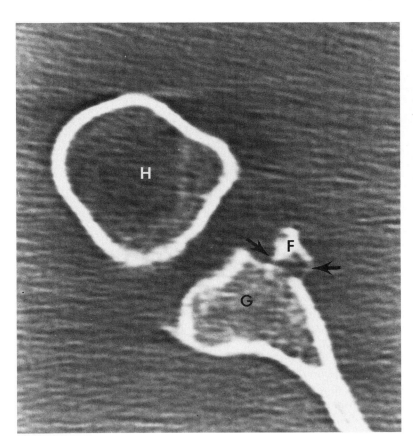

Figure 5-33   Bankart Fracture. *Axial CT scan through the inferior rim of the glenoid shows a fracture off the anterior rim caused by previous anterior dislocation of the humeral head from the glenoid. H = humerus; G = bony glenoid; F = Bankart fragment; arrows = fracture line.*

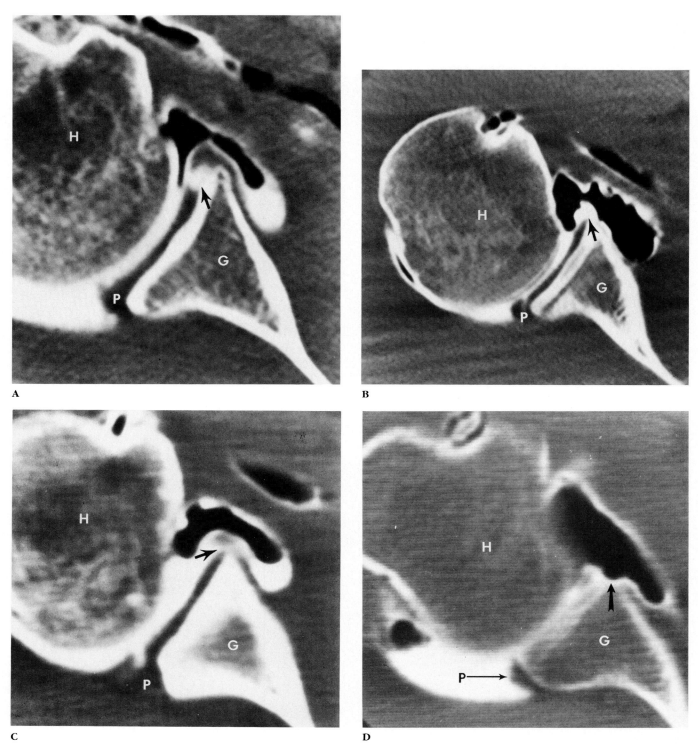

C

D

Figure 5-34   Anterior Bankart Lesions from Previous Anterior Dislocation. **A.** *CT arthrogram shows contrast staining the anterior glenoid labrum indicating a tear of that structure.* **B.** *The anterior labrum is deformed and radiodense. It has absorbed contrast* *through numerous fissures caused by tear from previous dislocation.* **C.** *A linear band of contrast within the anterior glenoid labrum represents tear from previous dislocation.* **D.** *CT scan following double-contrast arthrogram shows blunting and* *deformity of the anterior glenoid labrum indicating avulsion following previous anterior dislocation. Arrow = abnormality within anterior glenoid labrum; P = normal posterior glenoid labrum; G = bony glenoid; H = humerus.*

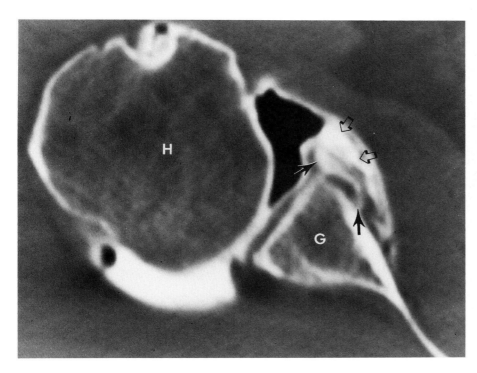

Figure 5-35 Bankart Fracture and Labral Tear. *Axial CT scan through the midglenoid shows a bony crescent representing a Bankart fracture. The overlying articular surface appears intact. The anterior rim of the glenoid is blunted. Contrast has leaked through a labral tear and is directed toward the anterior surface of the scapula. H = humerus; G = bony glenoid; arrows = Bankart bony fragment; open arrows = Bankart labral lesion.*

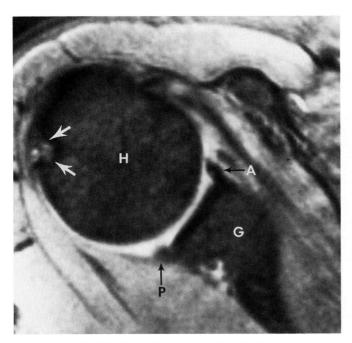

Figure 5-36 Hill-Sachs Deformity. *Axial MR scan at short TR gradient (FISP, 20°) sequence shows a defect involving the posterior/superior surface of the humeral head representing a Hill-Sachs compression fracture from previous anterior dislocation. H = humeral head; G = bony glenoid; arrows = Hill-Sachs defect; A = anterior glenoid labrum; P = posterior glenoid labrum.*

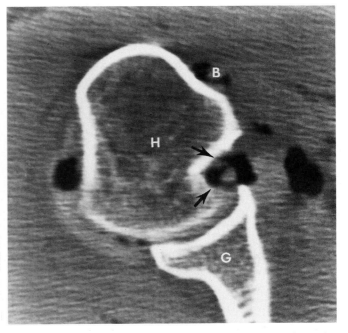

Figure 5-37 Hill-Sachs Deformity. *Axial CT scan through the midglenoid shows an area of cortical depression on the anterior surface of the humerus from previous posterior dislocation. This represents a reverse Hill-Sachs defect. H = humeral head; G = bony glenoid; arrows = Hill-Sachs defect; B = biceps tendon.*

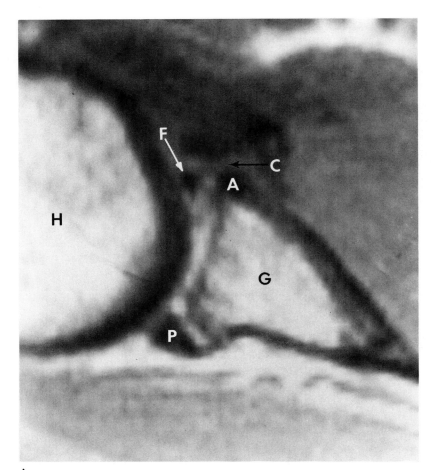

A

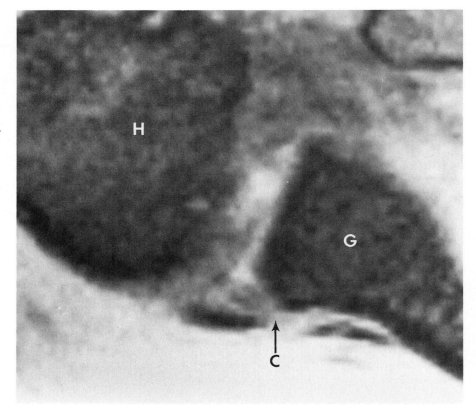

B

Figure 5-38   Bidirectional Instability with Tears of the Anterior and Posterior Glenoid Labra. **A.** *MR scan cranially through the glenohumeral joint shows tear of the anterior glenoid labrum and of the associated joint capsule.* **B.** *MR scan at T2-weighted sequence through the midglenoid shows tear of the posterior labrum from previous posterior dislocation. This individual, with bidirectional instability, had tears of the anterior and posterior labra. P = posterior glenoid labrum; A = anterior labrum; F = anterior labral fragment; C = capsule tear; H = humeral head; G = bony glenoid.*

"Normal" attrition of the labrum associated with advancing age has been noted. Up to 40 percent of individuals in the 40 to 50 age group have abnormalities of the anterior labrum.[69] Virtually all patients who are over 80 years of age have degenerative tears of the anterior labrum.[69] Anterior labral abnormalities are reported in 75 percent of baseball pitchers and are likely caused by chronic overuse. The findings which are seen on the combined CT arthrogram include the following labral abnormalities: marginal irregularity, deformity, contrast imbibition, and avulsion.

The glenoid labral abnormalities that may be recognized on MR include lines of increased signal, fragmentation, and labral absence. These features are easier to assess in the presence of joint effusion.

MR and CT both are useful in the evaluation of the shoulder afflicted with multidirectional instability. In that circumstance, there is combined abnormality of the anterior and posterior glenoid labra (Fig. 5-38). It is important to distinguish this entity from unidirectional instability since treatment for unidirectional instability will accentuate the symptoms of unrecognized multidirectional instability.[57]

CHRONIC PROBLEMS

Adhesive capsulitis and loose bodies (Figs. 5-39 and 5-40)

Among the entities responsible for chronic pain and disability about the shoulder include adhesive capsulitis (frozen shoulder), degenerative arthritis of either the acromioclavicular or glenohumeral joints (Fig. 5-39), posttraumatic cyst formation, intraarticular loose bodies, and abnormality of the biceps tendon. Loose bodies may be detected either on plain radiographs, on computed tomographic scans, or with magnetic resonance imaging (Fig. 5-40). The determination of mobile intraarticular loose bodies may require the injection of air and/or contrast into the shoulder joint. With freely mobile intraarticular bodies, the change in position of those structures and/or the complete encirclement of them by air or contrast allows distinction of intraarticular loose bodies from ossifications which are contained within the adjacent soft tissues.

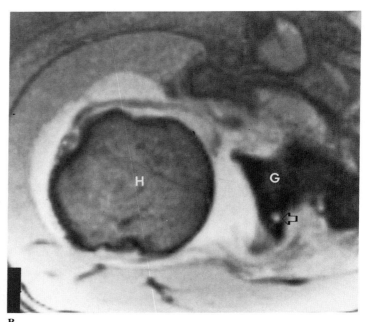

B

Figure 5-39 Degenerative Arthritis. **A.** *MR scan at T2-weighted sequence demonstrates narrowing of the articular cartilage of the glenoid.* **B.** *MR scan at short TR gradient echo (FISP, 20°) sequence shows joint effusion. A glenoid cyst is noted.* (Fig. 5-39C continues on next page.)

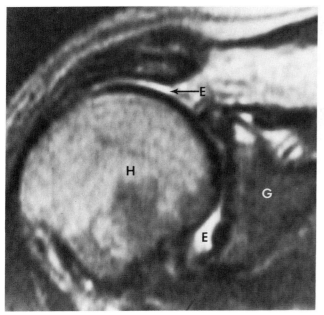

A

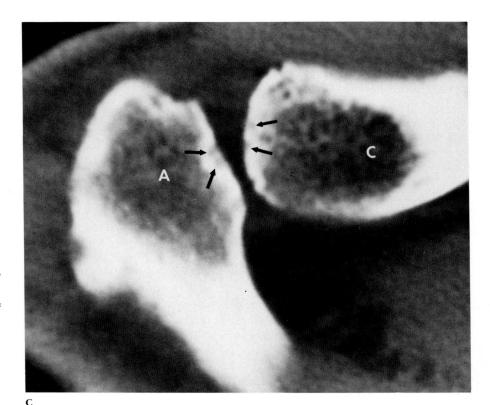

Figure 5-39 Degenerative Arthritis (Continued). **C.** *CT scan through the acromioclavicular joint shows subcortical cystic change. This degenerative feature represents overuse arthrosis. H = humeral head; G = bony glenoid; open arrow = cyst; E = effusion; C = clavicle; A = acromion process; arrows = subcortical cysts.*

C

A

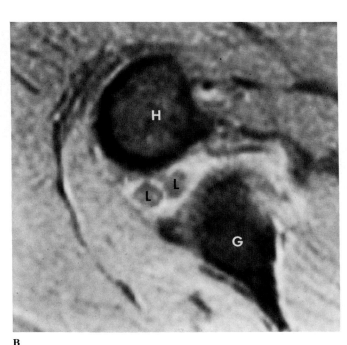

B

Figure 5-40 Intraarticular Loose Bodies. **A.** *CT scan following double-contrast shoulder arthrogram shows contrast and air surrounding several intraarticular loose bodies.* **B.** *MR scan in another patient at short TR gradient echo (FISP, 20°) sequence shows two intraarticular loose bodies to be present. L = loose body; H = humeral head; G = bony glenoid.*

Bicipital tendon abnormalities (Figs. 5-1 and 5-41)

Bicipital tendinitis is characterized by pain and crepitation over the biceps tendon and with the accumulation of fluid within the bicipital tendon sheath (Fig. 5-41). This can be detected either with sonography or with magnetic resonance imaging. Chronic medial subluxation of the biceps tendon from a congenitally flattened bicipital groove may be suspected if the plain film demonstrates deficiency of the lesser tuberosity, which normally defines the medial border of that groove. Single- or double-contrast arthrography can help to confirm bicipital tendon dislocation. A CT scan through the proximal humerus following shoulder arthrography is an effective way to assess the biceps tendon and to diagnose its medial dislocation[70] (Fig. 5-1). MR can demonstrate this condition without the need for contrast injection.

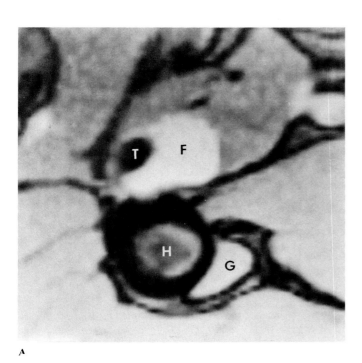

A

Figure 5-41 Bicipital Tendinitis. **A.** *Axial scan at short TR gradient echo (FISP, 20°) sequence shows fluid surrounding the biceps tendon. This indicates bicipital tendinitis.* **B.** *MR scan in the sagittal plane of another patient at T2-weighted sequence demonstrates fluid surrounding the biceps tendon. F = fluid within biceps tendon sheath; T = tendon; H = humerus; G = glenoid.*

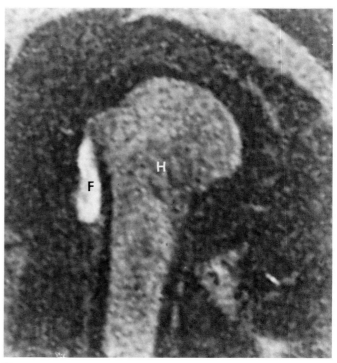

B

Avascular necrosis (Fig. 5-42)

The magnetic resonance scan can effectively confirm the diagnosis of avascular necrosis of the humeral head. Although the triple-phase bone scan is extremely sensitive, it is nonspecific when used to diagnose this entity. Magnetic resonance scanning characteristically shows a region of abnormal bone containing necrotic fat, which on T1 images contains intermediate signal intensity. This is surrounded by a rim of low-signal intensity, which, on T2-weighting, shows a peripheral border of high-signal intensity (Fig. 5-42). These features are characteristic for avascular necrosis and resemble the findings seen in other anatomic sites.

Stress fracture and periostitis (Figs. 5-43 and 5-44 and Drawing I)

TPBS is the imaging modality of choice in detecting stress fracture and periostitis (Fig. 5-43). In the upper extremity and thorax, one of the most common areas to develop stress fracture is the ribs and is associated with rowing, pitching, and golfing.[71-74] Stress fracture of the humerus is usually associated with tennis, weightlifting, gymnastics, javelin throwing, and baseball pitching.[9,30,75,76] Although rare, stress fracture of the sternum has been reported in wrestlers.[77]

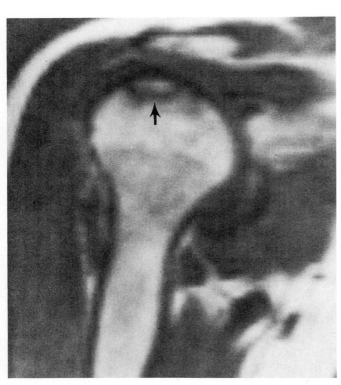

Figure 5-42 Avascular Necrosis. *MR scan at T1-weighted sequence in the coronal plane shows a ring of low signal (arrow) at the apex of the humeral head. This represents granulation tissue encircling a necrotic bony fragment.*

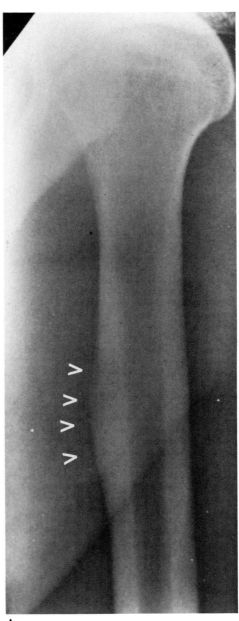

Figure 5-43 Stress Fracture, Left ▶ Humerus. *Male athlete with chronic left arm pain associated with throwing.* **A.** *Anteroposterior radiograph of the left humerus demonstrates cortical thickening medially (arrowheads).* (Fig. 5-43B continues on the opposite page.)

A

The extreme forces generated by upper extremity activity produce a wide variety of lesions. One of the more unusual is bilateral periostitis of the proximal to midhumerus, representing tearing at the insertion sites of the pectoralis major muscle (Fig. 5-44). This is found in gymnasts who use iron rings and in weightlifters who engage in repeated lateral curls. Both of these activities involve severe, forceful, repeated abduction of the upper arms from the torso, thereby fully stretching the pectoralis major muscle (Drawing I).

Heterotopic ossification (Figs. 5-45 to 5-48)

Heterotopic ossification is not always easily detectable by plain radiographs. Even when present, the clinician or radiologist may not be certain as to whether the positive finding is a new lesion that is metabolically active and, therefore, probably symptomatic, or old. Based on the nuclide activity, TPBS can help to localize the area of heterotopic ossification and to suggest its chronicity.[7–9] Patients who have undergone

bone or joint surgery with persistent postoperative pain should be evaluated with TPBS to identify the development of heterotopic ossification[78] (Fig. 5-45). CT scanning, either before or after TPBS, is a helpful adjunct to identify the three-dimensional extent of that abnormality. Posttraumatic myositis ossificans of the upper extremity, especially the humerus, is a common problem. TPBS is useful in identifying the region of involvement as well as in assessing the stage of development. This information is clinically important[9,79–81] (Figs. 5-46 to 5-48).

Posttraumatic intramuscular cyst (Fig. 5-49)

Posttraumatic cyst from degenerated intramuscular hematoma can cause a palpably worrisome mass which, when evaluated with sonograph, shows an echolucent collection to be present (Fig. 5-49). Sonographically guided cyst aspiration is both diagnostic and curative.

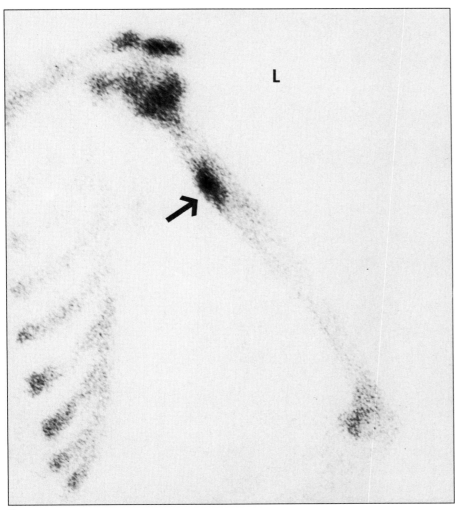

Figure 5-43 Stress Fracture, Left Humerus (Continued). **B.** *High-resolution anterior image of left shoulder and humerus from TPBS. A focus of increased nuclide activity is present (arrow), representing with a stress fracture of sufficient age to result in the corresponding radiographic changes.*

B

Figure 5-44 Bilateral Humeral Periostitis (Ringman's Lesion). *Male weightlifter with bilateral upper arm pain and normal radiographs. High-resolution delayed images of both shoulders and upper arms were taken with the extremity positioned in external rotation.* **A.** *Right shoulder shows mildly increased nuclide activity in the proximal third of the shaft of the right humerus (arrowheads).* **B.** *Left shoulder and humerus show increased nuclide activity which is significantly more intense (arrowheads) than present on the right. The area of involvement bilaterally represents the sites of attachment of the pectoralis major muscle. Increased nuclide activity represents periostitis at the attachment sites. (This mechanism is similar to that noted in the development of shin splints and thigh splints.) (See Drawing I.)*

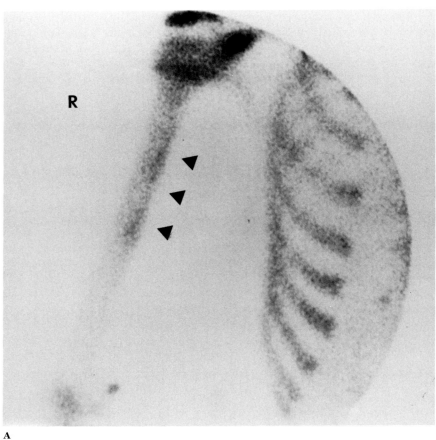

A

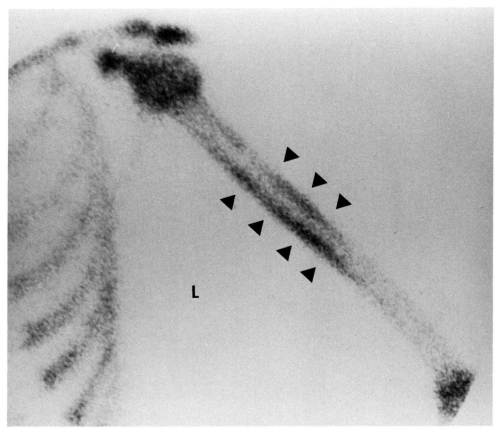

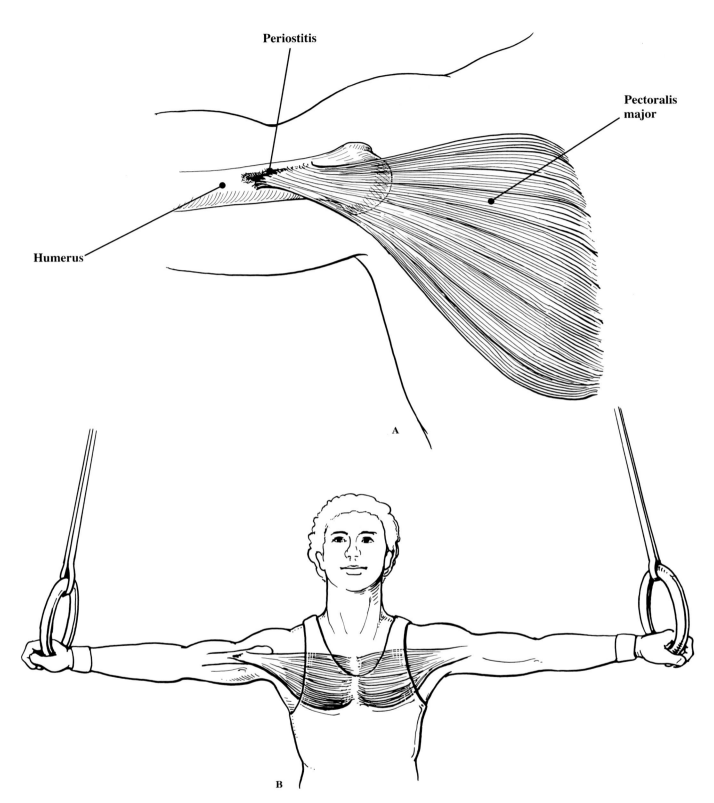

Drawing I   A. Pectoralis Major Periostitis. *Overuse injury of the pectoralis major muscle may result in tearing of muscle fibers at their periosteal insertion near the proximal to middle shaft of the humerus. This leads to focal periostitis with an associated inflammatory response.* **B.** Ringman's Lesion. *The iron cross position performed in gymnastics on the rings is a maneuver that creates maximal stress on the pectoralis major insertion and may result in focal periostitis. A weightlifting exercise, known as lateral curls, may produce similar stress and injury.*

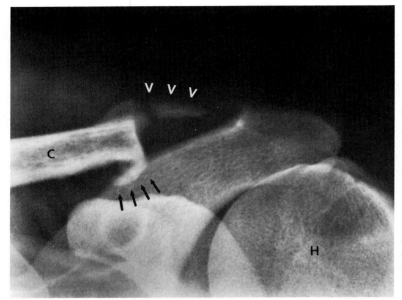

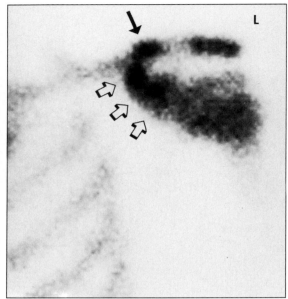

A

B

Figure 5-45 Postsurgical Heterotopic Ossification. *Male athlete following left distal clavicular resection has persistent pain.* **A.** *Anteroposterior radiograph of the left shoulder shows distal clavicular resection. Two abnormal foci of heterotopic ossification are present* adjacent to the clavicle [superiorly (white arrowheads) and inferiorly (black arrows)]. **B.** High-resolution delayed anterior image of left shoulder from TPBS. Foci of increased nuclide activity are present superiorly (black arrow) and inferiorly (open arrows). These correspond to the areas of heterotopic ossification and demonstrate them to be metabolically active and a likely cause of this patient's symptoms. C = clavicle; H = humeral head.

Figure 5-46 Myositis Ossificans of Right Upper Arm. *College lacrosse player hit by ball in upper arm almost three weeks prior to TPBS.* **A.** *Initial blood pool image of right humerus (in internal rotation) demonstrates a focal area of increased nuclide activity in the midshaft of the humerus (arrow).* **B.** *High-resolution image of right humerus in external rotation shows an area of intense nuclide activity (arrow) adjacent to the midshaft of the humerus. H = humerus.* (Fig. 5-46C continues on the opposite page.)

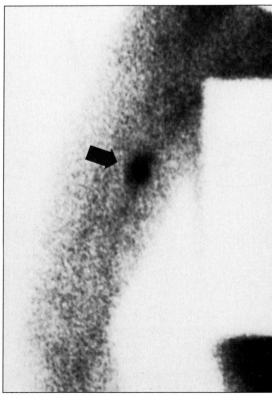

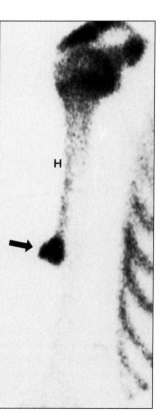

A

B

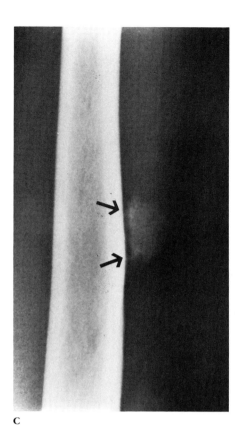

Figure 5-46 Myositis Ossificans of Right Upper Arm (Continued). **C.** *Coned down radiograph of the right humeral shaft in internal rotation. Soft tissue ossification representing a region of myositis ossificans is seen (arrows), which is clearly separated from the bony shaft.*

C

Figure 5-47 Myositis Ossificans of Upper Arm. *College lacrosse player hit by stick in left upper arm 10 days before first TPBS.* **A.** *High-resolution delayed image of left humerus in the anterior projection demonstrates a large area of intense nuclide activity (arrow) adjacent to the midshaft of the left humerus. Radiograph taken at that time was normal.* **B.** *High-resolution delayed image of left humerus in anterior position taken almost 4 weeks later shows a decrease in nuclide activity consistent with interval healing.* **C.** *Coned down radiograph of the left humerus taken on the same day as the second TPBS demonstrates soft tissue ossification (arrows) separated from the humeral shaft representing myositis ossificans. H = humerus.*

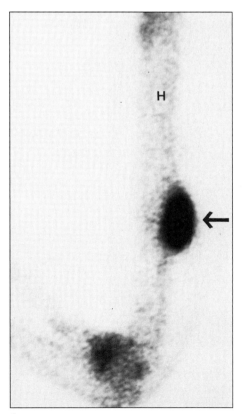

A

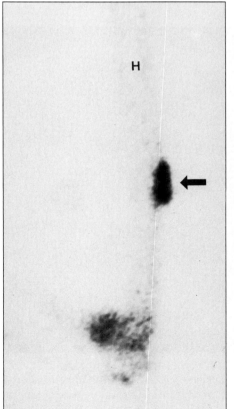

B

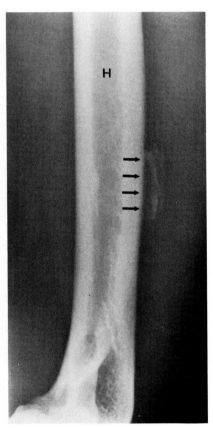

C

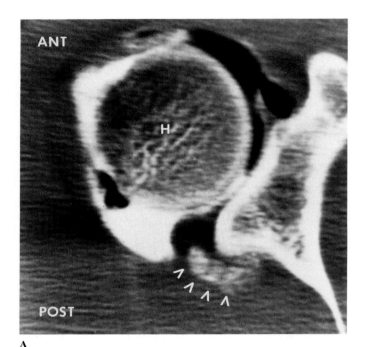

A

B

Figure 5-48 Heterotopic Calcification. *Professional baseball pitcher 6 months following shoulder surgery for rotator cuff repair has persistent right shoulder pain posteriorly. Routine radiographs were normal. CT scan and TPBS were then done.* **A.** *CT scan of the right shoulder demonstrates heterotopic calcification posteriorly (arrowheads) at the level of the humeral head (H) and glenoid.* **B.** *High-resolution delayed posterior image from TPBS performed approximately 2 weeks after the CT shows intense nuclide activity (arrow), which indicates that the calcification is metabolically active and is likely associated with this patient's symptoms.*

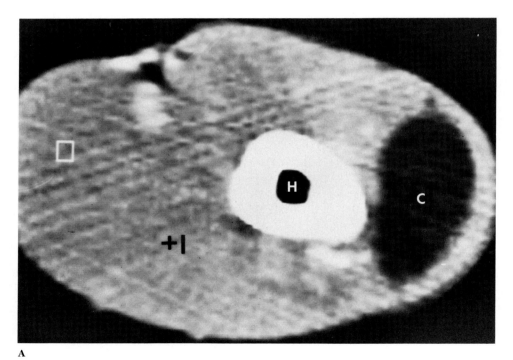

A

Figure 5-49 Posttraumatic Cyst. **A.** *CT scan at the level of the middle shaft of the humerus following injection of intravenous contrast material shows a nonenhancing lucent lesion in the brachioradialis muscle.* (Fig. 5-49B continues on the opposite page.)

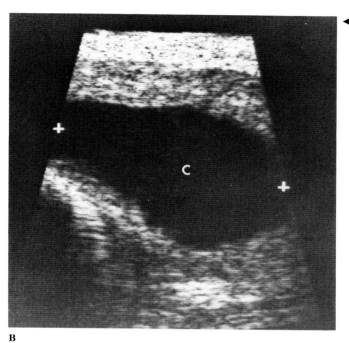

B

◄ **Figure 5-49** Posttraumatic Cyst (Continued). **B.** *Ultrasound demonstrates lack of internal echoes with enhanced through transmission indicating this to be a cyst. Previous trauma with hematoma formation has resulted in a posttraumatic cyst. C = cyst; H = humerus.*

Figure 5-50 RSD of Right Upper Extremity. *Male athlete with initial blunt trauma to right hand/wrist. Persistent right upper extremity pain, swelling, and decreased range of motion, despite normal radiographs, was evaluated with TPBS.* **A.** *High-resolution delayed images of both hands and wrists. Marked asymmetry is seen. Diffusely increased nuclide activity that involves the wrist, metacarpophalangeal, and interphalangeal joints is present on the right side.* (Fig. 5-50B and C continues on next page.)

▼

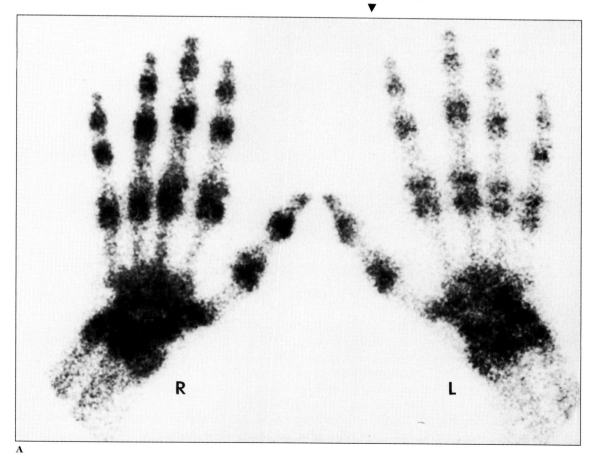

R   L

A

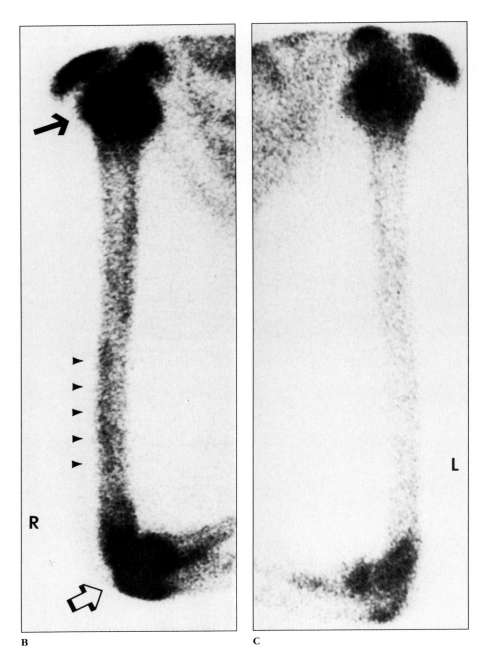

Figure 5-50 RSD of Right Upper Extremity (Continued). **B.** *High-resolution delayed image of entire right humerus, elbow, and proximal forearm demonstrates increased activity in the elbow and right humerus and mildly increased activity along the right humeral shaft. Black arrow = humeral head; open arrow = elbow joint; arrowheads = distal humeral shaft.* **C.** *Normal appearing left shoulder, humerus, and elbow for comparison.*

DIAGNOSTIC PROBLEMS

Not every abnormality is related to trauma or overuse.[82,83] Reflex sympathetic dystrophy (RSD), either focal or diffuse, is more frequent than often considered and is best detected with TPBS.[9,84,85] (Fig. 5-50). Any blunt or crush injury that results in persistent or chronic pain, swelling, decreased range of motion, or atrophic changes which cannot be explained by other radiographic findings should raise the clinician's index of suspicion for RSD.

As in other areas of the body, the physician must be alert to the possibility of infection (Figs. 5-51 and 5-52) or tumor. A wide variety of benign and malignant bone tumors that may mimic sports injury can be seen in the shoulder and ribs[82,83] (Figs. 5-53 to 5-56). For those patients who either fail to respond to appropriate treatment or who demonstrate atypical signs and symptoms, these entities should be considered.

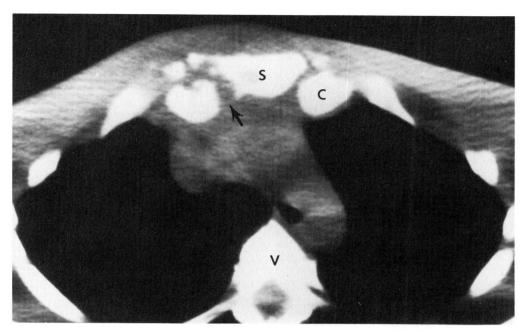

Figure 5-51 Septic Arthritis of the Sternoclavicular (SC) Joint. *CT scan through the sternoclavicular joints shows destructive arthropathy on the right side with bony fragmentation. The right first rib and the left sternoclavicular joint are normal. Arrow = septic right SC joint; S = sternum; C = normal left clavicle; V = vertebral body.*

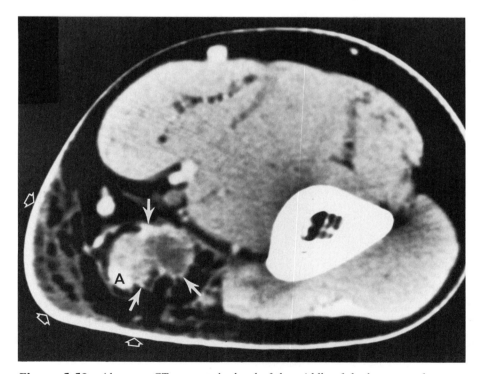

Figure 5-52 Abscess. *CT scan at the level of the middle of the humerus after dynamic contrast injection shows an ill-defined density adjacent to the brachial artery representing an abscess. Skin and fascial thickening is present indicating cellulitis. A = brachial artery; arrows = abscess; open arrows = skin and fascial plane thickening.*

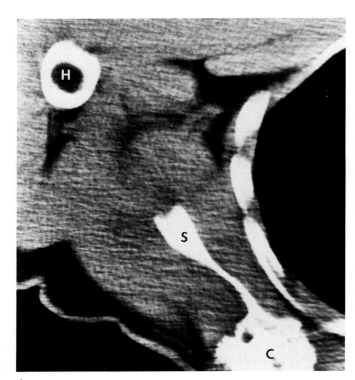

▲

Figure 5-53 Osteochondroma. *This athlete complained of a snapping sensation in his shoulder. CT scan demonstrates an osteochondroma of the scapula which impinged on the posterior ribs during certain motions. H = humerus; S = body of scapula; C = osteochondroma.*

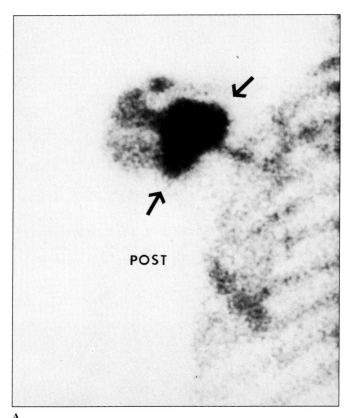

A

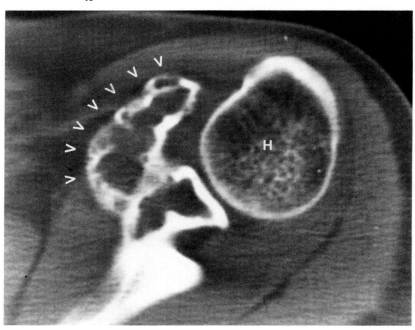

Figure 5-54 Fibrous Dysplasia of Left ▶ Scapula. *Female athlete with left shoulder pain.* **A.** *High-resolution delayed posterior image of the left shoulder demonstrates a large focus of increased nuclide activity in the left scapula (arrows).* **B.** *CT scan shows a corresponding lytic and expansile process (arrowheads) altering a large portion of the scapula representing a focus of fibrous dysplasia.*

B

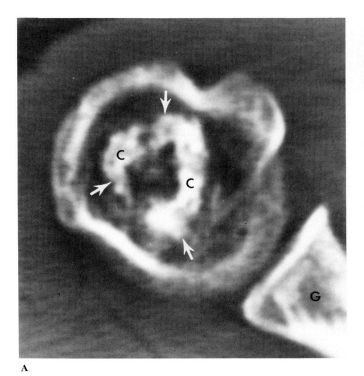

A

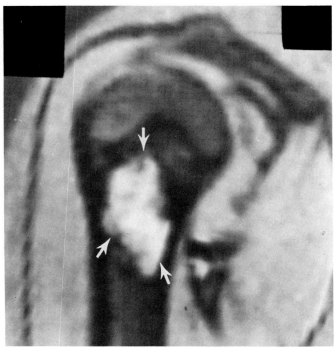

B

Figure 5-55 Cartilaginous Tumor.
A. *Axial CT scan demonstrates a focus of cartilaginous calcification within the medullary space of the humerus* *proximally.* **B.** *MR scan at T2-weighted sequence shows a high-signal lesion within the proximal metaphysis of the humerus. This represented a benign* *enchondroma. C = cartilaginous calcification; arrows = border to neoplasm; G = bony glenoid.*

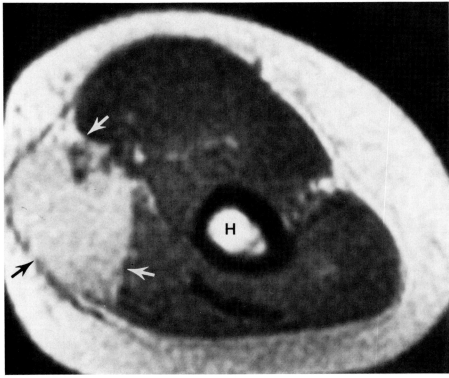

A

Figure 5-56 Infiltrating Neoplasm.
A. *MR scan at T1-weighted sequence through the midhumerus shows a region of high signal infiltrating the medial muscles.* (Fig. 5-56B and C continues on next page.)

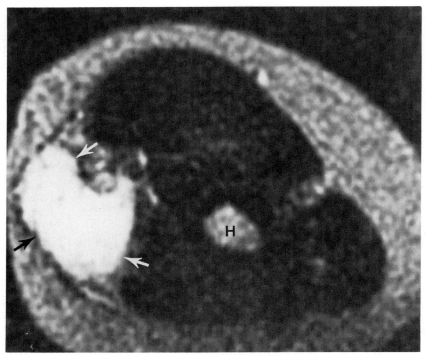

B

Figure 5-56 Infiltrating Neoplasm (Continued). **B.** *MR scan at T2-weighted sequence shows high signal within this abnormal region.* **C.** *MR scan in the coronal plane at T2-weighted sequence shows a soft tissue mass adjacent to the upper arm muscles extending into the adjacent fat. Blockage of venous channels distal to this mass is caused by extrinsic compression on the veins. Arrows = neoplasm; V = partially blocked vein; H = humerus.*

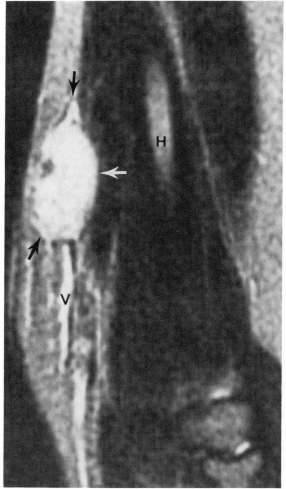

C

REFERENCES

1. Cox JS: The fate of the acromioclavicular joint in athletic injuries. Am J Sports Med 9:50–53, 1981.
2. Gundry CR, Schils JP, Resnick D, Sartoris DJ: Arthrography of the post-traumatic knee, shoulder, and wrist: current status and future trends. Radiol Clin North Am 27:957–971, 1989.
3. Crass JR, Craig EV, Bretzke C, Feinberg SB: Ultrasonography of the rotator cuff. RadioGraphics 5:941–953, 1985.
4. Middleton WD, Reinus WR, Totty WG, et al.: Ultrasonographic evaluation of the rotator cuff and biceps tendon. J Bone Joint Surg 68(A):440–450, 1986.
5. Callaghan JJ, McNiesh LM, Dehaven JP, et al.: A prospective comparison study of double contrast computed tomography (CT) arthrography and arthroscopy of the shoulder. Am J Sports Med 16:13–20, 1988.
6. Fogelman I (ed): *Bone Scanning in Clinical Practice*. Springer-Verlag, London, 1987.
7. Holder LE: Clinical radionuclide bone imaging. Radiology 176:607–614, 1990.
8. Holder LE, Matthews LS: The nuclear physician and sports medicine, in Freeman L, Weissman H (eds): *Nuclear Medicine Annual 1984*. Raven, New York, 1984, pp 88–140.
9. Martire JR: The role of nuclear medicine scans in evaluating pain in athletic injuries. Clin Sports Med 6:713–737, 1987.
10. Rupani HD, Holder LE, Espinola DA, et al.: Three phase radionuclide bone imaging in sports medicine. Radiology 156:187–196, 1985.
11. Hershman EB, Mailly T: Stress fractures. Clin Sports Med 1:183–214, 1990.
12. Kieft GJ, Sartoris DJ, Bloem JL, et al.: Magnetic resonance imaging of glenohumeral joint diseases. Skeletal Radiol 16:285–290, 1987.
13. Deutsch AL, Resnick D, Mink JH: Computed tomography of glenohumeral and sternoclavicular joints. Orthop Clin North Am 16:497–511. 1985.
14. Zlatkin MB, Bjorkengren AG, Gylys-Morin V, et al. Cross-sectional imaging of the capsular mechanism of the glenohumeral joint. AJR 150:151–158, 1988.
15. Seeger LL, Gold RH, Bassett LW: Shoulder instability: evaluation with MR imaging. Radiology 168:695–697, 1988.
16. McNiesh LM, Callaghan JJ: CT arthrography of the shoulder: variations of the glenoid labrum. AJR 149:963–966, 1987.
17. Pennes DR, Jonsson K, Buckwalter K, et al.: Computed arthrotomography of the shoulder: comparison of examinations made with internal and external rotation of the humerus. AJR 153:1017–1019, 1989.
18. Tehranzadeh J, Serafini AN, Pais MJ: *Avulsion and Stress Injuries of the Musculoskeletal System*. Karger, Basel, 1989.
19. Benton J, Nelson C: Avulsion of the coracoid process in an athlete. J Bone Joint Surg 53(A):356–358, 1977.
20. Boyer DW: Trapshooters shoulder: Stress fracture of the coracoid process: Case report. J Bone Joint Surg 57(A):862, 1975.
21. Derosa PG, KemalFamp DB: Fracture of the coracoid process of the scapula. J Bone Joint Surg 59(A):696–697, 1977.
22. Lasda NA, Murray DG: Fracture separation of the coracoid process associated with acromioclavicular dislocation. Clin Orthop 134:222–224, 1978.
23. Mariani PP: Isolated fracture of the coracoid process in an athlete. Am J Sports Med 8:129–130, 1980.
24. Montgomery SP, Loyd DR: Avulsion fracture of the coracoid epiphysis with acromioclavicular separation. J Bone Joint Surg 59(A):963–965, 1977.
25. Protess JJ, Spampfli FV, Osmer JC: Coracoid process fracture diagnosis in acromioclavicular separation. Radiology 116:61–64, 1975.
26. Sandrock AR: Another sports fatigue fracture: stress fracture of the coracoid process of the scapula. Radiology 117:274–275, 1975.
27. Smith DM: Coracoid fracture associated with acromioclavicular dislocation. Clin Orthop 108:165–167, 1975.
28. Rockwood CA, Odor JM: Spontaneous atraumatic anterior subluxation of the sternoclavicular joint. J Bone Joint Surg 71(A):1280–1288, 1989.
29. Levinsohn EM, Bunnell WP, Yuan HA: Computed tomography in the diagnosis of dislocations of the sternoclavicular joint. Clin Orthop 140:12–16, 1979.
30. Fulton MN, Albright JP, El-Khoury GY: Cortical desmoid-like lesion of the proximal humerus and its occurrence in gymnasts (Ringman's shoulder lesion). Am J Sports Med 7:57–61, 1979.
31. Baker BE: Current concepts in the diagnosis and treatment of musculotendinous injuries. Med Sci Sports Exerc 16:323–327, 1984.
32. Stoller DW (ed), Genant HK, Helms CA, Goumas CG (assoc eds): *Magnetic Resonance Imaging in Orthopaedics and Rheumatology*. Lippincott, Philadelphia, 1989, chap 6, pp 264–283.
33. Kilcoyne RF, Reddy PK, Lyons F, Rockwood CA: Optimal plain film imaging of the shoulder impingement syndrome. AJR 153:795–797, 1989.
34. Cofield RH: Current concepts review: rotator cuff disease of the shoulder. J Bone Joint Surg 67(A):974–979, 1985.
35. Kursunoglu-Brahme S, Resnick D: Magnetic resonance imaging of the shoulder. Rad Clin North Am 28:941–954, 1990.
36. Kieft GJ, Bloem JL, Rozing PM, Obermann WR: Rotator cuff impingement syndrome: MR imaging. Radiology 166:211–214, 1988.
37. Holt RG, Helms CA, Steinbach L, et al.: Magnetic resonance imaging of the shoulder: rationale and current applications. Skeletal Radiol 19:5–14, 1990.
38. Seeger LL: Magnetic resonance imaging of the shoulder. Clin Orthop 244:48–59, 1989.
39. Rafii M, Firooznia H, Sherman O, et al.: Rotator cuff lesions: signal patterns at MR imaging. Radiology 177:817–823, 1990.
40. Iannotti JP, Zlatkin MB, Esterhai JL, et al.: Magnetic resonance imaging of the shoulder. J Bone Joint Surg 73(A):17–29, 1991.
41. Zlatkin MB, Iannotti JP, Roberts MC, et al.: Rotator cuff tears: diagnostic performance of MR imaging. Radiology 172:223–229, 1989.
42. Buirski G: Magnetic resonance imaging in acute and chronic rotator cuff tears. Skeletal Radiol 19:109–111, 1990.
43. Beltran J, Gray LA, Bools JC, et al.: Rotator cuff lesions of the shoulder: evaluation by direct sagittal CT arthrography. Radiology 160:161–165, 1986.
44. Goldman AB, Ghelman B: The double-contrast shoulder arthrogram: a review of 158 studies. Radiology 127:655–663, 1978.

45. Schneider R, Ghelman B, Kaye JJ: A simplified injection technique for shoulder arthrography. Radiology 114:738–739, 1975.

46. Mink JH, Harris E, Rappaport M: Rotator cuff tears: evaluation using double-contrast shoulder arthrography. Radiology 157:621–623, 1985.

47. Kernwein GA, Roseberg B, Sneed WR: Arthrographic studies of the shoulder joint. J Bone Joint Surg 39(A):1267–1279, 1957.

48. Burk DL, Karasick D, Kurtz AB, et al.: Rotator cuff tears: prospective comparison of MR imaging with arthrography, sonography, and surgery. AJR 153:87–92, 1989.

49. Bangert BA, Pathria MN, Resnick D: Advanced imaging of the shoulder. Appl Radiology 18(7):33–37, 1989.

50. Kneeland JB, Middleton WD, Carrera GF, et al.: MR imaging of the shoulder: diagnosis of rotator cuff tears. AJR 149:333–337, 1987.

51. Evancho AM, Stiles RG, Fajman WA, et al.: MR imaging diagnosis of rotator cuff tears. AJR 151:751–754, 1988.

52. Flannigan B, Kursunoglu-Brahme S, Snyder S, et al.: MR arthrography of the shoulder: comparison with conventional MR imaging. AJR 155:829–832, 1990.

53. Hajek PC, Baker LL, Sartoris DJ, et al.: MR arthrography: anatomic-pathologic investigation. Radiology 163:141–147, 1987.

54. Pappas AM, Goss TP, Kleinman PK: Symptomatic shoulder instability due to lesions of the glenoid labrum. Am J Sports Med 11:279–288, 1983.

55. McGlynn FJ, Caspari RB: Arthroscopic findings in the subluxating shoulder. Clin Orthop 183:173–178, 1984.

56. Rafii M, Minkoff J, Bonamo J, et al.: Computed tomography (CT) arthrography of shoulder instabilities in athletes. Am J Sports Med 16:352–361, 1988.

57. Singson RD, Feldman F, Bigliani LU, Rosenberg ZS: Recurrent shoulder dislocation after surgical repair: double-contrast CT arthrography. Work in progress. Radiology 164:425–428, 1987.

58. Singson RD, Feldman F, Bigliani L: CT arthrographic patterns in recurrent glenohumeral instability. AJR 149:749–753, 1987.

59. Legan JM, Burkhard TK, Goff II WB, et al: Tears of the glenoid labrum: MR imaging of 88 arthroscopically confirmed cases. Radiology 179:241–246, 1991.

60. Haynor DR, Shuman WP: Double contrast CT arthrography of the glenoid labrum and shoulder girdle. RadioGraphics 4:411–421, 1984.

61. Kieft GJ, Bloem JL, Rozing PM, Obermann WR: MR imaging of recurrent anterior dislocation of the shoulder: comparison with CT arthrography. AJR 150:1083–1087, 1988.

62. Kinnard P, Tricoire JL, Levesque RY, Bergeron D: Assessment of the unstable shoulder by computed arthrography. Am J Sports Med 11:157–159, 1983.

63. Rafii M, Firooznia H, Golimbu C, et al.: CT arthrography of capsular structures of the shoulder. AJR 146:361–367, 1986.

64. Hall FM, Rosenthal DI, Goldberg RP, Wyshak G: Morbidity from shoulder arthrography: etiology, incidence, and prevention. AJR 136:59–62, 1981.

65. Hall FM, Goldberg RP, Wyshak G, Kilcoyne RF: Shoulder arthrography: comparison of morbidity after use of various contrast media. Radiology 154:339–341, 1985.

66. Deutsch AL, Resnick D, Mink JH, et al.: Computed and conventional arthrotomography of the glenohumeral joint: normal anatomy and clinical experience. Radiology 153:603–609, 1984.

67. Shuman WP, Kilcoyne RF, Matsen FA, et al.: Double-contrast computed tomography of the glenoid labrum. AJR 141:581–584, 1983.

68. Wilson AJ, Totty WG, Murphy WA, Hardy DC: Shoulder joint: arthrographic CT and long-term follow-up, with surgical correlation. Radiology 173:329–333, 1989.

69. Andrews JR, Carson WG, McLeod WD: Glenoid labrum tears related to the long head of the biceps. Am J Sports Med 13:337–341, 1985.

70. Levinsohn EM, Santelli ED: Bicipital groove dysplasia and medial dislocation of the biceps brachii tendon. Skeletal Radiol (in press).

71. Freiberger RH, Mayer V: Ununited bilateral fatigue fractures of the first ribs. J Bone Joint Surg 46(A):615–618, 1964.

72. Gurther R, Pavlov H, Torg JS: Stress fracture of the ipsolateral first rib in a pitcher. Am J Sports Med 13:277–279, 1985.

73. Holden D, Jackson D: Stress fracture of the ribs in female rowers. Am J Sports Med 13:342–348, 1985.

74. Rasad S: Golfer's fractures of the ribs. AJR 120:901–902, 1974.

75. Rettig AC, Beltz HF: Stress fracture in the humerus in an adolescent tennis tournament player. Am J Sports Med 13:55–58, 1985.

76. Tullos HS, Erwin WD, Woods GW, et al.: Unusual lesions of the pitching arm. Clin Orthop 88:169–182, 1972.

77. Keating TM: Stress fracture of the sternum in a wrestler. Am J Sports Med 15:92–93, 1987.

78. Orzel JA, Rudd TG: Heterotopic bone formation: clinical laboratory imaging correlation. J Nucl Med 26:125–132, 1984.

79. Huss CD, Puhl JJ: Myositis ossificans of the upper arm. Am J Sports Med 8:419–424, 1980.

80. Lipscomb AB, Thomas ED, Johnston RK: Treatment of myositis ossificans traumatica in athletes. Am J Sports Med 4:111–120, 1976.

81. Suzuki Y, Hisada K, Takeda M: Demonstration of myositis ossificans by ^{99m}Tc pyrophosphate bone scanning. Radiology 111:663–666, 1974.

82. Baker BE, Levinsohn EM, Coren AB: Pitfalls to avoid in diagnosing pain in the athlete. Clin Sports Med 6:921–934, 1987.

83. Lewis MM, Reilly JF: Sports tumors. Am J Sports Med 4:362–365, 1987.

84. Holder LE, MacKinnon SE: Reflex sympathetic dystrophy in the hands: strict clinical and scintigraphic criteria. Radiology 152:517–522, 1984.

85. MacKinnon SE, Holder LE: The use of three phase radionuclide bone scanning in the diagnosis of reflex sympathetic dystrophy. J Hand Surg 9(A):556–563, 1984.

Orthopedic overview

Injuries to the hand and wrist in athletics are extremely common. Many of these injuries are initially either overlooked or undertreated by the patient, coach, trainer, and/or even physician because of the multiplicity of joints, ligaments, tendons, and neurovascular structures potentially injured and therefore the complexity of the potential problems. Unfortunately, the diagnosis of a *sprain* (a term that is no longer used in describing athletic injuries to the knee) is still commonly used to describe athletic injuries to the hand and/or wrist. Considering the depth of knowledge that now exists in regard to anatomy, function, and injury patterns, athletic injuries to this area might better be described in terms of the specific bone and/or joint involved, ligament and/or tendon injured, degree of instability and/or resultant deformity. The long-term consequences of untreated bony or soft tissue injuries to the hand and wrist in the athlete run the gamut from an intermittent nuisance to career-ending disability.

Patients presenting with injuries to the hand and wrist should be thoroughly evaluated as soon as possible following the injury with careful clinical exam and appropriate radiographic studies. Often, as in the case of a knee injury, it is best to evaluate the athlete on the sideline immediately following the injury before limiting swelling and pain have developed. This is perhaps the best time to test for the severity of ligament injury. A careful clinical evaluation should include an assessment of the athlete's ability to move the injured joint through a complete range of motion, the neurovascular status of the extremity distal to the injury, tenderness about the injury site coinciding with ligamentous origin or insertion, instability to stress testing, swelling, and finally resting deformity. Following such a careful clinical evaluation, appropriate radiographic studies should be obtained.

A radiographic examination of the injured hand or wrist should begin with routine posteroanterior (PA), lateral, and oblique radiographs. These films should be analyzed for soft tissue swelling, fractures, subluxation/dislocations, and finally alignment. Often these routine radiographic studies will be all that is needed to make the appropriate diagnosis and initiate treatment. Routine radiographs with slight modifications are often helpful for detecting subtle injuries. Examples are an oblique film of the wrist or a carpal tunnel view of the wrist to detect a hamate hook fracture as might be seen in a golfer, an oblique view of the wrist to evaluate the pisotriquetral joint for a loose body or a small avulsion, an ulnarly deviated view of the wrist to profile the body of the scaphoid, a stress radiograph for assessing ligamentous injury to a collateral ligament such as about the proximal interphalangeal (PIP) or metacarpophalangeal (MC) joint, a neutral forearm rotation view of the wrist for measuring ulnar variance and assessing the possibility of ulnar impaction, an anteroposterior supinated view of the wrist to profile the scapholunate joint for rotary subluxation of the scaphoid, and finally a motion study of the wrist to detect abnormal carpal mobility in a patient with dynamic carpal instability. These rather routine radiographic studies and their modifications, in conjunction with a careful history and physical examination, should result in the clinician being able to diagnose the vast majority of athletic injuries to the hand and wrist.

CHAPTER 6

HAND, WRIST, FOREARM, AND ELBOW

The advent of special studies has allowed us to diagnose and recommend treatment for many more athletic injuries which may have, in the past, gone unrecognized or been misdiagnosed. Bone scans have proved to be extremely helpful in evaluating patients with a suggestive history for a fracture about the hand and wrist but normal routine radiographs. Although the bone scan tends not to be specific for injury pattern, it is rather specific for location of injury and is most helpful in identifying an occult fracture such as a fracture of the hook of the hamate or the body of the lunate. It is also useful in identifying acute soft tissue injuries such as a torn scapholunate or lunotriquetral ligament.

Tomograms, including trispiral or hypocycloidal tomography, are most helpful in evaluating the carpus for acute fractures as well as for assessing healing of fractures following prolonged immobilization.

The CT scan has found, to date, only limited use in the hand and wrist in the diagnosis and treatment of athletic injuries. It has been most helpful in evaluating the distal radioulnar joint for subluxation or dislocation. Its greatest merit in evaluating the distal radioulnar joint is its ability to assess congruency of the ulnar head in the sigmoid notch in various positions of forearm rotation, either in or out of plaster.

The arthrogram, and in particular the triple injection arthrogram, and in recent years magnetic resonance imaging have been most helpful in assessing carpal ligamentous injuries. When the plain film or motion study of the wrist reveals a carpal diastasis such as in rotary subluxation of the scaphoid, an arthrogram or MR of the wrist is not necessary, as the diagnosis is apparent to all. In patients, however, who have sustained a hyperextension injury to the wrist associated with pain in the region of the scapholunate or lunotriquetral junction without carpal malalignment or dissociation, an arthrogram and to a lesser extent an MR study are most helpful in elucidating a ligamentous perforation. Great caution, however, must be exercised by the clinician not to overread some of the arthrographic studies that erroneously have been interpreted as a tear but in fact are simple perforations that may be degenerative in nature.

As stated above, an individual sustaining an athletic injury to the hand and wrist should be evaluated carefully as soon as possible following the injury, with a careful history and physical examination as well as routine radiographic studies. Some have recommended, following this initial evaluation, prior to proceeding with more extensive radiographic evaluation, direct visualization of the injury site, i.e., arthroscopy. Wrist arthroscopy in the last few years has gained considerable acceptance and is now a commonly performed procedure. Arthroscopy of the small joints of the hand and wrist is still in its infancy. Although one can learn a lot by arthroscoping injuries acutely and at times one can learn more this way than with any other known study, I still believe that arthroscopy should be viewed as an operative procedure and considerably more invasive than many of the radiographic studies listed above. At the present time, I use arthroscopy in evaluating athletic injuries to the hand and wrist more for the chronic problems such as chondromalacia, carpal instability, and triangular fibrocartilage complex (TFCC) perforations.

The finger joints, and to a lesser extent the wrist joint, are small in comparison with the major joints of the lower extremity but of equal importance. What appears to be a minor injury radiographically to the hand and wrist very possibly can represent a potentially devastating injury to the patient if not properly diagnosed in treatment. An example might be an apparent simple fracture to the distal phalanx of the ring finger in a competitive football player which, in fact, represents an avulsion of the profundus tendon from its insertion at the base of the distal phalanx. Untreated, this profundus tendon avulsion would result in loss of terminal flexion of the ring finger, weakness of grasp of that hand, potentially an interference with the function of the other tendons of the hand and limited motion, and chronic pain. Careful evaluation of routine radiographic studies of the hand and wrist and their interpretation in light of the known anatomic structures which lie in proximity to the area being evaluated are imperative if we are to do away with the antiquated term *sprain* when referring to athletic injuries of the hand and wrist. The sophisticated imaging studies that are now available to us will only serve to heighten our ability to diagnose what have become very common injuries in today's society.

ANDREW K. PALMER, M.D.
Professor of Orthopedic Surgery and Director, Hand Surgery Service
SUNY Health Science Center
Syracuse, New York

TRAUMA TO THE HAND and wrist makes up one-fourth of all athletic injuries and is an important cause of disability.[1] The relative frequency of hand injury varies significantly from one sport to another (Table 6-1). If overlooked, injuries to the hand and wrist may result in serious long-term complications leading to functional impairment, deformity, and permanent incapacity. Appropriate management of athletic injuries requires prompt and accurate assessment, and advanced imaging techniques play a key role in their diagnosis.

In addition to the standard plain film radiographic evaluation, special views are useful in visualizing such hidden areas as the hook of the hamate and the articulation of the pisiform with the triquetrum.[2,3] Ligamentous assessment may require stress examination as well as fluoroscopic and arthrographic evaluation.[4–7] Tears of the triangular fibrocartilage complex (TFCC) as well as diagnosis and localization of ganglia and of muscle, nerve, and tendinous disorders may be best recognized with either arthrography or magnetic resonance imaging (MRI).[8,9] The advent of high-resolution thin section computed tomography (CT) is proving itself to be a valuable tool in the detection of occult carpal bone fracture and in the assessment of osseous healing.[10–14] The development of three-dimensional CT holds promise for potentially useful carpal tunnel and spatial analyses as well as for the assessment and treatment planning of complex fractures and dislocations.[15]

TABLE 6-1

Relative frequency of hand injuries compared with total injuries[a]

Sport	Percentage
Boxing	31
Handball	30
Volleyball	23
Basketball	19
Gymnastics	17
Skiing	16
Judo	10
Soccer	10
Ice hockey	5

[a] *Adapted from Amadio PC: Epidemiology of hand and wrist injuries in sports. Hand Clinics 6:379–381, 1990; with permission.*

MR imaging can provide important information in the diagnosis of avascular necrosis as well as in less common problems such as infiltrative marrow disorders caused by either neoplasm or infection. Additionally, MR is especially helpful in the identification of soft tissue abnormalities including focal overuse synovitis, carpal tunnel syndrome, TFCC injury, ganglia, and neoplasms.[16,17]

Triple-phase bone scanning (TPBS) is useful in demonstrating normal nuclide activity (Fig. 6-1) as well as in assessing both acute and chronic problems.[18–21] Specific entities that can be clearly identified by TPBS include occult and stress fractures, reflex sympathetic dystrophy (RSD), and vascular lesions such as aneurysm and thrombosis. TPBS

can also be helpful in the evaluation of posttraumatic synovitis, acute avulsion injuries, and fracture healing.[22–24]

In the forearm and elbow, the most problematic injuries involving stress and overuse include such entities as tendinitis, epicondylitis, bursitis, stress fracture, osteochondritis dissecans, and traction spur.[25–30] TPBS is especially helpful in evaluating overuse problems in this region, first by demonstrating the early degree of hyperemia or inflammation (blood flow and blood pool phases), followed by demonstrating nuclide activity accumulating focally, which indicates a local abnormality (high-resolution delayed images).[20,31] MR is effective in the elbow in the detection and evaluation of osteochondritis dissecans.[32]

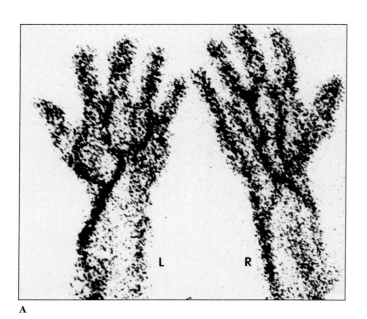

A

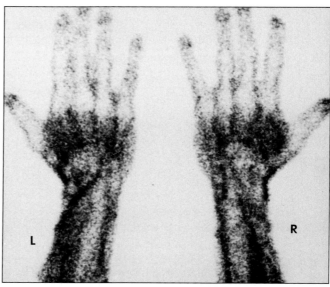

B

Figure 6-1   Normal TPBS of Hand and Wrist. **A.** *Dynamic flow study of the hand and wrist demonstrates isotope in the radial and ulnar arteries with symmetric perfusion of the digits.*
B. *The blood pool phase several minutes after injection demonstrates isotope accumulation in the soft tissues. Note that in the hand and wrist the greatest accumulation is in the thenar region.*
C. *High-resolution delayed images taken several hours after injection show a normal distribution of isotope with the greatest activity seen in the carpal bones as well as the metacarpophalangeal and interphalangeal joints.*

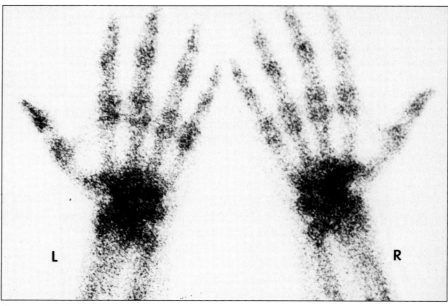

C

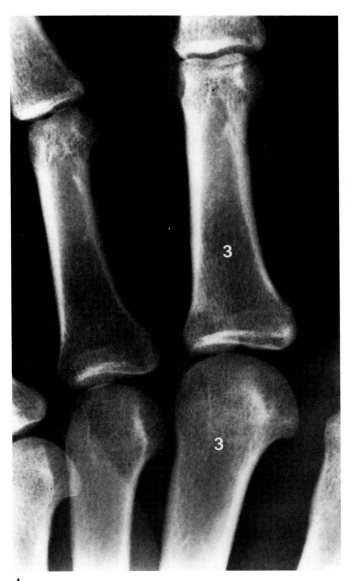

A

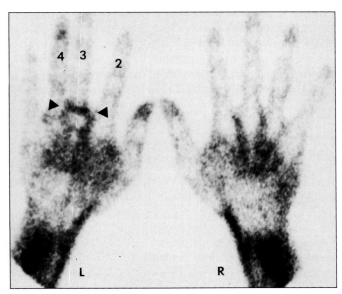

B

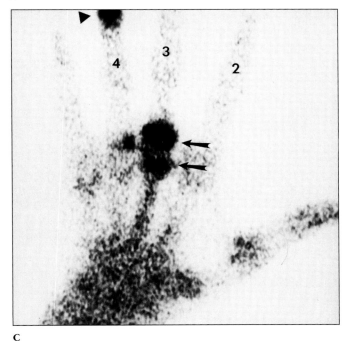

C

Figure 6-2   Phalangeal and Metacarpal Fractures. *Top-ranked professional boxer with healing fracture of left fourth distal interphalangeal joint (DIP) joint also has acute pain at the base of the proximal phalanx of the third metacarpophalangeal joint.* **A.** *Coned radiographs of the left third metacarpophalangeal joint are normal.* **B.** *Blood pool image of the TPBS demonstrates a horizontal area of increased nuclide activity at the base of the proximal phalanx of the left third finger. Arrowheads = isotope at base of left middle finger.* **C.** *High-resolution delayed image of TPBS shows increased activity on both sides of the left third metacarpophalangeal joint (most intense at the base of the proximal phalanx of the middle finger). These combined findings (positive on both blood pool and delayed images) suggest an acute fracture. The increased activity of the left third metacarpal head on delayed images only is not consistent with an occult fracture but rather a ''bone bruise.'' Increased activity at the left fourth DIP joint is again noted (old healing fracture). Arrowhead = fourth left DIP joint; arrows = increased activity, left third metacarpophalangeal joint.*

ACUTE PROBLEMS

There is a broad spectrum of acute hand and wrist injuries that occur in the athlete. Physicians unfamiliar with the complex nature of hand and wrist problems may tend to minimize their severity and importance.[33] Acute fractures of the wrist and hand account for nearly 8 percent of all fractures that occur in organized athletic activities.[34]

Fractures of the phalanges, metacarpals, and carpals (Figs. 6-2 to 6-12)

Fractures of the phalanges and metacarpals are most common in sports such as boxing, handball, and gymnastics, where the hand is the main point of contact.[1] A large study of hand and wrist injuries associated with boxing demonstrated that the most common site of fracture involved the thumb and represented 39 percent of the hand and wrist fractures sustained by boxers. This was followed by fractures involving the bases of the second through fifth metacarpals (35 percent). Fractures of the phalanges and metacarpal shafts accounted for the remaining 26 percent.[35] TPBS is especially helpful in detecting occult fractures and in separating acute fractures from healing fractures (Fig. 6-2).

Fracture and dislocation of a carpal bone are common athletic injuries; one report demonstrates carpal fracture in 1 percent of football players.[36] The scaphoid is the most commonly fractured carpal bone (70 to 80 percent), usually resulting from a fall on the outstretched hand forcing the scaphoid against the styloid process of the radius.[2] The location of the fracture is critical in determining the prognosis for healing and the likelihood of developing avascular necrosis. Seventy percent of scaphoid fractures involve the scaphoid waist, 20 percent the proximal pole, and 10 percent the distal pole.[2] One study estimates that 30 percent of scaphoid waist fractures and 100 percent of proximal pole fractures will develop avascular necrosis. Other problems associated with scaphoid fracture include delayed union, nonunion, fragment displacement, and the late development of carpal instability.[36]

Often, routine radiographs do not reveal the presence of carpal fracture. Not infrequently, the presumption of a nondisplaced scaphoid fracture may be confirmed by taking radiographs after a delay of 7 to 10 days. Should more aggressive imaging be indicated, TPBS can determine acute fracture in greater than 95 percent of the cases within 24 h of injury. The blood flow and blood pool images show a generalized increase in nuclide activity in the area of injury, with delayed images showing an intense focus of activity (''hot spot'') localizing the occult carpal fracture[18,20,21] (Fig. 6-3).

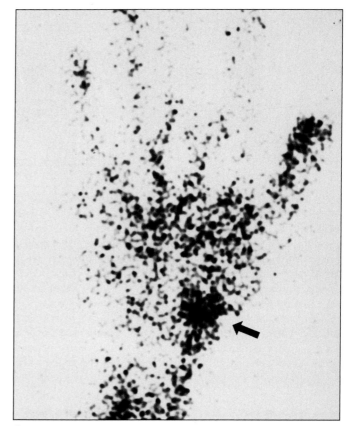

Figure 6-3 Scaphoid Fracture. *Lacrosse player with wrist trauma, pain, and normal radiographs.* **A.** *Blood flow phase of TPBS shows focal accumulation of isotope in the proximal carpal row radially. Arrow = area of increased isotope flow.* (Fig. 6-3B and C continues on the opposite page.)

A

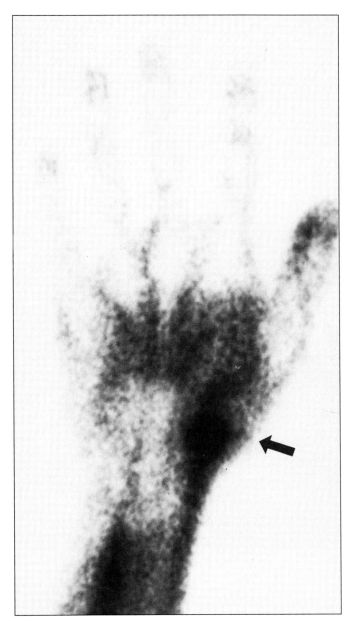

B

Figure 6-3   Scaphoid Fracture (Continued). **B.** *Blood pool phase of TPBS shows increased isotope in the same area as shown in the blood flow phase. Arrow = scaphoid activity.* **C.** *High-resolution delayed image of TPBS shows focally intense activity in the region of the scaphoid representing an occult fracture. Arrow = scaphoid fracture. (From Martire JR: The role of nuclear medicine scans in evaluating pain in athletic injuries. Clinics in Sports Medicine 6:713–737, 1987. Reprinted with permission.)*

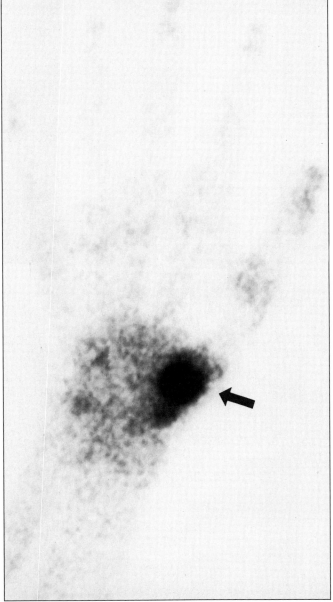

C

Once a scaphoid fracture is identified, a high-resolution thin section CT examination may prove useful in analyzing the alignment and position of fragments. In performing the CT examination, it is most useful to align the fracture such that the axis of the CT scan crosses perpendicularly to the fracture line. In this way, the fracture line and the position of the bony fragments will best be seen (Fig. 6-4). Following scaphoid fracture, volar rotation of the distal pole of the scaphoid with posterior displacement of the proximal aspect of that fragment leads to a "humpback" deformity which, if uncorrected, will result in malunion or nonunion (Fig. 6-5). Although MR imaging may demonstrate the fracture line (Fig. 6-6), the CT exam provides more detailed visualization of fine bony structure. MR is effective in showing bony contusion and intraosseous hemorrhage.[37] Stress fracture of the scaphoid is uncommon and appears to be the result of repeated compressive and dorsiflexion loads. It is not surprising that the most scaphoid stress fractures have been found in gymnasts who perform maneuvers requiring repeated dorsiflexion.[38,39] TPBS is a sensitive modality in detecting both stress and occult fractures of the scaphoid.

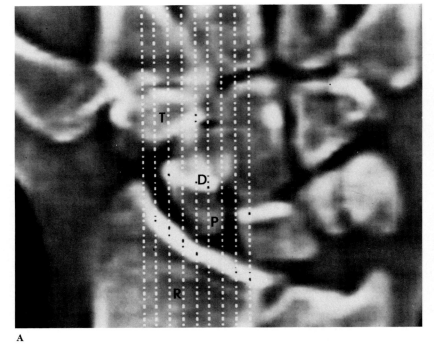

A

Figure 6-4 Scaphoid Fracture. **A.** *Antero-posterior projection of the wrist obtained as a "scout scan" from the CT scanner demonstrates the hand positioned such that the axis of each scan intersects perpendicularly to the fracture line, which, in this case, traverses the waist of the scaphoid bone.* **B.** *Direct sagittal CT scan shows an acute scaphoid fracture without displacement of bony fragments. Arrow = fracture line; P = proximal fragment; D = distal fragment; R = radius; T = trapezium.*

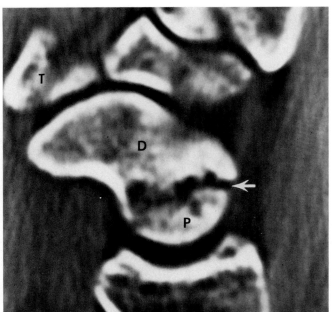

B

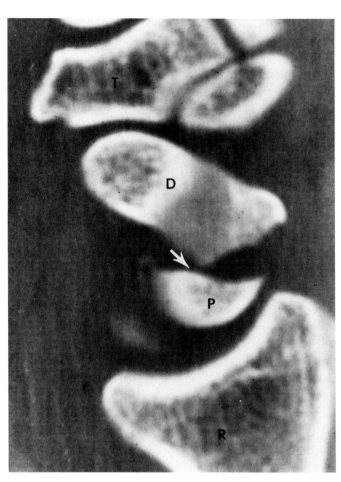

◄ **Figure 6-5**   Scaphoid Fracture (displaced). *Direct sagittal scan through the scaphoid demonstrates a displaced fracture through the proximal pole of the scaphoid causing a "humpback" deformity. Arrow = fracture line; P = proximal fragment; D = distal fragment; R = radius; T = trapezium.*

Figure 6-6   Scaphoid Fracture. *MR scan in the coronal plane at T2-weighted sequence demonstrates a band of low-signal intensity (arrow) representing a fracture within the midportion of the scaphoid. High-signal intensity in the proximal (P) and distal (D) fragments indicates bone viability in both areas. (From Levinsohn EM: Evaluation of wrist pain.* Radiology Report *2:60–68, 1989. Reprinted with permission of CV Mosby.)*
▼

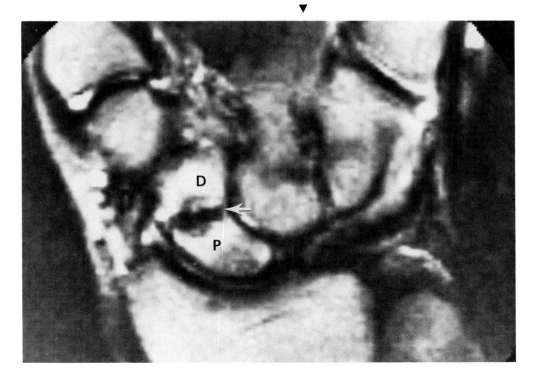

Fractures of carpal bones other than the scaphoid occur with much less frequency. Occult lunate fractures can be shown both by CT and TPBS (Figs. 6-7 and 6-8). Hook of the hamate fractures result from blunt trauma to the hamate hook and occur typically in those sports where a direct blow against the hook of the hamate is caused by the handle of a tennis racquet, golf club, or baseball bat during a swing[40] (Drawing I). High-resolution CT provides greater image detail and is more diagnostically useful at a lower radiation dose than is routine tomography when used to visualize subtle carpal fractures. These fractures may be visualized on radiographs taken in the carpal tunnel projection as well as on oblique views of the wrist. If some doubt still remains following those exposures, high-resolution CT and TPBS are quite accurate in securing their diagnosis[2,41-43] (Figs. 6-9 and 6-10). Bilateral fractures of the hook of the hamate have also been reported.[44] Using multiple views of the delayed images of a TPBS, one can accurately recognize the individual carpal bones and localize the site of virtually any carpal fracture[20] (Figs. 6-11 and 6-12).

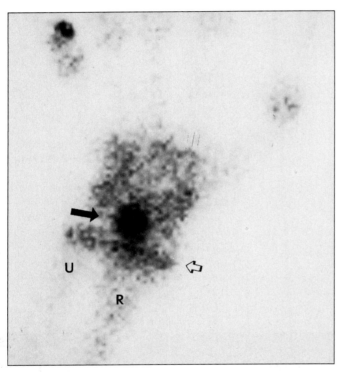

Figure 6-7 Lunate Fracture. *High-resolution delayed image from TPBS of right wrist in the palmar projection shows a focal area of increased activity (black arrow) corresponding to a lunate fracture. Radiographs were normal. U = distal ulna; R = distal radius; black arrow = lunate activity; open arrow = normally increased activity in distal physis of the radius in an adolescent.*

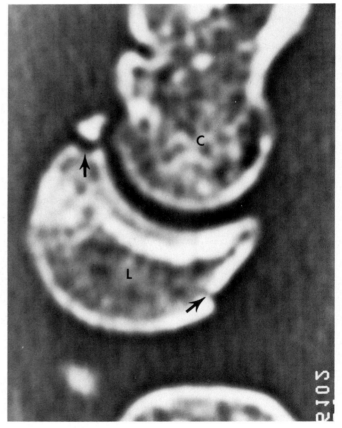

Figure 6-8 Lunate Fractures. *Direct sagittal CT scan through the lunate demonstrates a tiny avulsion fracture off the volar pole distally as well as cortical interruption dorsally. These fractures were not visible on plain radiographs. Arrows = fracture lines; L = lunate; C = capitate.*

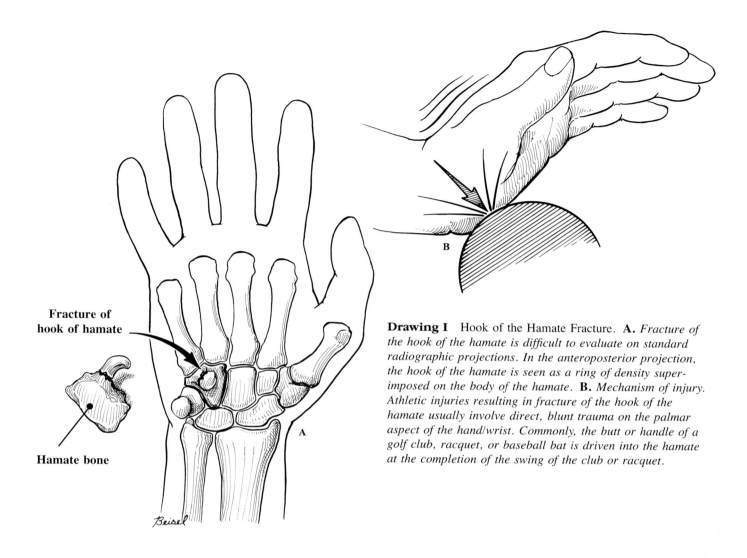

Fracture of hook of hamate

Hamate bone

Beisel

Drawing I Hook of the Hamate Fracture. **A.** *Fracture of the hook of the hamate is difficult to evaluate on standard radiographic projections. In the anteroposterior projection, the hook of the hamate is seen as a ring of density superimposed on the body of the hamate.* **B.** *Mechanism of injury. Athletic injuries resulting in fracture of the hook of the hamate usually involve direct, blunt trauma on the palmar aspect of the hand/wrist. Commonly, the butt or handle of a golf club, racquet, or baseball bat is driven into the hamate at the completion of the swing of the club or racquet.*

Figure 6-9 Hook of Hamate Fracture. **A.** *Blood pool images of TPBS demonstrate mildly increased activity in the distal carpal row corresponding to hamate bone hyperemia. Black arrow = hamate activity.* (Fig. 6-9B and C continues on next page.)

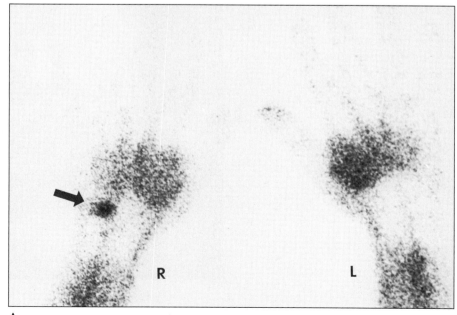

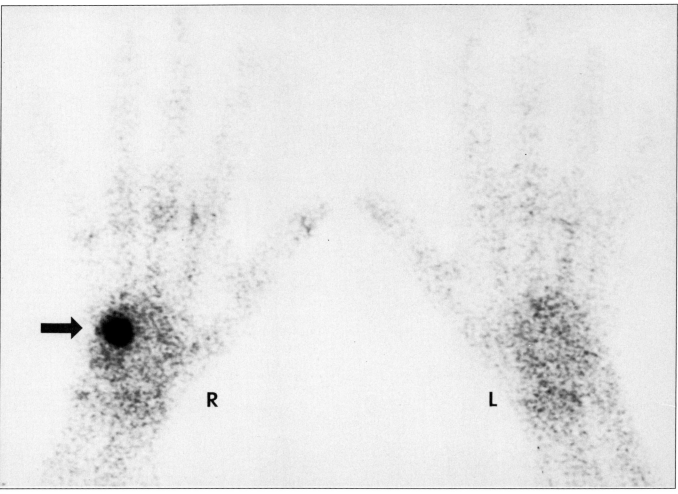

B

Figure 6-9 Hook of Hamate Fracture (Continued). **B.** *High-resolution delayed image of TPBS shows a region of focally intense activity corresponding to an occult hamate fracture in a tennis player with wrist pain and normal radiographs. Black arrow = hamate activity. C. CT scan through the hook of the hamate shows the fracture line. Black arrowheads = fracture line through the hook of the hamate (see Drawing I).*

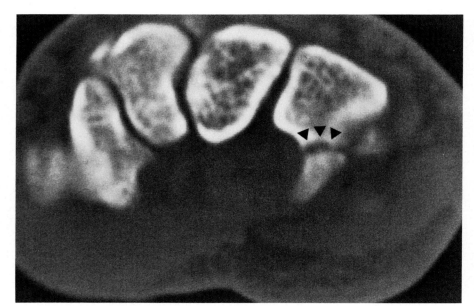

C

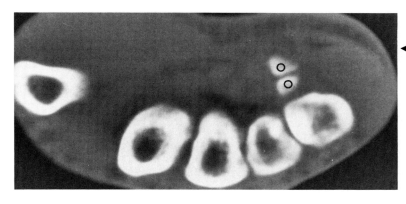

◀ **Figure 6-10**   Hamate Hook Ossicles. *CT scan in the axial plane at the level of the hook of the hamate shows two small ossicles. The smooth borders indicate these to be accessory centers of ossification rather than fractures. O = accessory ossicles.*

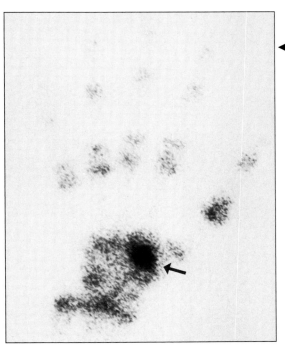

◀ **Figure 6-11**   Trapezoid Fracture. *High-resolution delayed image of TPBS shows focally increased activity in the distal carpal row of the right hand corresponding to an occult fracture of the trapezoid bone. Black arrow = increased trapezoid activity consistent with fracture.*

Figure 6-12   Triquetrum ▶
Fracture. *High-resolution delayed images of both hands and wrists show focally intense activity in the proximal row of the right wrist representing an occult fracture of the triquetrum in an athlete with normal radiographs. Black arrow = increased triquetral activity/ fracture.*

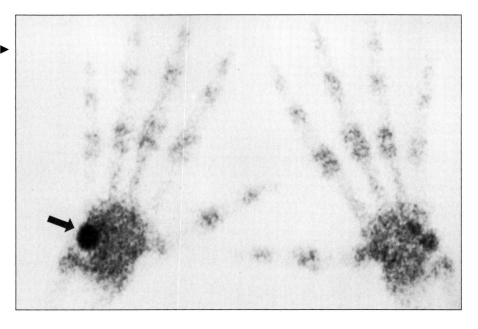

Radial-ulnar fractures and TFCC injuries (Figs. 6-13 to 6-25)

Avulsion injuries at the sites of insertion of tendons and ligaments are often difficult to visualize with routine radiographs unless a small piece of avulsed bone can be seen. TPBS gives us the ability to find these subtle injuries. Characteristically, these avulsion injuries show increased activity on the early blood flow and blood pool images in the most superficial portion of the injured long bone. On delayed views, we typically see a linear, vertical focus of increased activity (in contrast to the more common rounded focus of activity) in the region which corresponds to the insertion site of the tendon or ligament[20] (Fig. 6-13, Drawing II).

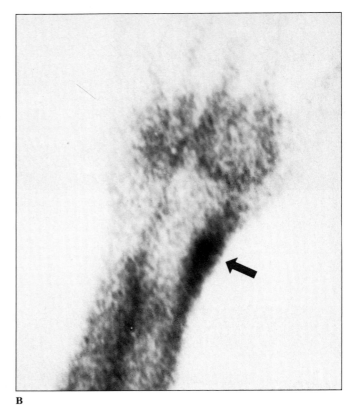

B

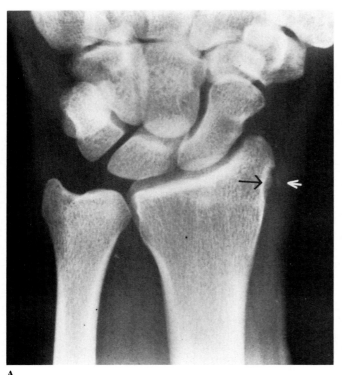

A

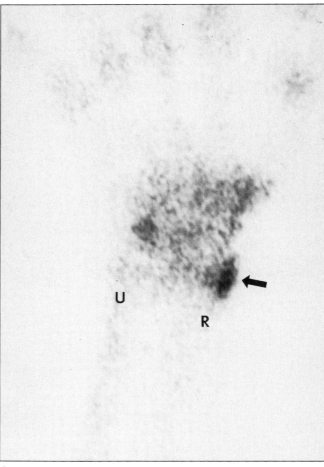

C

Figure 6-13 Insertional/Avulsion Injury of Radial Styloid. **A.** *Anteroposterior radiograph of left wrist in a 50-year-old male golfer with left wrist pain brought on by driving golf balls. Black arrow = cortical irregularity of the radial styloid process;* white arrow = *tiny calcification or avulsion fragment in the adjacent soft tissues.* **B.** *Blood pool phase of TPBS shows increased activity in the region of the styloid process. Black arrow = radial styloid activity.* **C.** *High-resolution delayed image of TPBS shows increased activity linearly and peripherally in the region of the radial styloid corresponding to the insertion site of the brachioradialis tendon. Black arrow = activity at site of avulsion injury (see Drawing II).*

Although fractures of the long bones of the forearm are usually easily recognized and evaluated with standard radiographs, assessment in and around joints may be difficult and TPBS may prove diagnostic[6,11–14] (Fig. 6-14). Fracture with intraarticular extension is an important entity requiring anatomic restoration for a good functional result. High-resolution CT is an ideal tool to make that diagnosis and to determine the location of bony fragments (Fig. 6-15).

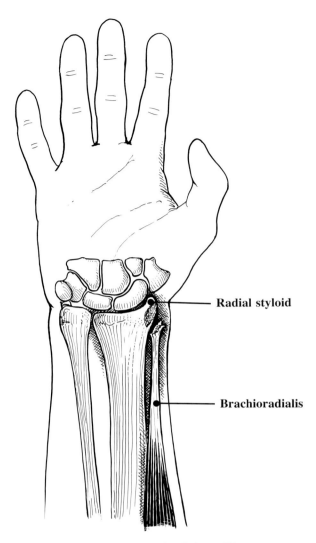

Drawing II   Radial Styloid Insertion Injury. *The brachioradialis tendon inserts at the level of the styloid process of the radius. Athletes with point tenderness localized to that area should be suspected of having an insertional injury which may be associated with a tiny avulsed fragment.*

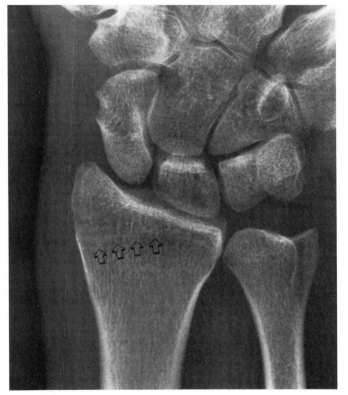

A

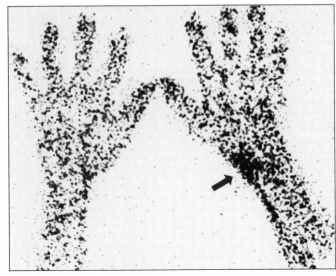

B

Figure 6-14   Distal Radius Fracture. *Male racquetball player complained of persistent left wrist pain.* **A.** *Posteroanterior radiograph of the left wrist in ulnar deviation shows a faint sclerotic line in the distal portion of the radius felt to represent possibly an occult fracture. Open arrows = subtle fracture line.* **B.** *Blood flow phase of TPBS shows mildly increased activity in the region of the distal portion of the left radius. Black arrow = increased nuclide activity.* (Fig. 6-14C and D continues on next page.)

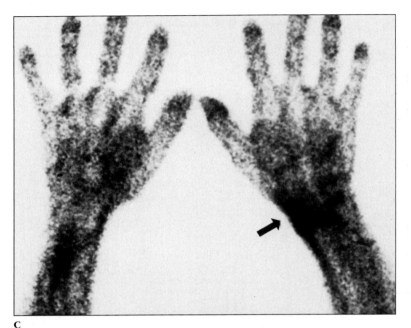

C

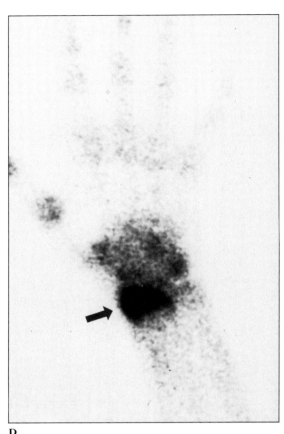

D

Figure 6-14 Distal Radius Fracture (Continued). **C.** *Blood pool phase of TPBS shows increased activity adjacent to the distal portion of the left radius. Black arrow = increased activity, distal left radius.* **D.** *High-resolution delayed image of TPBS shows focally increased activity in the distal portion of the radius representing an occult fracture. Black arrow = site of occult fracture.*

Figure 6-15 Radius Fracture. **A.** *Direct sagittal CT through the radius shows a fracture of the volar corner with anterior displacement of the bony fragment.* **B.** *Direct sagittal scan through the midradius to include the lunate and capitate bones shows fragment displacement with volar subluxation of the lunate. Arrow = fracture line; F = bony fragment; S = scaphoid; L = lunate; R = radius; C = capitate.*

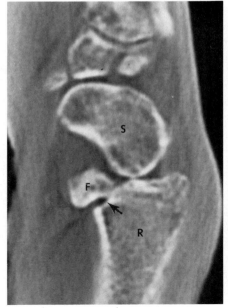

A

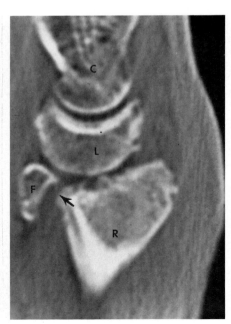

B

Fracture-dislocation of the ulna in the region of the distal radioulnar joint can best be assessed with CT[45-48] (Figs. 6-16 and 6-17). Normally, the distal articulating surface of the ulna congruently articulates with the sigmoid notch of the distal radius. That relationship is constant with the hand positioned in either pronation or supination[46] (Fig. 6-18). Although disruption of the distal radioulnar joint (DRUJ) is usually posttraumatic, rarely may this present as a congenital abnormality.[49]

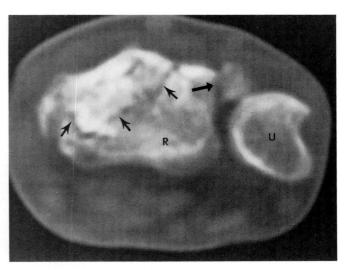

Figure 6-17   Radius Fracture with Intraarticular Extension. *Axial CT scan through the distal radius at the DRUJ shows fractures of the radius with intraarticular extension and DRUJ incongruity. R = radius; U = ulna; arrows = fracture lines.*

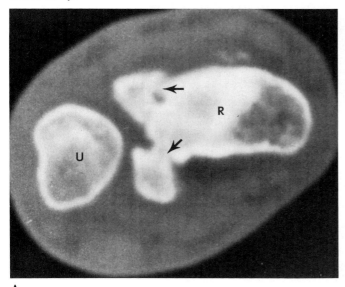

A

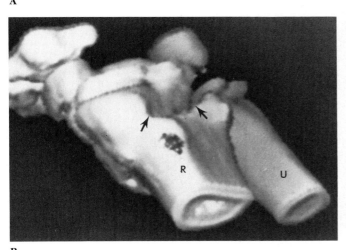

B

Figure 6-16   Radius Fracture with Intraarticular Extension. **A.** *CT scan in the axial plane through the distal metaphysis of the radius shows a fracture with volar displacement and incongruity of the articulating surface at the distal radioulnar joint (DRUJ).* **B.** *Three-dimensional reconstructed image derived from thin section continuous axial scans shows a fracture of the distal metaphysis of the radius with intraarticular extension and DRUJ incongruity. R = radius; U = ulna; arrows = fractures. (From Levinsohn EM: Imaging of the wrist.* Radiologic Clinics of North America *28(5):905–921, 1990. Reprinted with permission.)*

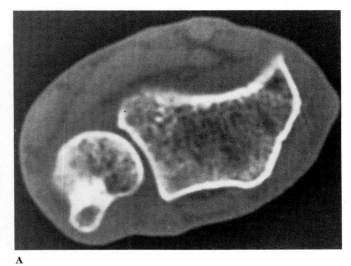

A

Figure 6-18   Normal Articulation at DRUJ. **A.** *Axial CT scan with the wrist supinated shows congruent articulation of the distal ulna within the sigmoid notch of the radius.* (Fig. 6-18B and C continues on next page.)

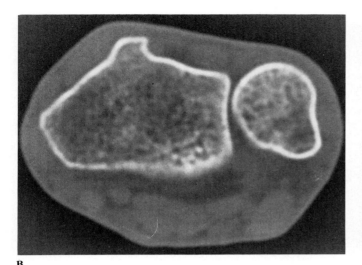

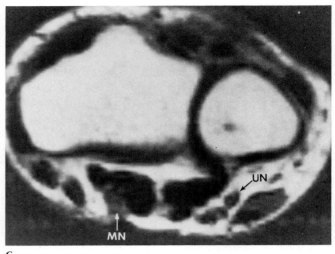

B

C

Figure 6-18 Normal Articulation at DRUJ (Continued). **B.** *Axial scan with wrist pronated shows persisting congruent articulation. Normally this joint remains congruent both in* *pronation and in supination. Subluxation or dislocation does not normally occur.* **C.** *MR scan with the wrist pronated shows normal articulation at the DRUJ. The low-signal volar* *structures represent the flexor tendons, and the dorsally located low-signal structures represent extensor tendons. The median nerve (MN) and ulnar nerve (UN) are indicated.*

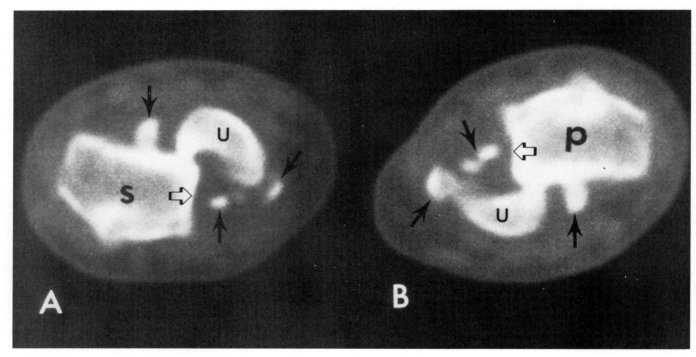

Figure 6-19 Fracture Dislocation of the Ulna at DRUJ. **A.** *Axial CT scan through the DRUJ with the wrist supinated (S) shows volar dislocation of the ulna from the sigmoid notch of the radius.* **B.** *Axial scan with the wrist pronated (P) shows persisting volar dislocation of a fragmented ulna. Arrows = bony fragments; U = ulna; open arrow = sigmoid notch of radius. (From Mino DE, Palmer AK, Levinsohn EM: Radiography and computerized tomography in the diagnosis of incongruity of the distal radio-ulnar joint. The Journal of Bone and Joint Surgery 67(A):247–212, 1985. Reprinted with permission.)*

With DRUJ instability, pronation forces may result in dorsal displacement of the ulna and supination forces in volar displacement. Although this diagnosis can occasionally be made on lateral radiographs of the wrist in neutral rotation, CT of the DRUJ is an accurate and easily obtainable examination for securing that diagnosis.[50] Since subluxation or dislocation of the distal ulna from the sigmoid notch may be positionally dependent, the CT examination should be designed to provide images with both hyperpronation and hy-persupination (Figs. 6-19 and 6-20). In addition to the dorsal or the volar subluxation or dislocation which may occur, distal dislocations may follow radial shaft fracture with shortening.[51,52] The CT examination in this setting may demonstrate the shaft of the ulna to articulate with the sigmoid notch, and dorsal or volar displacement may not be present (Fig. 6-21). Finally, occult fractures of the distal ulna or ulnar styloid process, with normal or equivocal radiographs, can be confirmed with TPBS (Fig. 6-22).

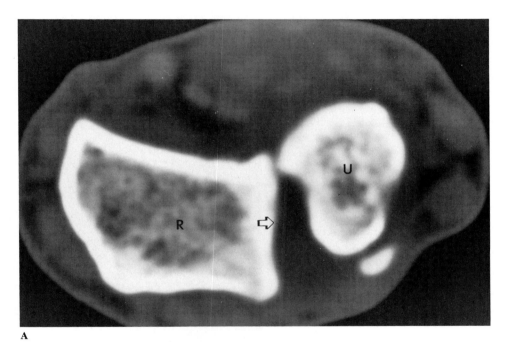

A

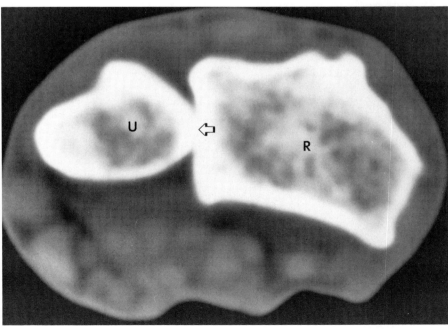

B

Figure 6-20   Dislocation of the Ulna at the DRUJ. **A.** *Axial CT scan with the wrist fully supinated shows volar dislocation of the ulna from the sigmoid notch of the radius.* **B.** *With pronation, the ulna articulates normally within the sigmoid notch. R = radius; U = ulna; open arrow = sigmoid notch.*

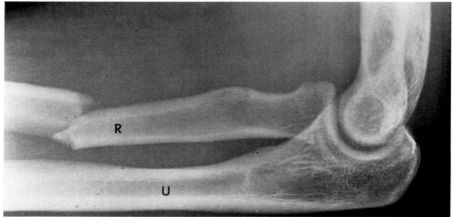

A

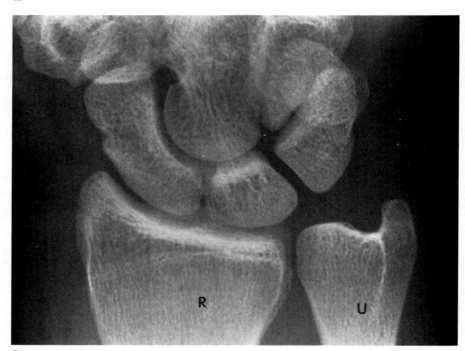

B

Figure 6-21 Fractured Radius with Distal Dislocation of Ulna. **A.** *Lateral radiograph of the proximal forearm shows a fracture of the radius with shortening.* **B.** *Posteroanterior radiograph of the wrist shows 2-mm ulna plus variance to be present.* **C.** *Axial CT scan through the DRUJ shows the ulna to be congruently located within the sigmoid notch of the radius.* **D.** *Coronal reconstruction derived from the axial examination shows marked ulna plus variance to be present. R = radius; U = ulna; open arrow = sigmoid notch of radius.*

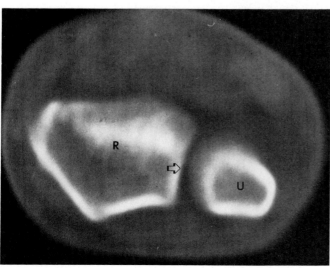

C

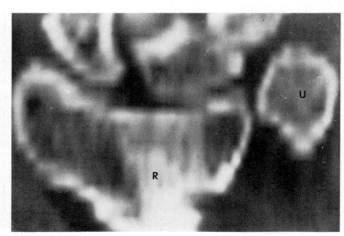

D

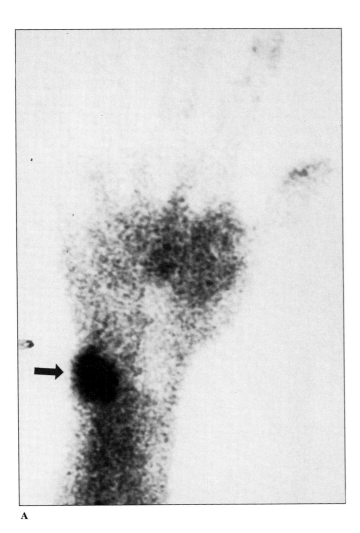

A

Figure 6-22   Fracture, Ulnar Styloid Process. *High school football player complained of pain in the region of the ulnar styloid process following a fall. Radiographs were normal.* **A.** *Blood pool phase of TPBS demonstrates focally intense activity overlying the right ulnar styloid process. Black arrow = increased ulnar styloid activity.* **B.** *High-resolution delayed image of TPBS shows focally intense activity corresponding to the left ulnar styloid process suggestive of an occult fracture of the styloid process. Black arrow = ulnar styloid fracture site; U = distal ulna; R = distal radius.*

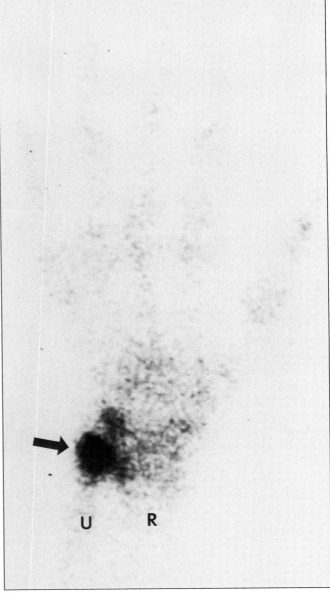

B

Wrist arthrography is generally considered to be a highly accurate examination when used to assess the triangular fibrocartilage complex (TFCC) as well as the intracarpal ligaments.[6,9,53–58] The traditional single-compartment examination performed by injecting contrast into the radiocarpal joint has in recent years been replaced by the three-compartment examination. Separate injections of contrast into the midcarpal compartment, radiocarpal joint, and DRUJ show up to 30 percent additional abnormality when compared with a single injection into only the radiocarpal joint.[59–61] The addition of CT to the wrist arthrogram has as yet not been shown to provide additional useful information.[62] Although MR accurately demonstrates the normal TFCC (Fig. 6-23) as well as tears of that structure (Figs. 6-24 and 6-25), the accuracy of the MR exam has not yet reached that of three-compartment wrist arthrography.[63]

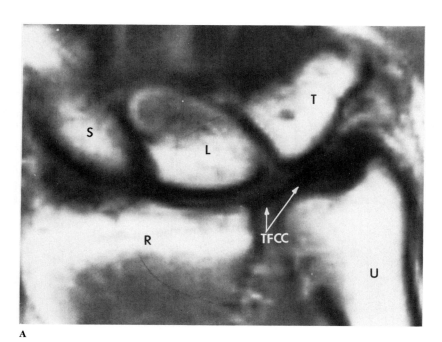

A

Figure 6-23 Normal Triangular Fibrocartilage Complex (TFCC). **A.** *MR scan in the coronal plane at T1-weighted sequence shows a low-signal structure representing an intact TFCC.* **B.** *A focus of intermediate signal lying between the TFCC and radius represents articular cartilage of the radius and is a normal anatomic feature in this location. This should not be mistaken for a TFCC perforation or tear. R = radius; U = ulna; S = scaphoid; L = lunate; T = triquetrum; TFCC = triangular fibrocartilage complex; arrow = normal articular cartilage between radius and TFCC.*

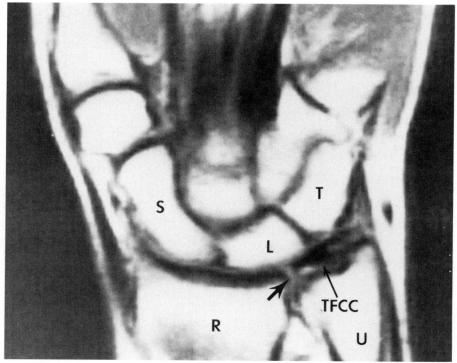

B

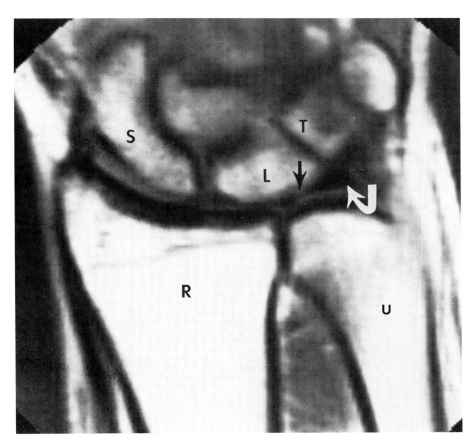

Figure 6-24 TFCC Tear. *MR scan in the coronal plane at T1-weighted sequence shows a focus of intermediate signal representing a tear within the midsubstance of the TFCC. Normally the TFCC shows uniformly low signal intensity throughout. Arrow = TFCC tear; R = radius; U = ulna; S = scaphoid; L = lunate; T = triquetrum; curved arrow = normal residual TFCC. (From Levinsohn EM: Imaging of the wrist. Radiologic Clinics of North America 28(5):905–921, 1990. Reprinted with permission.)*

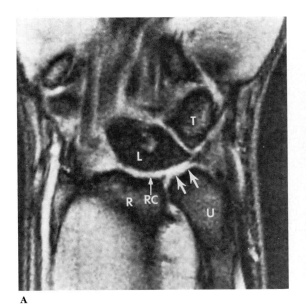

A

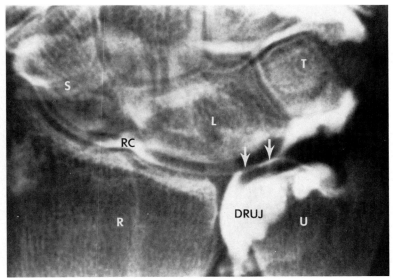

B

Figure 6-25 TFCC Tear. **A.** *MR scan in the coronal plane at a short TR gradient echo sequence shows a focus of high signal in the region of the TFCC representing a tear.* **B.** *Arthrogram shows communication of the radiocarpal joint with the distal radioulnar joint. This indicates TFCC perforation. Arrows = TFCC perforation; U = ulna; R = radius; S = scaphoid; T = triquetrum; L = lunate; RC = contrast in radiocarpal joint; DRUJ = contrast in distal radioulnar joint.*

CHRONIC PROBLEMS

Posttraumatic and inflammatory lesions of the hand and wrist (Figs. 6-26 to 6-36)

Complications of carpal bone fracture include delayed union, nonunion, instability, and avascular necrosis.[2,36,64,65] Scaphoid fracture notoriously may be complicated by nonunion and avascular necrosis. CT and MR both are useful diagnostic tools in helping to make these diagnoses. With CT, one sees a persisting fracture line with sclerosis of the bony margins at the fracture interface as evidence of nonunion (Fig. 6-26). CT may prove useful in assessing nonunion of a fracture despite the presence of a metallic screw stabilizing the proximal and distal fragments. In that situation, the axis of the CT scan should be directed parallel to

that of the screw in order to minimize the metallic artifact (Fig. 6-27). CT may provide sufficiently detailed images to clearly identify healing of a scaphoid fracture (Fig. 6-28). If avascular necrosis develops, increased density, often with fragmentation of the proximal fragment of the scaphoid, occurs. On MR imaging, loss of the normal high signal from the marrow space on T1- and T2-weighted sequences develops. Furthermore, a linear band of low signal at the fracture line on T1-weighted images may be accompanied by an adjacent high-signal line seen on the T2-weighted images (Figs. 6-29 and 6-30).

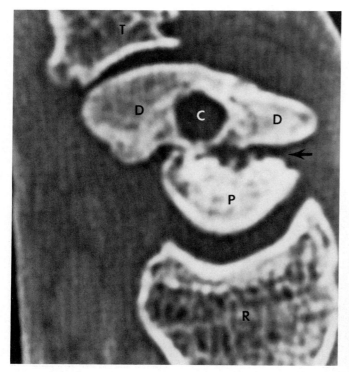

Figure 6-26   Scaphoid Fracture with Nonunion. *Direct sagittal CT scan through the scaphoid with the scan axis positioned perpendicular to the fracture line shows persisting fragment displacement without healing. A cyst has developed within the distal fragment. Arrow = fracture line; P = proximal fragment; D = distal fragment; R = radius; T = trapezium; C = cyst.*

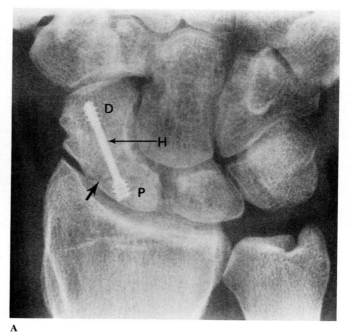

A

Figure 6-27   Scaphoid Fracture with Nonunion.
A. *Anteroposterior radiograph shows a fracture (arrow) through the midscaphoid stabilized with a Herbert screw (H). D = distal pole; P = proximal pole.* (Fig. 6-27B and C continues on the opposite page.)

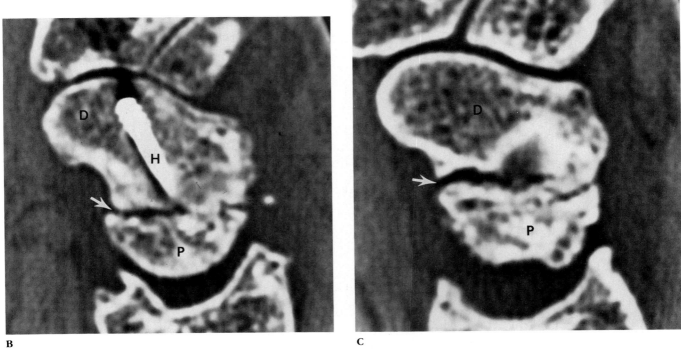

B   **C**

Figure 6-27   Scaphoid Fracture with Nonunion (Continued). **B.** *Direct sagittal CT scan parallel to the axis of a Herbert screw shows the position of that screw and demonstrates persisting fracture line.* **C.** *Direct sagittal CT scan just medial to the Herbert screw shows persisting fracture line without healing.*

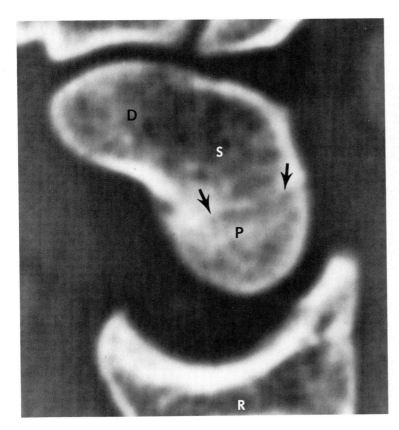

Figure 6-28   Scaphoid Fracture (Healed). *Direct sagittal CT scan through the midscaphoid shows a vague intraosseous lucency representing the site of a healed fracture without avascular necrosis. S = scaphoid; R = radius; arrows = healed fracture line; D = distal pole; P = proximal pole.*

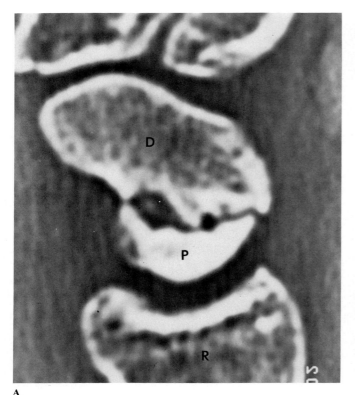

A

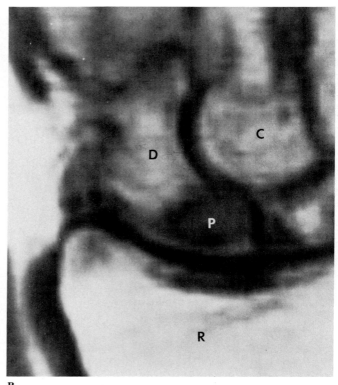

B

Figure 6-29 Scaphoid Fracture with Nonunion and Avascular Necrosis.
A. *Direct sagittal CT scan through the scaphoid shows a fracture line crossing the waist of the scaphoid without evidence for healing. Sclerosis of the proximal bony fragment indicates the*
development of avascular necrosis.
B. *MR scan of another patient with a transscaphoid fracture done in the coronal plane at T1-weighted sequence shows intermediate to low-signal intensity within the proximal scaphoid fragment representing avascular*
necrosis. The marrow space of the distal fragment and of the capitate and radius shows normally high signal. P = proximal fragment; D = distal fragment; R = radius; C = capitate.

Figure 6-30 Avascular Necrosis of the Scaphoid. **A.** *MR scan in the coronal plane at T1-weighted sequence demonstrates intermediate signal intensity diffusely involving the scaphoid with a band of low signal across the waist and focal areas of low signal within the proximal pole of the scaphoid. Normal signal is present within the adjacent bones.* (Fig. 30B continues on the opposite page.)

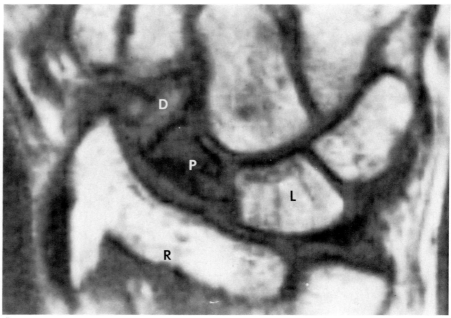

A

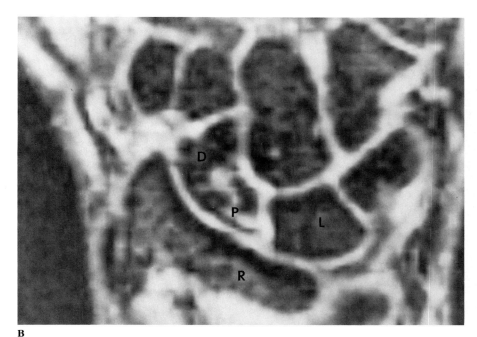

B

Figure 6-30   Avascular Necrosis of the Scaphoid (Continued). **B.** *MR scan in the coronal plane at a short TR gradient echo sequence shows focal areas of high signal within the proximal and midportions of the scaphoid. These changes represent avascular necrosis of the scaphoid with areas of revascularization. D = distal pole of scaphoid; P = proximal pole of scaphoid; L = lunate; R = radius.*

Figure 6-31   Avascular Necrosis of the Lunate. *MR scan in ▶ the sagittal plane at T1-weighted sequence through the lunate shows focal areas of low signal and intermediate signal within the lunate. Normal high-signal fat has been replaced by low-signal granulation tissue and dead fat cells. L = lunate; C = capitate; R = radius.*

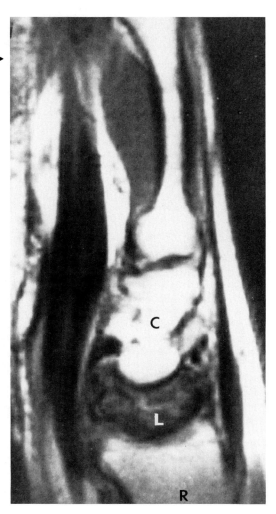

Avascular necrosis of the lunate is a somewhat more insidious problem, since preexisting trauma, which may have led to this complication, often is unrecognized (Fig. 6-31). One large prospective study showed MR imaging to be more specific than radiography or TPBS in making the diagnosis of ischemic necrosis of the lunate. Two patterns of lunate signal alteration were seen on MR imaging, demonstrating either focal or generalized signal loss on T1- and T2-weighted images.[66]

Cysts of the scaphoid (Fig. 6-32) or of the lunate (Figs. 6-33 and 6-34) may present with pain and weakness. This entity is easily recognized on CT as a well-defined lucency, sometimes with a communicating tract to the adjacent joint. On MR scans, the lucent defect shows intermediate signal on T1-weighted images and high-signal intensity with T2-weighting.

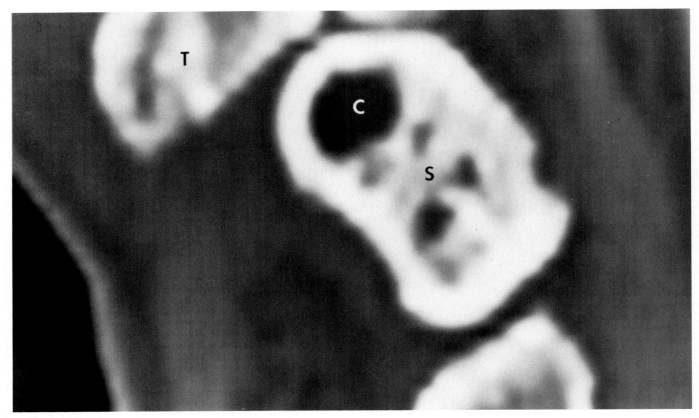

Figure 6-32   Scaphoid Cyst. *Sagittal CT scan through the scaphoid demonstrates a lucent defect within the distal pole representing a scaphoid cyst. The overlying bony cortex appears intact. S = scaphoid; C = cyst; T = trapezium.*

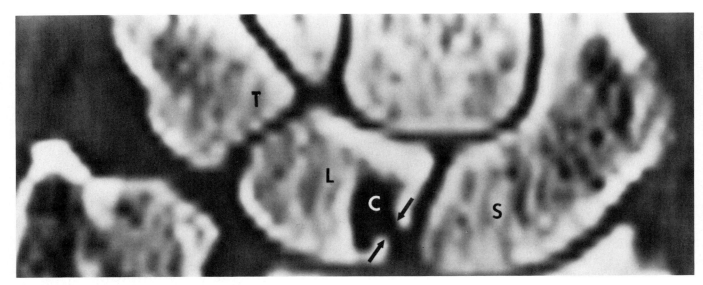

Figure 6-33   Lunate Cyst. *Coronal reconstruction derived from contiguous CT axial scans through the wrist demonstrates a lucency within the lunate representing a cyst. Interruption of the radial cortex of the lunate has occurred allowing communication of that cyst with the adjacent joint space. L = lunate; C = cyst; arrows = cortical interruption; S = scaphoid; T = triquetrum.*

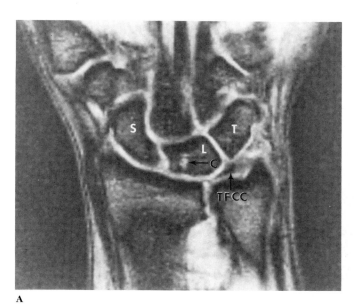

A

Figure 6-34 Lunate Cyst. **A.** *MR scan in the coronal plane at short TR gradient echo sequence shows a focal area of increased signal within the lunate representing a cyst. The hyalin cartilage shows high signal throughout. The low-signal TFCC is normal.* **B.** *MR scan in the coronal plane at T2-weighted sequence shows high signal within the lunate cyst.* **C.** *MR scan in the coronal plane at T2-weighted sequence through the volar aspect of the wrist shows high signal surrounding the pisiform indicating a joint effusion. L = lunate; S = scaphoid; T = triquetrum; P = pisiform; C = cyst; E = effusion; TFCC = triangular fibrocartilage complex.*

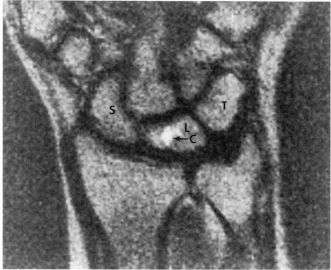

B

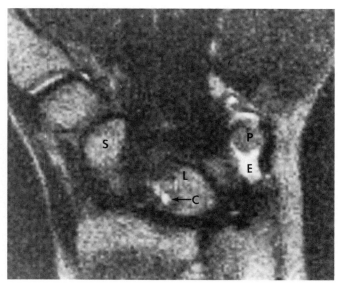

C

Posttraumatic synovitis is usually a clinical diagnosis based on history and physical exam. MR and TPBS can both help to confirm this diagnosis.[6,20] Joint effusion (Fig. 6-35), often related to posttraumatic synovitis, is easily identified on MR scans. Following trauma, persistent pain, despite normal radiographs, may indicate a posttraumatic synovitis. The TPBS is useful in helping exclude other causes of pain such as occult fracture, stress fracture, and RSD.[20] On TPBS, suspected posttraumatic synovitis is characterized by mildly to moderately increased blood flow in the involved area as well as generalized increased uptake on the delayed images corresponding to the hyperemia and inflammation of this entity (Fig. 6-36).

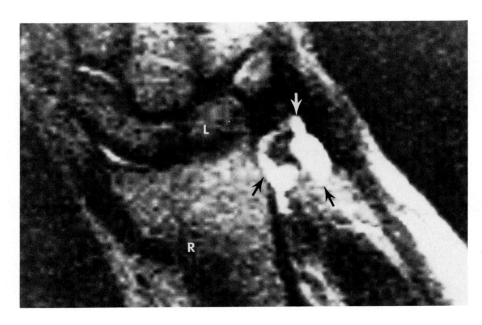

Figure 6-35 DRUJ Effusion. *MR scan in the coronal plane at T2-weighted sequence shows high signal within the DRUJ indicating an effusion. R = radius; L = lunate; arrows = effusion.*

Figure 6-36 Posttraumatic Tenosynovitis. *Twenty-five-year-old male weightlifter complained of chronic wrist pain despite normal radiographs. High-resolution delayed image of TPBS shows increased activity in the right wrist (when compared with the normal left wrist). This pattern of accumulation is most suggestive of an inflammatory process in the wrist such as tenosynovitis. Black arrows = increased nonspecific activity, right wrist.*

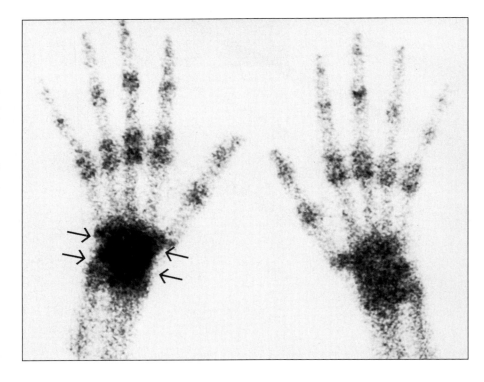

Overuse and stress problems (Figs. 6-37 to 6-47)

Wrist

Chronic wrist problems in the gymnast may result from a wide variety of causes (Table 6-2). The incidence of chronic injuries in gymnastics ranges from 17 to 43 percent overall, but dysfunction resulting from chronic overuse is estimated to account for 80 to 90 percent of these problems.[67–69] Some of the entities that must be considered include physeal stress reaction of the distal radius, tenosynovitis, and ganglia.[67,70] Although ganglia may be diagnosed arthrographically, the communicating track between the joint and the ganglion does not usually opacify sufficiently to demonstrate the ganglion.[71,72] Ganglia which are larger than 2 mm may be detectable by either sonography or MR[67] (Figs. 6-37 and 6-38). Additionally, premature closure of the distal radial growth plate leading to ulnar positive variance has been reported commonly in gymnasts and is best evaluated with plain film radiography.[73]

In general, CT and MR both provide tools to image the soft tissues and bones of the wrist.[74] Additionally, MR may show abnormalities in the carpal tunnel that are associated with the carpal tunnel syndrome.[75–77]

TABLE 6-2

Chronic gymnastic wrist injuries[a]

Bony
    Avascular necrosis capitate
    Scaphoid stress fracture
    Acquired Madelung's deformity
    Carpal chondromalacia
    Triquetrohamate impingement
    Ulnar impaction syndrome
    Scaphoid impaction syndrome
    Distal radius physeal stress reaction (compressive)
    Distal radius and ulnar physeal stress reaction (traction)
    Distal radius physeal arrest

Soft tissue
    Wrist capsulitis
    Wrist splints
    TFCC tear
    Ganglia
    Carpal instability
    Distal radioulnar joint instability

[a] Adapted from Dobyns JH, Gadel GT: Gymnast's wrist. Hand Clinics 6:493–505, 1990; with permission.

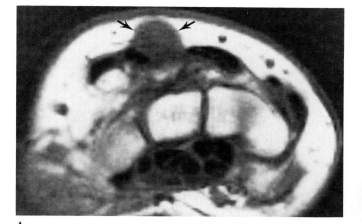

A

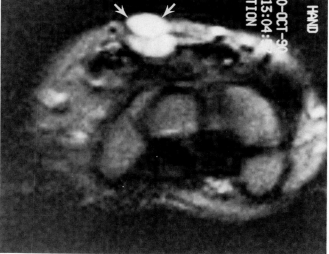

B

Figure 6-37 Dorsal Ganglion. **A.** *MR scan in the axial plane at T1-weighted sequence through the wrist shows a globular region of intermediate signal protruding dorsally.* **B.** *Similar image at T2-weighted sequence shows the globular protrusion to show high signal. These features are characteristic for a dorsal ganglion (arrows).*

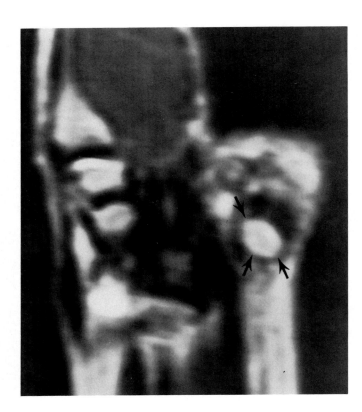

Figure 6-38 Volar Ganglion. *Coronal image through the palmar aspect of the wrist at T2-weighted sequence shows a globular high-signal focus corresponding to a volar ganglion (arrows).*

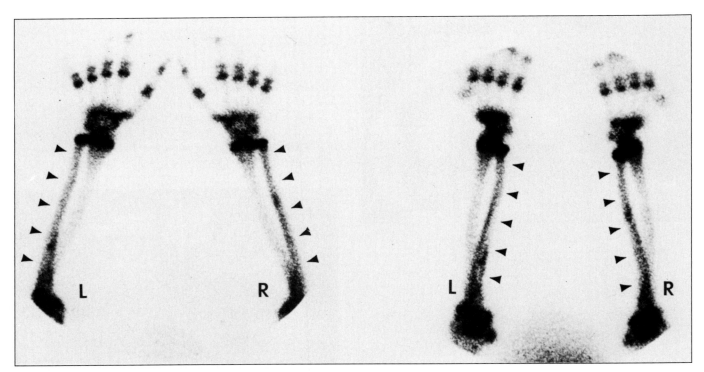

Figure 6-39 Bilateral Ulnar Stress Fracture. *High school football player complained of forearm pain caused by repeated curls associated with weightlifting. High-resolution delayed images of TPBS in the anterior and posterior projections show diffusely increased activity along the entire shaft of the ulna in both forearms when compared with the normal activity in the radius. This pattern suggests bilateral ulnar stress fractures. Black arrowheads = bilaterally increased activity in the ulnar shafts.*

Forearm

Stress fractures of the ulna are thought to be due to heavy overuse of the flexor muscles. Case reports have been noted in a variety of throwing, racquet, and lifting activities including tennis, baseball, and weightlifting and less commonly in volleyball and Kendo martial arts.[78-86] The dramatic increase in weight training, weightlifting, and bodybuilding has accounted for virtually all the ulnar stress fractures seen at our facility. The most common exercises associated with repeated overloading of the flexor muscles leading to ulnar stress fracture include curls (either long bar or dumbbell curls) and use of the preacher board (Figs. 6-39 and 6-40).

Elbow

In athletes the most common elbow symptoms that require advanced imaging tools for diagnosis include pain, swelling, and/or restricted motion. These are usually caused by chronic elbow overuse. Osteochondritis dissecans (OCD), if untreated, can lead to intraarticular loose bodies, degenerative joint disease, and locking. The most frequent site for elbow OCD is the capitellum. This condition results from repetitive compressive force between the radial head and the capitellum. When seen between the ages of 5 and 10 years, it is commonly referred to as *Panner's disease*. OCD is most commonly associated with those activities such as throwing, racquet sports, and gymnastics, in which there is a valgus stress across the elbow.[26,28-30,32,87] The radiographic workup should include routine plain films of the elbow, followed, if necessary, by fluoroscopy to identify the presence and location of suspected intraarticular loose bodies. Additionally, it may be helpful to supplement these examinations with a combined CT arthrogram. This combined examination can outline the intraarticular surfaces displaying calcified or cartilaginous loose bodies[32] (Figs. 6-41 and 6-42). Alternatively, MR imaging provides exquisite detail of the articular and periarticular surfaces.[88] Unossified cartilage can clearly be seen, and on short TR gradient echo images cartilaginous abnormalities may become apparent. Additionally, MR and CT imaging are quite helpful in identifying focal areas of synovitis and tendinitis (Figs. 6-43 and 6-44).

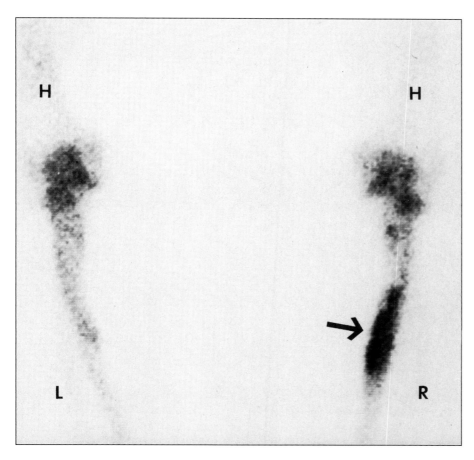

Figure 6-40 Unilateral Ulnar Stress Fracture. *Weightlifter complained of forearm pain caused by dumbbell curls. High-resolution delayed image of TPBS shows increased activity in the midshaft of the right ulna. This pattern represents stress fracture of the ulna. Black arrow = right ulnar shaft activity; H = humerus.*

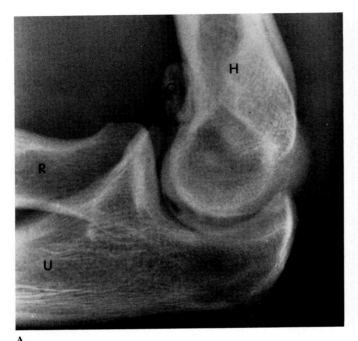

A

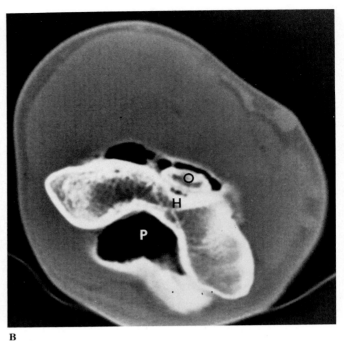

B

Figure 6-41 Intraarticular Loose Body/Elbow. **A.** *Lateral radiograph shows ossification superimposed over the anterior joint space.* **B.** *Axial CT scan* *following the injection of contrast and air into the elbow joint demonstrates a loose bony fragment within the anterior joint space. O = loose intraarticular* *ossicle; H = humerus; R = radius; U = ulna; P = posterior joint space.*

Figure 6-42 Osteochondritis Dissecans of the Trochlea. **A.** *Antero-posterior radiograph shows a lucent defect within the trochlea laterally.* (Fig. 42B and C continues on the opposite page.)

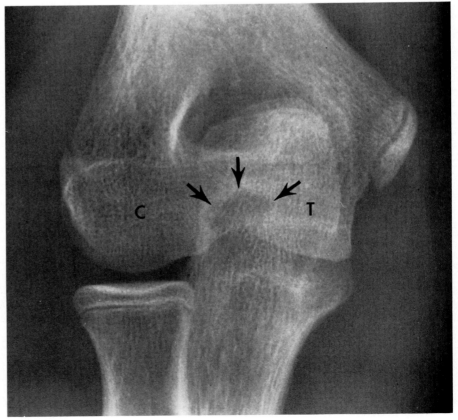

A

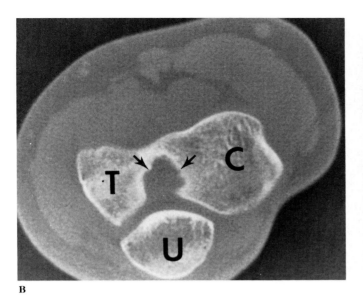

B

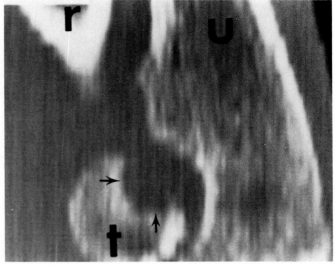

C

Figure 6-42   Osteochondritis Dissecans of the Trochlea (Continued). **B.** *Axial CT scan shows a well-defined lucent defect near the junction of* *the trochlea and capitellum.* **C.** *Sagittal reconstruction derived from contiguous thin section axial scans shows a defect in the articulating surface of trochlea. T =* *trochlea; C = capitellum; U = ulna; arrows = defect.*

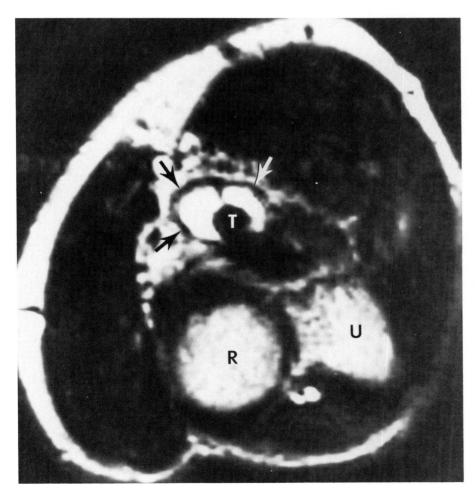

Figure 6-43   Biceps Tendinitis. *Axial MR scan at T2-weighted sequence shows the normally low-signal biceps tendon to be surrounded by high-signal fluid. These features represent bicipital tendinitis. Arrows = fluid within bicipital tendon sheath; T = biceps tendon; R = radius; U = ulna.*

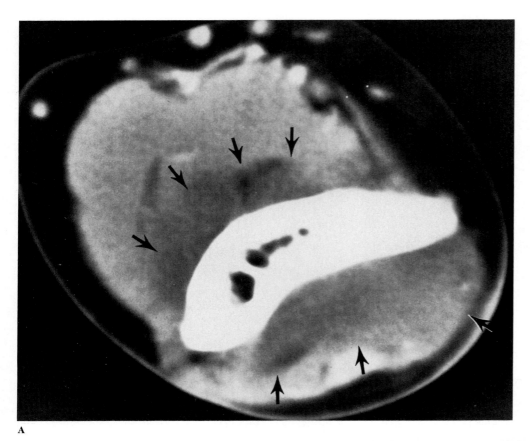

A

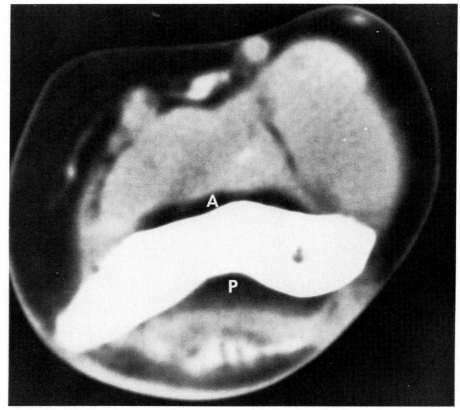

B

Figure 6-44   Focal Synovitis/ Elbow. **A.** *Axial CT scan shows diffuse thickening of the intraarticular synovial structures consistent with synovitis. Adjacent muscles and bones are otherwise normal.* **B.** *CT scan through opposite extremity at a similar location shows normal anterior and posterior fat pads. Arrows = synovial hypertrophy; A = anterior fat pad; P = posterior fat pad.*

Overuse injuries of the elbow include epicondylitis, bursitis, and hypertrophic traction spurs.[26,28,29] "Tennis elbow" (lateral epicondylitis) is associated with overuse at the origin of the extensor carpi radialis brevis. Repeated microtrauma at this location can be associated with calcification adjacent to the lateral humeral epicondyle, which can best be seen with CT.[28] On the medial side of the elbow, stress injury at the insertions of the flexor and pronator muscle groups can lead to medial epicondylitis ("Little Leaguer's elbow"). On plain radiographs, irregularity or separation of the medial epicondyle with associated soft tissue swelling can be seen. In young baseball pitchers, the medial epicondyle is susceptible to stress injury until it unites with the humerus between 18 and 20 years of age. With normal or equivocal radiographs, TPBS may be helpful in localizing the site of injury (Fig. 6-45). Similarly, repeated trauma to the olecranon bursa creates an inflammatory and hyperemic response, which can be detected by TPBS (Fig. 6-46).

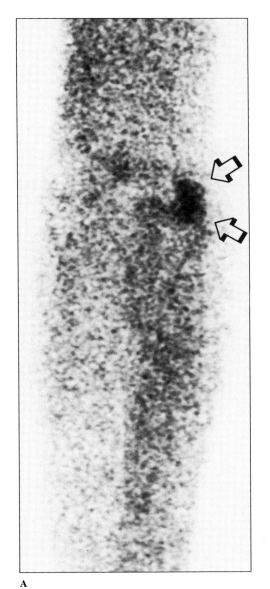

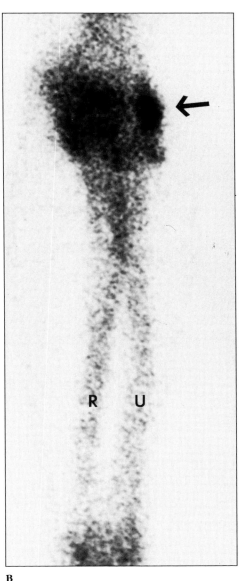

A   B

Figure 6-45   Medial Epicondylitis.
A. *Blood flow image of TPBS demonstrates focally increased activity on the ulnar side of the elbow consistent with focal hyperemia. Open arrows = medial epicondyle.* **B.** *High-resolution delayed image of TPBS (elbow and forearm) shows focally asymmetric, mildly increased activity in the medial aspect of the right elbow corresponding to medial epicondylitis in an athlete with elbow pain and normal radiographs. Arrow = medial epicondyle activity; R = radius; U = ulna.*

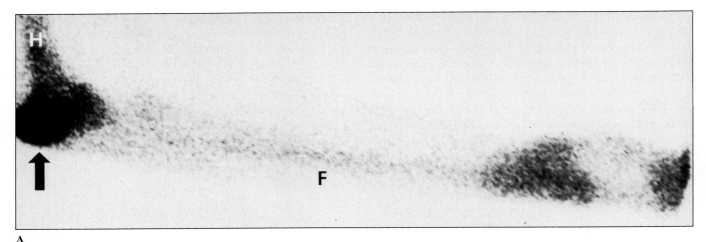

A

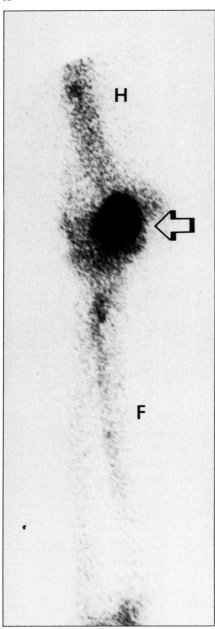

B

Figure 6-46   Olecranon Bursitis. *Male ice skater sustained repeated trauma to his left elbow and complained of pain and swelling. Radiographs were normal.* **A.** *Lateral view of high-resolution delayed images from TPBS shows focally increased activity covering a large portion of the elbow posteriorly extending within the soft tissues to the skin. This uptake in the region of the olecranon bursa represents posttraumatic bursitis. Black arrow = olecranon bursitis; F = forearm; H = humeral shaft.* **B.** *High-resolution anterior projection of delayed images from TPBS of distal arm. This single projection demonstrates the need for multiple views, especially in the region of the elbow, to localize a focus of abnormal activity, which in this case corresponds to the olecranon bursa. Open arrow = olecranon bursitis; H = humerus; F = forearm.*

Repetitive stress to the elbow results in a variety of injuries which are dependent on the type of activity and the age of the athlete. In young children and adolescents, there is sufficient ligamentous laxity so that muscles absorb the valgus strain associated with throwing. In the adult, however, the ulnar collateral ligament and the joint capsule are the primary elbow stabilizers. The most common focal bony stress change seen in adult baseball pitchers and tennis players is the development of hypertrophic traction spurs arising from the medial aspect of the coronoid tubercle[28] (Fig. 6-47).

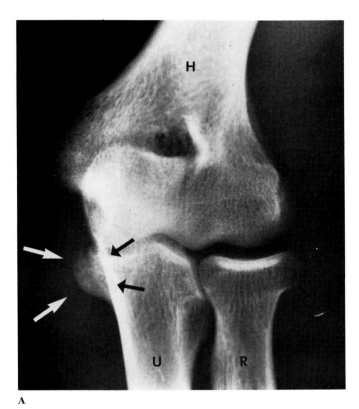

A

Figure 6-47 Hypertrophic Spurring of Coronoid Process. *College baseball pitcher with persistent elbow pain for 6 months.* **A.** *Oblique plain film of the right elbow demonstrates hypertrophic spurring originating from the medial aspect of the elbow (ulnar side) corresponding to the coronoid process. Black and white arrows = hypertrophic spurring.* **B.** *High-resolution delayed image of TPBS was obtained of both elbows in the flexed position (forearm flexed over the upper arm). Focally increased activity is noted in the medial aspect of the right elbow. Arrow = increased activity in the medial aspect of the right elbow representing the coronoid process of the ulna. H = humerus; U = ulna; R = radius. (Fig. 6-47C continues on next page.)*

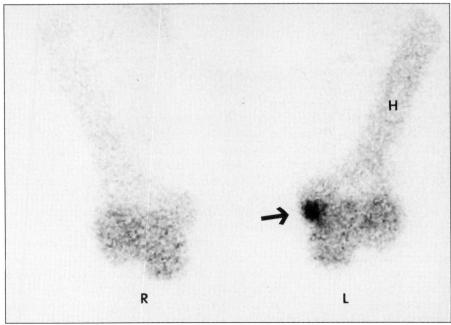

B

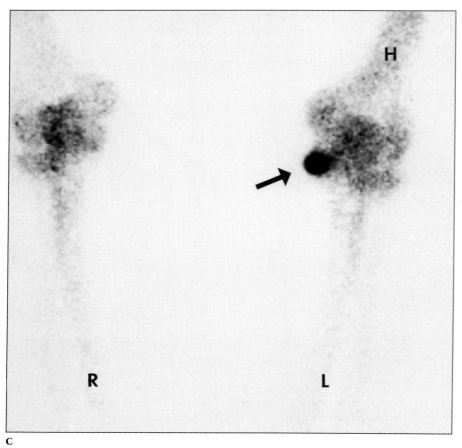

C

Figure 6-47 Hypertrophic Spurring of Coronoid Process (Continued). **C.** *High-resolution delayed images from TPBS with the elbows and forearms fully extended. Focally increased activity is present in the medial aspect of the ulna proximally, corresponding to overuse injury at the attachment of the medial ligament. H = humerus; black arrow = inflammatory reaction at the left coronoid process corresponding to the hypertrophic spurring at the attachment of medial ligament.*

Neurovascular injuries of hand-wrist-forearm (Figs. 6-48 to 6-50)

Neurovascular injuries of the hand, wrist, and forearm of athletes are uncommon when compared with the number of bony, ligamentous, tendinous, and muscular injuries encountered. Neurovascular dysfunction is usually the result of a repetitive motion, position, grip, or trauma leading to neuropraxia or ischemia.[89,90] Posttraumatic RSD may result from blunt trauma, crush injury, or fracture. Several etiologic theories have been postulated for the development of RSD of the hand and wrist in patients presenting with swelling, pain, tenderness, limited motion, and atrophic changes.[22,23] Any athlete suffering blunt trauma to or fracture of the hand or wrist is potentially at risk for the development of RSD. Previously, this had been a clinical diagnosis with radiographs usually showing only various degrees of osteoporosis.

Recent studies, however, have shown that TPBS is an accurate method of confirming a suspected diagnosis of RSD. The specificity, sensitivity, and negative predictive value of TPBS for RSD are all in the range of 96 to 98 percent.[19,20,22,23] When compared with the asymptomatic hand and wrist, the affected extremity will show diffusely increased uptake on delayed images in the metacarpophalangeal, interphalangeal, and carpal joints. The severity and extent of involvement are quite variable with some cases affecting only part of the hand and wrist and others involving the entire forearm, elbow, and upper arm (Fig. 6-48).

Sports-related arterial injury of the upper extremity is well documented in the literature.[90] In the hand, wrist, and forearm, blunt trauma of an acute or chronic nature can lead to vasospasm, arterial thrombosis, and aneurysm. The arterial tree of the hand is most susceptible to blunt trauma in those regions that are not protected by overlying fascia.

Digital vessels are most vulnerable to blunt trauma as they exit from under the protection of the palmar fascia.[91–94] For example, the radial artery is vulnerable in that region from the distal border of the transverse carpal ligament to the region where it enters the protective palmar fascia. Likewise, the ulnar artery is most susceptible in the hypothenar region where blunt trauma to the ulnar aspect of the palm forcefully pushes the ulnar artery against the hook of the hamate.

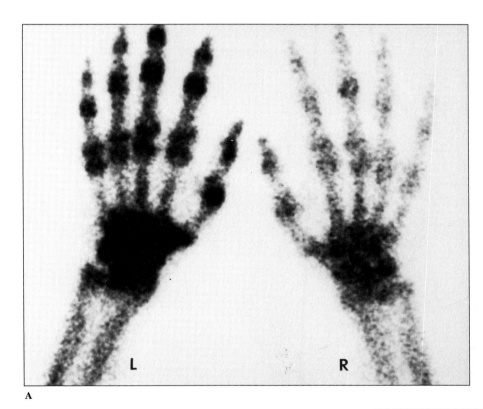

A

Figure 6-48   Reflex Sympathetic Dystrophy (RSD) of the Left Upper Extremity (Hand, Wrist, Forearm, and Elbow). **A.** *High-resolution delayed image of TPBS shows asymmetrically increased activity in all the joints of the left hand and wrist.* **B.** *High-resolution delayed image of TPBS shows increased activity in the left wrist, forearm, and elbow when compared with the right side, consistent with the clinical diagnosis of RSD. Black arrowheads = increased activity in the left wrist and elbow when compared with the right side.*

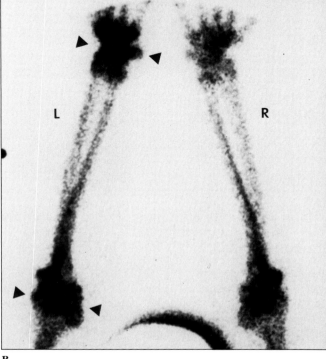

B

Traumatic aneurysms are of two types: *true* and *false*. False aneurysms develop following a penetrating injury that perforates a vessel wall. True aneurysms follow nonpenetrating trauma and are associated either with a single direct blow or repetitive injury. Digital aneurysms have been reported in lacrosse, volleyball, football, and martial arts.[90–94] TPBS is an easy, accurate, and noninvasive screening test to localize and confirm the presence of aneurysm. This is usually apparent on the blood flow and/or blood pool phase of the TPBS study[20,24,92] (Fig. 6-49).

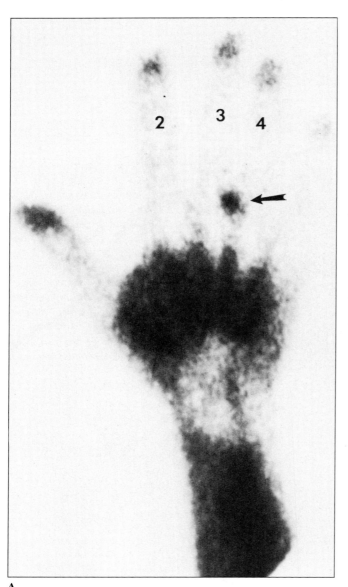

A

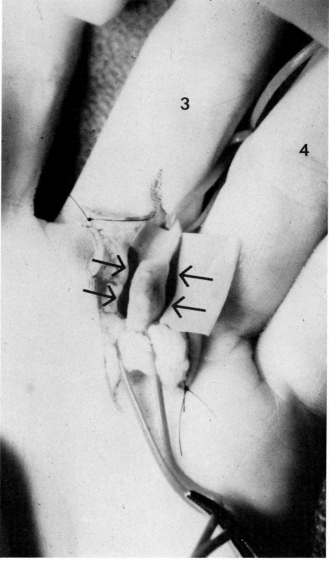

B

Figure 6-49 Digital Artery Aneurysm. *Lacrosse player was hit on the palmar aspect of his hand by a lacrosse stick.*
A. *Blood pool image of TPBS demonstrates focally intense area of increased activity at the base of the middle finger. Black arrow = focus of increased activity at the base of the left third digit.* **B.** *Surgical picture shows an aneurysm of the digital artery at the base of the left third digit. Black arrows = digital artery aneurysm. (From Ho PK, Dellon AL, Wilgis EFS.[92] Reproduced with permission.)*

Thrombosis of the ulnar artery has been reported in players of multiple sports including baseball, handball, hockey, and martial arts.[90,92] These share the features of repetitive trauma to the ulnar artery, usually at the level of the wrist. Clinical and Doppler tests may be diagnostic. TPBS is quite sensitive in identifying the site of thrombosis as well as the degree of delayed filling or ischemia noted in the ulnar digits (fourth and fifth) of the hand[20,24,90,95] (Fig. 6-50).

Baseball players are particularly prone to a wide variety of vascular injuries, which include venous thrombosis, ulnar artery thrombosis, and digital ischemia.[89,90,95–98] Although also reported in athletes who engage in martial arts, handball, and volleyball, baseball players (especially catchers) characteristically develop digital ischemia in the index finger of their catching hand. The main focus of impact of the baseball is directly over the area of the metacarpal head of the index finger, causing direct trauma to the digital artery at that location.[98]

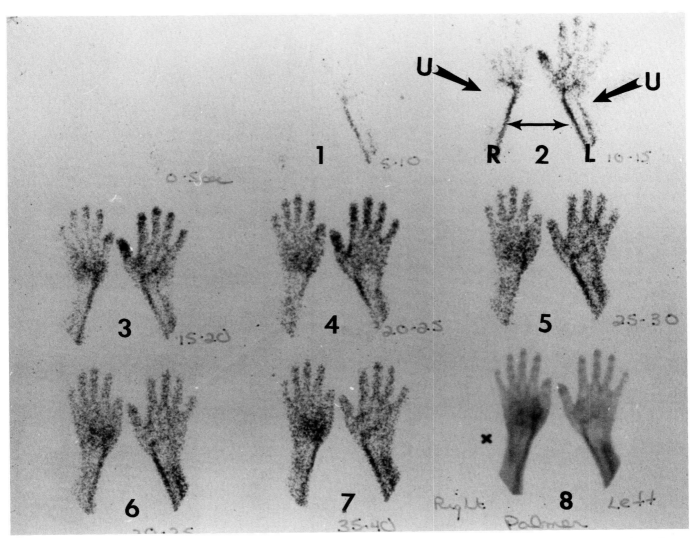

Figure 6-50 Ulnar Artery Thrombosis. *Dynamic flow phase of TPBS in the palmar projection taken at 5-s intervals (1 = 5- to 10-s interval following nuclide injection, 2 = 10- to 15-s interval following the injection, etc.). Frame 2 demonstrates nuclide activity within the radial and ulnar arteries of the left hand. There is symmetric perfusion of the digits. In the right hand and wrist, there is absent perfusion in the right ulnar artery and very minimal filling of the right ulnar digits (fourth and fifth fingers) when compared with the radial digits of the same hand. This dynamic flow study clearly shows early asymmetric perfusion. Doubleheaded arrow = radial arteries; black arrow = course of ulnar artery, which is patent on the left and absent on the right.*

DIAGNOSTIC PROBLEMS

As in other regions of the body, neoplasms and entities unrelated to previous trauma may mimic the pain, swelling, and disability that we usually associate with athletic injury.[99–101] In this circumstance, the physician should maintain a high index of suspicion for the presence of a nonathletic problem, particularly if that problem seems to be more persistent or atypical of athletic injury (Figs. 6-51 to 6-55).

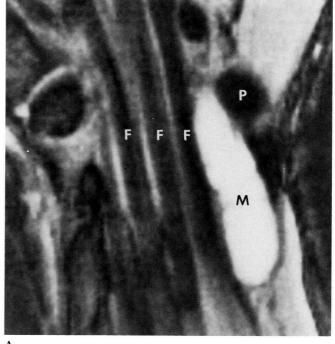

A

Figure 6-51 Neurofibroma of Wrist. **A.** *MR scan in the coronal plane at a short TR gradient echo sequence shows an elongated area of high signal lying medial to the flexor tendons and lateral to the pisiform.* **B.** *Axial MR scan at T1-weighted sequence through the DRUJ shows a globular density of intermediate signal adjacent to the ulnar artery and the flexor carpi ulnaris and flexor digitorum profundus tendons.* (Fig. 6-51C and D continues on the opposite page.)

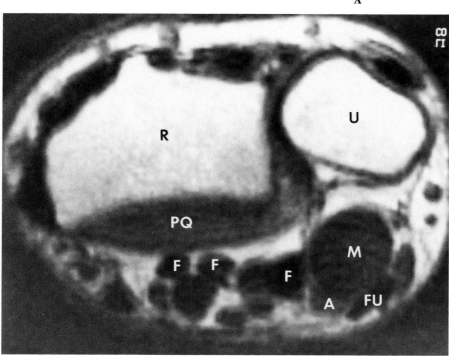

B

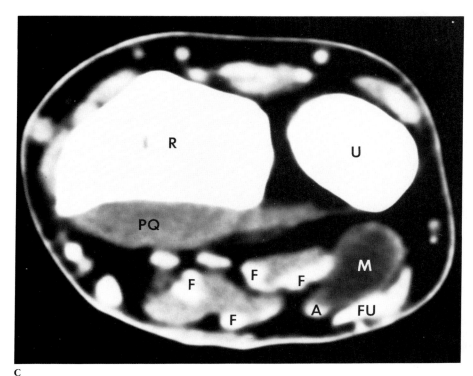

C

Figure 6-51   Neurofibroma of Wrist (Continued). **C.** *CT scan in the axial plane following intravenous contrast administration shows a nonenhancing globular mass in the region of the ulnar nerve.* **D.** *Ultrasound shows the mass to be uniformly hypoechoic. M = mass; F = flexor tendons; A = ulnar artery; FU = flexor carpi ulnaris; U = ulna; R = radius; P = pisiform; PQ = pronator quadratus muscle.*

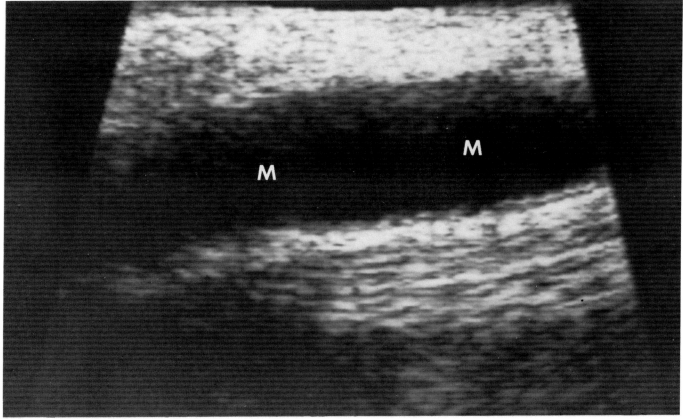

D

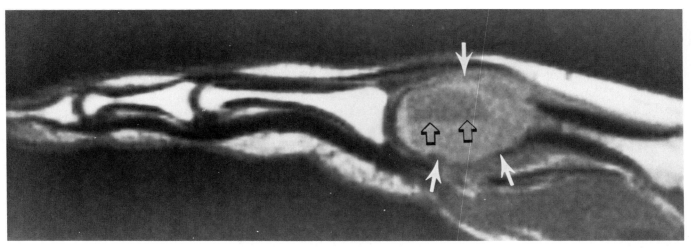

Figure 6-52 Aneurysmal Bone Cyst of Metacarpal. *MR scan in the sagittal plane at T1-weighted sequence shows an* *expansile destructive lesion of the distal half of the index metacarpal. A low signal fluid layer is present within this* *intermediate signal neoplasm. Open arrows = fluid layer; arrows = expansile mass.*

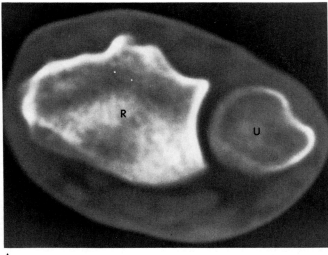

A

Figure 6-53 Radioulnar Synostosis. **A.** *This patient with inability to pronate or supinate the wrist has a normally congruent distal radioulnar articulation.* **B.** *Axial CT scan in the midforearm shows solid radioulnar synostosis accounting for his immobility. R = radius; U = ulna. (From Levinsohn EM: Imaging of the wrist.* Radiologic Clinics of North America 28(5):905–921, 1990. *Reprinted with permission.)*

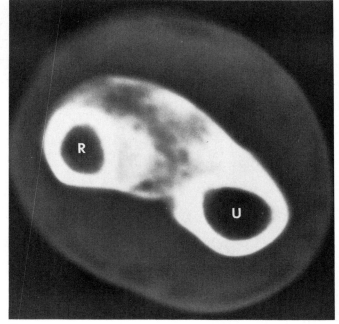

B

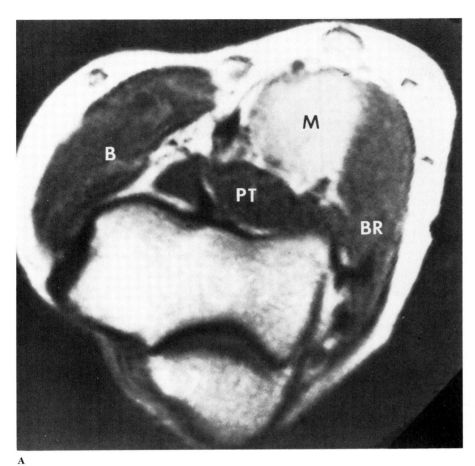

A

Figure 6-54   Synovial Sarcoma of Brachioradialis Muscle. **A.** *Axial MR scan at T1-weighted sequence shows a high-signal mass infiltrating the brachioradialis muscle. The underlying brachialis muscle seems unaffected.* **B.** *Axial MR scan at T2-weighted sequence shows similar findings. The invasion of the brachioradialis muscle is strong evidence for a malignant process. M = infiltrating mass; BR = brachioradialis muscle; B = brachialis muscle; PT = pronator teres muscle.*

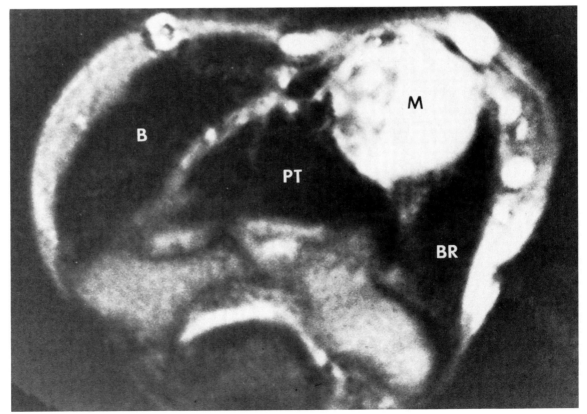

B

Figure 6-55   Lipoma of Brachio-radialis Muscle. **A.** *Axial CT scan shows a well-defined fatty mass within the brachioradialis muscle. This appearance is characteristic for benign lipoma.* **B.** *Coronal MR scan at T1-weighted sequence in another patient shows focal enlargement of the medial subcutaneous tissues representing a subcutaneous lipoma. At this sequence, the ossification center of the capitellum can be seen developing within its cartilaginous center. The trochlea and radial head have not yet ossified. L = lipoma; BR = brachioradialis muscle; C = capitellum; R = radius; RH = cartilaginous radial head.*

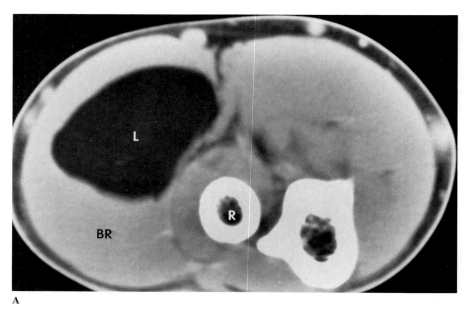

A

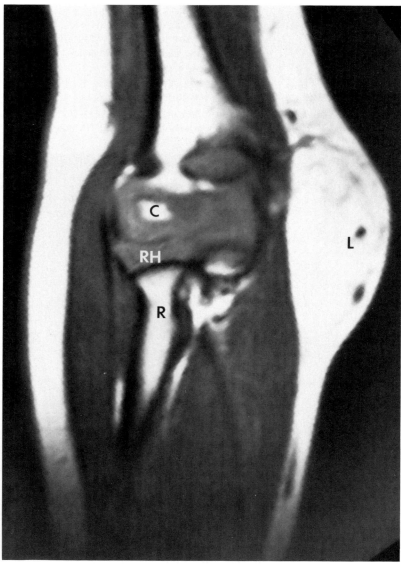

B

REFERENCES

1. Amadio PC: Epidemiology of hand and wrist injuries in sports. Hand Clin 6:379–381, 1990.
2. Recht MP, Burk DL, Dalinka MK: Radiology of wrist and hand injuries in athletes. Clin Sports Med 6:811–828, 1987.
3. Stark HH, Chao E-K, Zemel NP, et al.: Fracture of the hook of the hamate. J Bone Joint Surg 71(A):1202–1207, 1989.
4. Braunstein EM, Louis DS, Greene TL, Hankin FM: Fluoroscopic and arthrographic evaluation of carpal instability. AJR 144:1259–1262, 1985.
5. Gilula LA, Weeks PM: Post-traumatic ligamentous instabilities of the wrist. Radiology 129:641–651, 1978.
6. Levinsohn EM: Imaging of the wrist. Radiol Clin North Am 28:905–921, 1990.
7. Taleisnik J: Current concepts review carpal instability. J Bone Joint Surg 70(A):1262–1268, 1988.
8. Binkovitz LA, Ehman RL, Cahill DR, Berquist TH: Magnetic resonance imaging of the wrist: normal cross sectional imaging and selected abnormal cases. RadioGraphics 8:1171–1202, 1988.
9. Golimbu CN, Firooznia H, Melone CP, et al.: Tears of the triangular fibrocartilage of the wrist: MR imaging. Radiology 173:731–733, 1989.
10. Kursunoglu-Brahme S, Gundry CR, Resnick D: Advanced imaging of the wrist. Radiol Clin North Am 28:307–320, 1990.
11. Bush CH, Gillespy T III, Dell PC: High-resolution CT of the wrist: initial experience with scaphoid disorders and surgical fusions. AJR 149:757–760, 1987.
12. Hindman BW, Kulik WJ, Lee G, Avolio RE: Occult fractures of the carpals and metacarpals: demonstration by CT. AJR 153:529–532, 1989.
13. Quinn SF, Belsole RJ, Greene TL, Rayhack JM: Advanced imaging of the wrist. RadioGraphics 9:229–246, 1989.
14. Quinn SF, Murray W, Watkins T, Kloss J: CT for determining the results of treatment of fractures of the wrist. AJR 149:109–111, 1987.
15. Bresina SJ, Vannier MW, Logan SE, Weeks PM: Three dimensional wrist imaging: evaluation of functional and pathologic anatomy by computer. Clin Plast Surg 13:389–405, 1986.
16. Zlatkin MB, Chao PC, Osterman AL, et al.: Chronic wrist pain: evaluation with high-resolution MR imaging. Radiology 173:723–729, 1989.
17. Baker LL, Hajek PC, Bjorkengren A, et al.: High-resolution magnetic resonance imaging of the wrist: normal anatomy. Skeletal Radiol 16:128–132, 1987.
18. Holder LE: Clinical radionuclide bone imaging. Radiology 176:607–614, 1990.
19. Holder LE, Matthews LS: The nuclear physician and sports medicine, in Freeman L, Weissman H (eds): *Nuclear Medicine Annual*. Raven, New York, 1984, pp 88–140.
20. Martire JR: The role of nuclear medicine scans in evaluating pain in athletic injuries. Clin Sports Med 6:713–737, 1987.
21. Matin PM: Bone scintigraphy in the diagnosis and management of traumatic injury. Semin Nucl Med 13:104–122, 1983.
22. Holder LE, MacKinnon SE: Reflex sympathetic dystrophy in the hands: strict clinical and scintigraphic criteria. Radiology 152:517–522, 1984.
23. MacKinnon SE, Holder LE: The use of three phase radionuclide bone scanning in the diagnosis of reflex sympathetic dystrophy. J Hand Surg 9(A):556–563, 1984.
24. Maurer AH, Holder LE, Espinola DA, et al.: Three phase radionuclide scintigraphy of the hand. Radiology 146:761–775, 1983.
25. Baker BE: Current concepts in the diagnosis and treatment of musculotendinous injuries. Med Sci Sports Exerc 16:323–327, 1984.
26. Hotchkiss RN: Common disorders of the elbow in athletes and musicians. Hand Clin 6:507–515, 1990.
27. Miller JE: Javelin thrower's elbow. J Bone Joint Surg 42(B):788–792, 1960.
28. Newburg AH: The radiographic evaluation of shoulder and elbow pain in the athlete. Clin Sports Med 6:785–809, 1987.
29. Singer KM, Roy SP: Osteochondrosis of the humeral capitellum. Am J Sports Med 12:351–360, 1984.
30. Woodward AH, Binko AJ Jr.: Osteochondritis dissecans of the elbow. Clin Orthop 110:35–41, 1975.
31. Rupani HD, Holder LE, Espinola DA, et al.: Three phase radionuclide bone imaging in sports medicine. Radiology 156:187–196, 1985.
32. Dalinka MK, Kricum ME, Zlatkin MB, Hibbard CA: Modern diagnostic imaging in joint disease. AJR 152:229–240, 1989.
33. McCue FC, Baugher WH, Kulund DN, et al.: Hand and wrist injuries in the athlete. Am J Sports Med 7:275–286, 1979.
34. Posner MA: Injuries to the hand and wrist in athletes. Orthop Clin North Am 8:593–618, 1977.
35. Noble C: Hand injuries in sports. Am J Sports Med 15(4):342–346, 1987.
36. Zemel NP, Stark HH: Fractures and dislocations of the carpal bones. Clin Sports Med 5:709–724, 1986.
37. Mink JH, Rosenfeld RT: MR views sports-related bony, muscular injuries. Diagn Imaging 13(2):108–114, 1191.
38. Hanks GA, Kalenak A, Bowman LS, et al.: Stress fractures of the carpal scaphoid: a report of four cases. Bone Joint Surg 71(A):938–941, 1988.
39. Manzione M, Pizzutillo PD: Stress fracture of the scaphoid waist: a case report. Am J Sports Med 9:268–269, 1981.
40. Stark HH, Jobe FW, Boyes JH, et al.: Fracture of the hook of the hamate in athletes. J Bone Joint Surg 59(A):575–582, 1977.
41. Norman A, Nelson J, Green S: Fractures of the hook of the hamate: radiographic signs. Radiology 154:49–53, 1985.
42. Ogunro O: Fracture of the body of the hamate bone. J Hand Surg 8:353–355, 1983.
43. Polivy KD, Millender LH, Frank G: Fractures of the hook of the hamate: failure of clinical diagnosis. J Hand Surg 10:101–104, 1984.
44. Bray TJ, Swafford AR, Brown RL: Bilateral fracture of the hook of the hamate. J Trauma 25:174–175, 1985.
45. Cone RO, Szabo R, Resnick D, et al.: Computed tomography of the normal radioulnar joints. Invest Radiol 18:541–545, 1983.
46. Mino DE, Palmer AK, Levinsohn EM: The role of radiography and computerized tomography in the diagnosis of subluxation and dislocation of the distal radioulnar joint. J Hand Surg 8:23–31, 1983.

47. Mino DE, Palmer AK, Levinsohn EM: Radiography and computerized tomography in the diagnosis of incongruity of the distal radio-ulnar joint. J Bone Joint Surg 67(A):247–252, 1985.

48. Wechsler RJ, Wehbe MA, Rifkin MD, et al.: Computed tomography diagnosis of distal radioulnar subluxation. Skeletal Radiol 16:1–5, 1987.

49. Fulkerson JP, Watson HK: Congenital anterior subluxation of the distal ulna: a case report. Clin Orthop 131:179–182, 1978.

50. Alexander AH: Bilateral traumatic dislocation of the distal radioulnar joint, ulna dorsal: case report and review of the literature. Clin Orthop 129:238–244, 1977.

51. Weseley MS, Barenfeld PA, Bruno J: Volar dislocation distal radioulnar joint. J Trauma 12:1083–1088, 1972.

52. Demos TC: Galeazzi fracture-dislocation. Orthop 3:432–435, 1980.

53. Ganel A, Engel J, Ditzian R, et al.: Arthrography as a method of diagnosing soft-tissue injuries of the wrist. J Trauma 19:376–380, 1979.

54. Kricun ME: Wrist arthrography. Clin Orthop 187:65–71, 1984.

55. Levinsohn EM, Palmer AK: Arthrography of the traumatized wrist. Radiology 146:647–651, 1983.

56. Palmer AK, Levinsohn EM, Kuzma GR: Arthrography of the wrist. J Hand Surg 8:15–23, 1983.

57. Shigematsu S, Abe M, Onomura T, et al.: Arthrograpy of the normal and posttraumatic wrist. J Hand Surg 14(A):410–412, 1989.

58. Tirman RM, Weber ER, Snyder LL, Koonce TW: Midcarpal wrist arthrography for detection of tears of the scapholunate and lunotriquetral ligaments. AJR 144:107–108, 1985.

59. Levinsohn EM, Palmer AK, Coren AB, Zinberg EM: Wrist arthrography: the value of the three compartment injection technique. Skeletal Radiol 16:539–544, 1987.

60. Levinsohn EM, Rosen D, Palmer AK: Wrist arthrography: value of the three-compartment injection method. Radiology 179:231–239, 1991.

61. Zinberg EM, Palmer AK, Coren AB, Levinsohn EM: The triple injection wrist arthrogram. J Hand Surg 13(A):803–809, 1988.

62. Quinn SF, Belsole RS, Greene TL, Rayhack JM: Work in progress: postarthrography computed tomography of the wrist: evaluation of the triangular fibrocartilage complex. Skeletal Radiol 17:565–569, 1989.

63. Gundry CR, Kursunoglu-Brahme S, Schwaighofer B, et al.: Is MR better than arthrography for evaluating the ligaments of the wrist? In vitro study. AJR 154:337–341, 1990.

64. Parker RD, Berkowitz MS, Brahms MA, et al.: Hook of the hamate fractures in athletes. Am J Sports Med 14:517–523, 1986.

65. Reister JN, Baker BE, Mosher JF, et al.: A review of scaphoid fracture healing in competitive athletes. Am J Sports Med 13:159–161, 1985.

66. Sowa DT, Holder LH, Patt PG, et al.: Application of magnetic resonance imaging to ischemic necrosis of the lunate. J Hand Surg 14(A):1008–1016, 1989.

67. Dobyns JH, Gabel GT: Gymnast's wrist. Hand Clin 6:493–505, 1990.

68. Dobyns JH, Sim FH, Linscheid RL: Sports stress syndromes of the hand and wrist. Am J Sports Med 6:236–253, 1978.

69. Mandelbaum BR, Bartolozzi AR, Davis CA, et al.: Wrist pain syndrome in the gymnast. Am J Sports Med 17:305–317, 1989.

70. Carter SR, Aldridge MJ, Fitzgerald R, et al.: Stress changes of the wrist in adolescent gymnasts. Br J Radiol 61:109–112, 1988.

71. Andren L, Eiken O: Arthrographic studies of wrist ganglions. J Bone Joint Surg 53(A):299–302, 1971.

72. Nelson CL, Sawmiller S, Phalen GS: Ganglions of the wrist and hand. J Bone Joint Surg 54(A):1459–1464, 1972.

73. Albanese SA, Palmer AK, Kerr DR, et al.: Wrist pain and distal growth plate closure of the radius in gymnasts. J Pediatr Orthop 9:23–28, 1989.

74. Cone RO, Szabo R, Resnick D, et al.: Computed tomography of the normal soft tissues of the wrist. Invest Radiol 18:546–551, 1983.

75. Mesgarzadeh M, Schneck CD, Bonakdarpour A: Carpal tunnel: MR imaging. Part I. Normal anatomy. Radiology 171:743–748, 1989.

76. Middleton WD, Kneeland JB, Kellman GM, et al.: MR imaging of the carpal tunnel: normal anatomy and preliminary findings in the carpal tunnel syndrome. AJR 148:307–316, 1987.

77. Zeiss J, Skie M, Ebraheim N, Jackson WT: Anatomic relations between the median nerve and flexor tendons in the carpal tunnel: MR evaluation in normal volunteers. AJR 153:533–536, 1989.

78. Evans DL: Fatigue fracture of the ulna. J Bone Joint Surg 37(B):618–621, 1955.

79. Hamilton HK: Stress fracture of the diaphysis of the ulna in a body builder. Am J Sports Med 12:405–406, 1984.

80. Heinrichs EH, Senske BJ: Stress fracture of the ulnar diaphysis in athletes: a case report and a review of the literature. South Dakota J Med 41(2):5–8, 1988.

81. Kitchin ID: Fatigue fracture of the ulna. J Bone Joint Surg 30(B):622–623, 1948.

82. Mutoh Y, Mori T, Suzuki Y, et al.: Stress fractures of the ulna in athletes. Am J Sports Med 10:365–367, 1982.

83. Pascale MS, Grana WA: Stress fracture of the ulna. Orthopedics 11:830–832, 1988.

84. Rettig AC: Stress fracture of the ulna in an adolescent tournament tennis player. Am J Sports Med 11:103–106, 1983.

85. Sakai N, Sumiya A, Watanuki C: A case with fatigue fracture of the bilateral ulnae in school girl Kendo player. J West Jpn Clin Sports Med 1:7–11, 1980.

86. Tehranzadeh J, Serafini AN, Pais MJ: *Avulsion and Stress Injuries of the Musculoskeletal System*. Karger, Basel, 1989.

87. Brown R, Blazina ME, Kerlan RK, et al.: Osteochondritis of the capitellum. Am J Sports Med 2:27–46, 1974.

88. Stoller DW: Musculoskeletal applications of magnetic resonance imaging. Appl Radiol 17:39–46, 1988.

89. Tullos HS, Erwin WD, Woods GW, et al.: Unusual lesions of the pitching arm. Clin Orthop 88:169–182, 1972.

90. Aulicino PL: Neurovascular injuries in the hands of athletes. Hand Clin 6:455–466, 1990.

91. Green DP: True and false traumatic aneurysms in the hand. J Bone Joint Surg 55(A):120–128, 1973.

92. Ho PK, Dellon AL, Wilgis EFS: True aneurysms of the hand resulting from athletic injury. Am J Sports Med 13:136–139, 1985.

93. McCarthy WJ, Yao JS, Schafer MF, et al.: Upper extremity arterial injury in athletes. J Vasc Surg 9:317–327, 1989.

94. Mousavi SM: Aneurysms and arterial thromboses of the hand. J Vasc Surg 12:294–305, 1978.

95. Porubsky GL, Brown SI, Urbaniak JR: Ulnar artery thrombosis: a sports related injury. Am J Sports Med 14:170–175, 1986.

96. Buckhout BC, Warner MA: Digital perfusion of handball players. Am J Sports Med 8:206–207, 1980.

97. Dawson WJ, Tullos N: Baseball injuries to the hand. Ann Emerg Med 10:302–306, 1981.

98. Sugawara M, Ogino T, Minami A, et al.: Digital ischemia in baseball players. Am J Sports Med 14:329–334, 1986.

99. Baker BE, Levinsohn EM, Coren AB: Pitfalls to avoid in diagnosing pain in the athlete. Clin Sports Med 6:921–934, 1987.

100. Lewis MM, Reilly JF: Sports tumors. Am J Sports Med (15):362–365, 1987.

101. Wood MB, Dobyns JH: Sports-related extraarticular wrist syndromes. Clin Orthop 202:93–101, 1986.

Orthopedic overview

The athlete presumably is an individual who is in good physical condition. In recent decades however, athletes have crossed the age barrier, resulting in individuals participating in sports-related activities well into the middle through retirement years. These athletes, because of age-related secondary changes such as decreased mineral content and increased ligamentous stiffness, are at increased risk of spine injury.

Initial evaluation of an athlete with a possible spinal injury includes inspection of the involved region, palpation for areas of local tenderness and deformity, and careful neurologic examination. The initial examination can usually be done without moving the patient. In patients in whom a serious spinal injury is suspected, transportation to a facility that allows more than just a cursory physical examination is needed. The spine should always be splinted during transportation. Splinting may range from simply a soft towel wrapped around the neck to the incorporation of specially designed backboards with transportation supervised by an emergency medical transport unit.

Full evaluation of the spine can commence once the patient has been transported to an appropriate facility. Suspected cervical spine injury should be evaluated radiologically by initially obtaining a cross-table lateral radiograph of the cervical spine. Care must be taken that the entire cervical spine down to and including the C7-T1 junction be visualized. This can be difficult particularly in well-muscled individuals. If voluntary depression of the shoulders is not possible, then gentle traction on the arms by the physician may be required. If the lateral radiograph is normal, an anteroposterior view and an open mouth odontoid view should be obtained. Both can be done without moving the patient.

Patients without neurologic deficit and with normal lateral, anteroposterior, and odontoid radiographs of the cervical spine can then be mobilized, as needed, to obtain a complete set of radiographs, which includes both oblique views (or pillar views) and flexion and extension lateral views, to confirm ligamentous stability. The presence of radicular pain necessitates further examination by either computed tomography (CT) or magnetic resonance imaging (MRI). MRI is preferable, since it allows the demonstration of the spine in three planes, a feature not directly achieved with CT. It also allows identification of soft tissue injury of the supra and interspinous ligaments, anterior and posterior longitudinal ligaments, and epidural tissues. In patients with radicular symptoms, flexion and extension lateral radiographs should not be done until an MR or CT examination is first performed. Although a nondisplaced vertebral body fracture may not be visible on either plain radiographs or CT scan, an MR examination will show marrow changes suggesting this diagnosis. Similarly, radionuclide bone scans will be positive within 48 h of fracture.

Cervical spine fractures that are documented on the initial radiographs almost always require additional evaluation with further studies. The CT scan is the most useful modality for delineating bony pathology. Scans should be performed with thin (1 to 2 mm) cuts across the injured area and

CHAPTER 7

SPINE

Edwin D. Cacayorin
Leo Hochhauser
John J. Wasenko
Jeffrey A. Winfield

*State University of New York
Health Science Center at Syracuse
Syracuse, New York*

281

should include both coronal and sagittal reconstructions. Multidirectional tomography is occasionally useful in the rare patient with a transverse fracture such as a type II odontoid fracture. The added risk of moving a patient onto a tomographic unit can often be avoided by obtaining thin section overlapping CT scans with sagittal and coronal reconstuctions.

The thoracic spine, especially from T1 to T7, is particularly difficult to assess on plain radiographs. If an injury is suspected in this area on the basis of the patient's complaints and the physical examination, then particular attention must be paid to obtaining high-quality anteroposterior and lateral radiographs of the area in question. If the suspected pathology cannot be adequately visualized, then either magnetic resonance or CT scanning of that area is essential. In those cases where the clinical suspicion is high and the radiographic studies are inconclusive, a nuclear medicine bone scan may prove diagnostic. The CT examination continues to be the gold standard for determining the appropriate treatment of a thoracic or thoracolumbar injury. In those circumstances where spinal cord visualization is necessary, the magnetic resonance scan is preferable to the myelogram.

Because there are no overlying ribs, the lumbar portion of the spine is easiest to inspect, palpate, and radiograph. A majority of lumbar fractures are identified on plain radiographs. The CT scan is used to augment that examination and is particularly useful in demonstrating canal compromise by bony fragments. MRI is helpful in visualizing the soft tissues in this region, particularly the neural elements and interspinous ligaments.

The sacrum should be included in the evaluation of all spinal injuries. Unless radiographs of this area are examined carefully, significant fractures may be missed. CT is of particular value in this area in assessing possible bone injury. MRI effectively demonstrates the sacral nerve roots, allowing inspection of these structures as they pass through specific neural foramina. In those problem cases where a suspected fracture is not seen on routine radiographs, the radionuclide bone scan may be diagnostic.

With the advent of CT and MRI, the imaging armamentarium available to the orthopedic surgeon in assessing injuries to the spine has improved significantly. The use of routine tomography can identify up to 30 percent more fractures than can plain radiographs. CT, MRI, and modern bone scanning have enhanced and clarified these diagnoses even more. Despite the enormous aid which these imaging tools provide, the need for a careful and accurate clinical examination remains paramount. A high index of suspicion for possible injury to the spine and a systematic evaluation of these injuries need to be maintained for the optimal management of athletic injury.

HANSEN YUAN, M.D.
Professor of Orthopedic Surgery
Chief, Division of Spinal Surgery
SUNY Health Science Center at Syracuse
Syracuse, New York

THE SPINAL CORD is inherently protected from traumatic injury by its central location and by its strong bony, ligamentous, and muscular surroundings. Thus athletes, because of their mobility and well-developed musculature, would seem to be less prone to serious spinal injury than are nonathletes, and indeed a majority of spine injuries are minor. Nevertheless, serious neurologic injuries have been sustained, particularly by those active in contact sports. Sports that entail repeated and severe flexion, extension, positional change, spinal loading, or torque have an increased incidence of significant neurologic injuries. These sports include football, diving, gymnastics, ballet, weightlifting, wrestling, and tennis.[1–9] To a lesser extent, even such sports as jogging, ice hockey, and lacrosse have been associated with spinal injury.[10–12] It is important to remember that young and old athletes alike are susceptible to spinal injury.[13–18]

The athlete with possible spinal injury requires rapid and systematic performance of radiographic studies. Certainly, the neurologic status heavily influences the choice of the initial imaging study and the sequence of complementary examinations. Nonetheless, the clinical suspicion of fracture, subluxation or dislocation, spinal instability, and spinal cord injury should be addressed.[19]

Given the complex nature of the spine, spinal cord, and supporting muscular, tendinous, and ligamentous structures, imaging of this region is complicated. As in others parts of the body, an adequate plain film examination should be performed first. CT and MR imaging are particularly suited to assess spinal injury because of their cross-sectional and multiplanar imaging capabilities. Because of its high-contrast resolution in the depiction of soft tissues, MR imaging has become the major tool for evaluating the disk, ligaments, and spinal cord, whereas CT is superior for evaluation of the bony structures. Triple-phase bone scanning (TPBS) may provide important complementary information to the plain radiographic examination, whether those studies were positive or negative (Figs. 7-1 to 7-3). Following a positive radiographic examination, TPBS may be helpful in determining whether the abnormal area shows increased nuclide uptake, which would indicate an active or acute lesion[11,20] (Figs. 7-4 and 7-5). Despite normal radiographs, TPBS may successfully demonstrate the site of an occult bony injury of the spine.[6,11]

The major diagnostic modalities for evaluation of spinal injuries include the following:

1. Plain radiograph
2. Pleuridirectional tomography (polytomography)
3. Computed tomography (CT)
4. Magnetic resonance imaging (MRI)
5. Myelography usually performed with CT (CTM)
6. Radionuclide bone scanning (TPBS and SPECT)

Knowledge of the merits and limitations of these diagnostic modalities is essential in optimally determining their individual role in the evaluation of spine injuries.

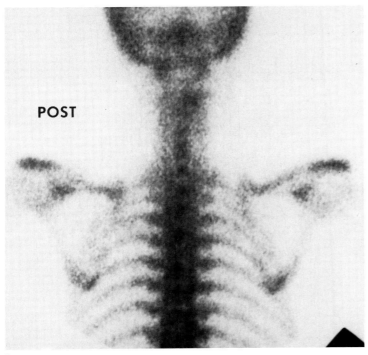

Figure 7-1 High-Resolution Delayed Images from TPBS of the Normal Spine. **A.** *Posterior projection. In the thoracic region, the vertebrae, uncovertebral junctions, and posterior aspects of the ribs are clearly seen.* (Fig. 7-1B and C continues on next page.)

A

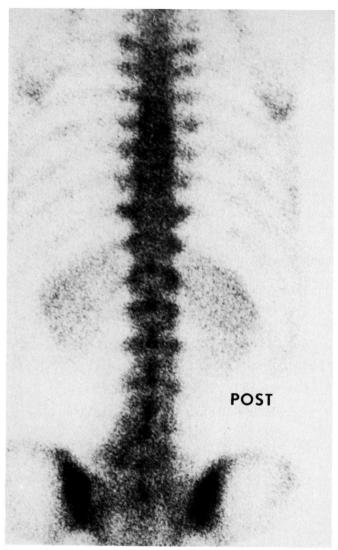

B

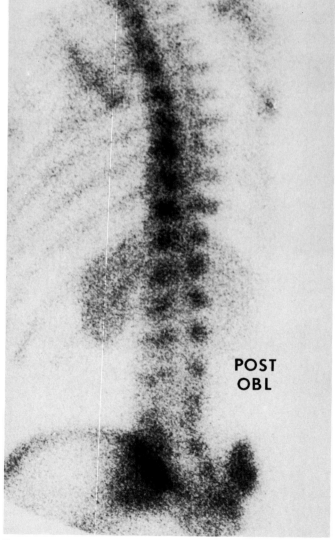

Figure 7-1   High-Resolution Delayed Images from TPBS of the Normal Spine (Continued). **B.** *Posterior projection. Nuclide activity is noted in the kidneys, reflecting this primary excretion site for the technetium bone scanning agent.* **C.** *Right posterior oblique projection. Supplemental views such as this are needed to identify pars abnormalities. This view demonstrates the posterior elements of the spine as well as the posterior aspects of the ribs.*

C

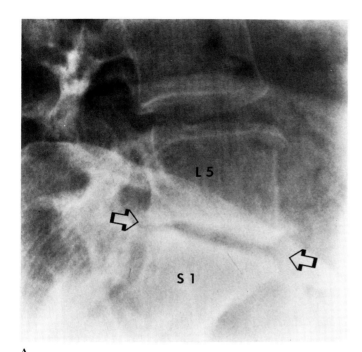

A

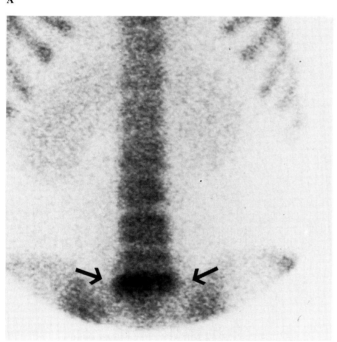

B

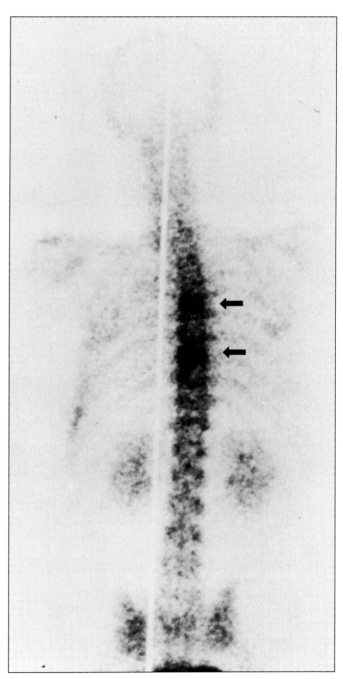

A

Figure 7-2   Degenerative Disk Disease (L5-S1 Level).
A. *Coned lateral radiograph at the L5-S1 level. Marked disk space narrowing with small anterior and posterior hypertrophic osteophytes. Open arrows = narrowed L5-S1 disk space.* **B.** *High-resolution delayed anterior image from TPBS at the thoracolumbar level. Minimally to mildly increased activity (arrows) at the L5-S1 level consistent with the radiographic abnormality. This study helps to confirm the clinical impression of degenerative disk disease and exclude other more serious possibilities (such as tumor or occult fracture) in this 56-year-old recreational athlete with low back pain.*

Figure 7-3   Vertebral Body Fracture. *Two thoracic vertebral body fractures are present which were not visible on plain radiographs.* **A.** *Radionuclide bone scan shows increased activity corresponding to underlying fractures.* (Fig. 7-3B continues on next page.)

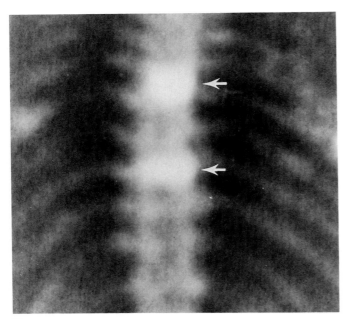

B

Figure 7-3   Vertebral Body Fracture (Continued). **B.** *SPECT scan is confirmatory. Arrows = increased nuclide activity corresponding to fractured vertebral bodies.*

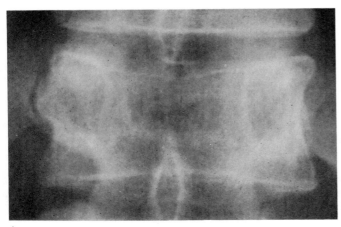

A

Figure 7-4   Acute Fracture of Vertebral Body (T12). *This world-class bobsledder developed acute back pain with transient bilateral lower extremity weakness and numbness. There was clinical need to date the chronicity of this abnormality. (Martire,[11] used with permission.)* **A.** *Coned anteroposterior radiograph of the thoracic spine demonstrates mild concavity of the upper endplate of the T12 vertebral body.* **B.** *High-resolution delayed image from TPBS of the thoracolumbar region of the spine demonstrates intense nuclide activity, positive on all three phases, involving the entire T12 vertebral body representing an acute fracture. Arrow = abnormal nuclide activity in T12 vertebral body.*

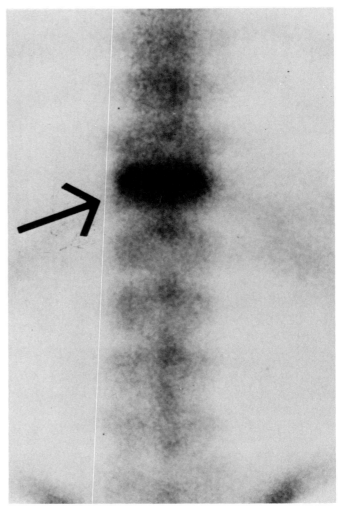

B

The selection and sequence of performance of multiple complementary diagnostic modalities should be heavily influenced by the type and localization of suspected injury, and associated neurologic manifestations.

Acute spine injuries may be classified by the following basic mechanisms:[21–24]

1. Flexion
2. Extension
3. Compression
4. Rotatory, frequently in combination with hyperflexion and hyperextension
5. Combination of the above

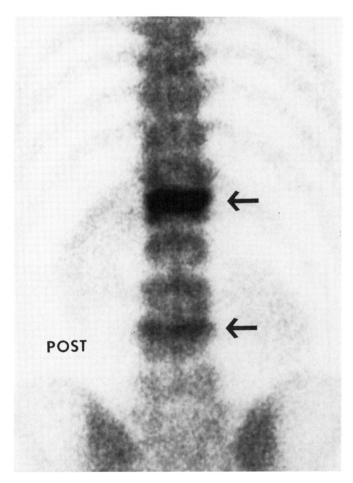

Figure 7-5 Acute Fracture of Vertebral Body (L1). *High-resolution delayed posterior image from TPBS of the thoraco-lumbar spine. Minimal nuclide activity is noted in the superior end plate of L4. Intense activity is seen in the superior half of L1 vertebral body. Sixty-nine-year-old female tennis player with acute and chronic back pain. These findings represent osteoporotic insufficiency fractures, chronic at L4 and acute at L1. Arrows = abnormal nuclide uptake in L1 and L4 vertebral bodies.*

ACUTE PROBLEMS

Ligamentous injuries (Figs. 7-6 and 7-7)

Ligamentous tears are the most frequently overlooked and least emphasized injuries to the spine in the acute setting of trauma. They commonly result in ligamentous instability leading to a high incidence of prolonged morbidity and debilitating pain.[36,37] These injuries include sprain, tear, and intraligamentous hemorrhage. Inadequately treated ligamentous disruption, particularly in the cervical spine, precipitates the development of degenerative hypertrophic spurs and erosive synovial and cartilaginous changes that eventually lead to vertebral and synovial joint subluxation and instability. Severe ligamentous disruptions are usually associated with flexion injuries.[37,38] Clinically, there is persistent pain and tenderness over the involved region. Radiographs taken dynamically in flexion and extension are usually accurate in determining the presence of significant ligamentous disruption and typically show the following:

1. Disproportionate widening of the interspinous distance with flexion (Fig. 7-6)
2. Widening of the injured uncovertebral joints and facet joints
3. Widening of the disk space posteriorly
4. Vertebral malalignment and malrotation

MR imaging allows recognition of associated ligamentous injury by the demonstration of hyperintense (edematous and hyperemic) ligamentous areas on T2-weighted sequences (Fig. 7-7).

Flexion injuries (Figs. 7-6 to 7-10)

This mechanism of injury is frequently characterized by the demonstration of severe pain and point tenderness over the involved interspinous space(s) and is often associated with marked limitation of flexion and extension. The more serious injuries are often associated with disruption of the posterior ligament complex (Figs. 7-6 to 7-8) and facet articulations, of which 50 percent develop delayed instability. Furthermore, this type of injury is associated with a high incidence of spinal cord damage.[23,24] The typical radiographic findings include the following:

1. Kyphotic angulation at the level of injury
2. Widening of the interspinous distance
3. Widening of the posterior disk space
4. Compression fracture (Fig. 7-9)
5. Facet dislocation, locked facets
6. "Teardrop" fracture (Fig. 7-10)

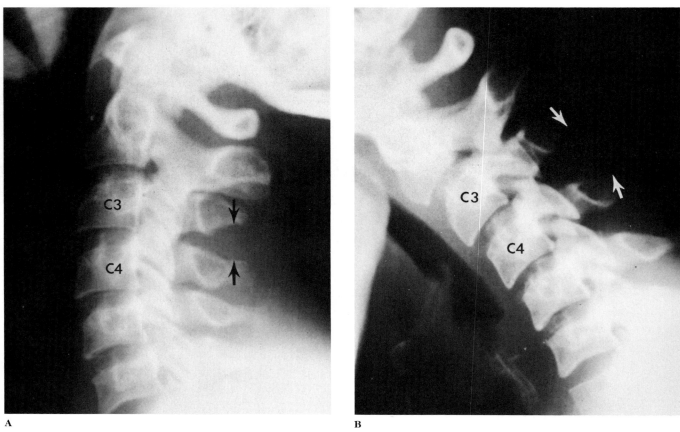

A   B

Figure 7-6 Ligamentous Injury C3-C4. **A.** *Widening of the C3-C4 interspinous distance (arrows) caused by ligamentous injury is evident on lateral radiograph with the neck held in the neutral position.* **B.** *With flexion there is additional widening of the interspinous distance (arrows).*

Figure 7-7 Flexion Injury of the Lower Thoracic Spine. *Sagittal T2-weighted image shows findings typical of severe flexion injury. There is posterior ligamentous disruption shown as a hyperintense area (closed arrows) and widening of the disk space posteriorly (open arrow). Edema or hemorrhage in the T12 vertebral body can be readily appreciated as an area of hyperintensity. Slight kyphosis can also be noted.*

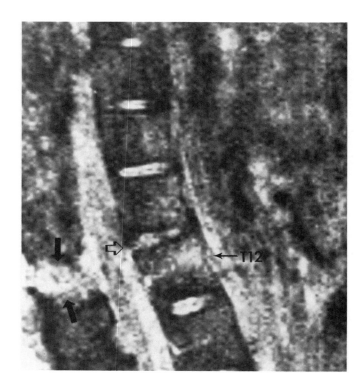

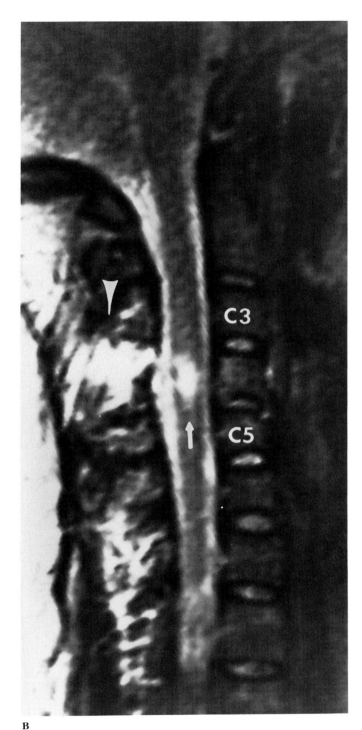

A

B

Figure 7-8 Subacute Posttraumatic Cord Cyst, Posterior Ligamentous Injury and Fracture. **A.** *Sagittal T1-weighted MR image demonstrates slight fusiform expansion of the midcervical cord from C3 to C5. The cyst can be appreciated as a focal hypointensity (arrow) in the central portion of the spinal cord at the* *level of C4. Decreased signal within posterior half of the C5 vertebral body reflects the presence of a fracture.* **B.** *Sagittal T2-weighted image shows the posttraumatic cyst as an oval region of hyperintensity (arrow). Adjacent edema contributes to and enlarges the hyperintense region. An irregular zone* *of hyperintensity (arrowhead) in the region of the posterior spinal ligaments indicates ligamentous disruption with edema and hemorrhage. The fractured and wedged C4 vertebral body shows hyperintense signal.*

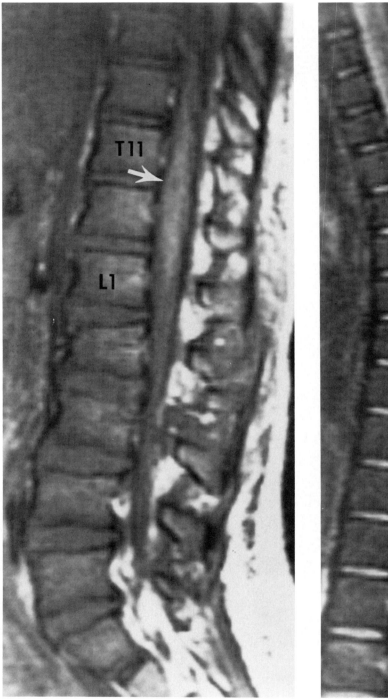

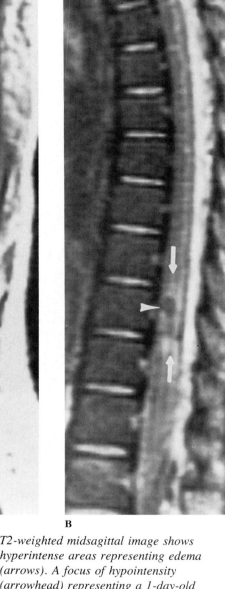

A

B

Figure 7-9   Spinal Cord Hematomas. **A.**
*T1-weighted midsagittal image shows slight
fusiform enlargement of the conus
medullaris. A subtle small focal
hypointensity (arrow) is noted at the T11-
T12 level. The L1 and L2 vertebral bodies
show anterior compression fractures.* **B.**

*T2-weighted midsagittal image shows
hyperintense areas representing edema
(arrows). A focus of hypointensity
(arrowhead) representing a 1-day-old
hematoma containing deoxyhemoglobin is
present.* (Fig. 7-9C through E continues on
the opposite page.)

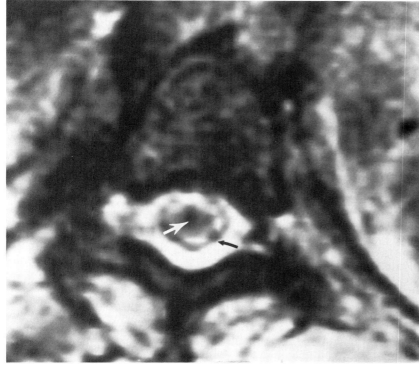

C

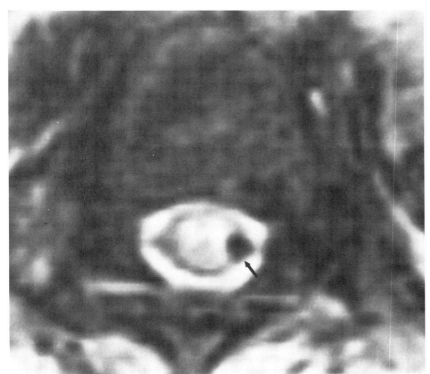

D

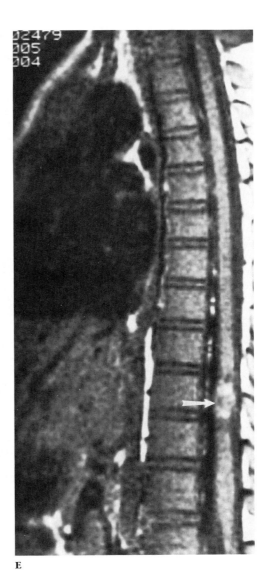

E

Figure 7-9 Spinal Cord Hematomas (Continued). **C, D.** *Gradient-recalled echo images in the axial plane sharply define the hemorrhagic foci with greater conspicuity, compared to the T1- and T2-weighted images. On these axial images central (white arrow) and peripheral (black arrow) hemorrhagic foci are readily delineated. **E.** T1-weighted sagittal image obtained almost 3 weeks later clearly defines the hematoma (arrow). The predominance of methemoglobin, which is now present, causes increased signal intensity.*

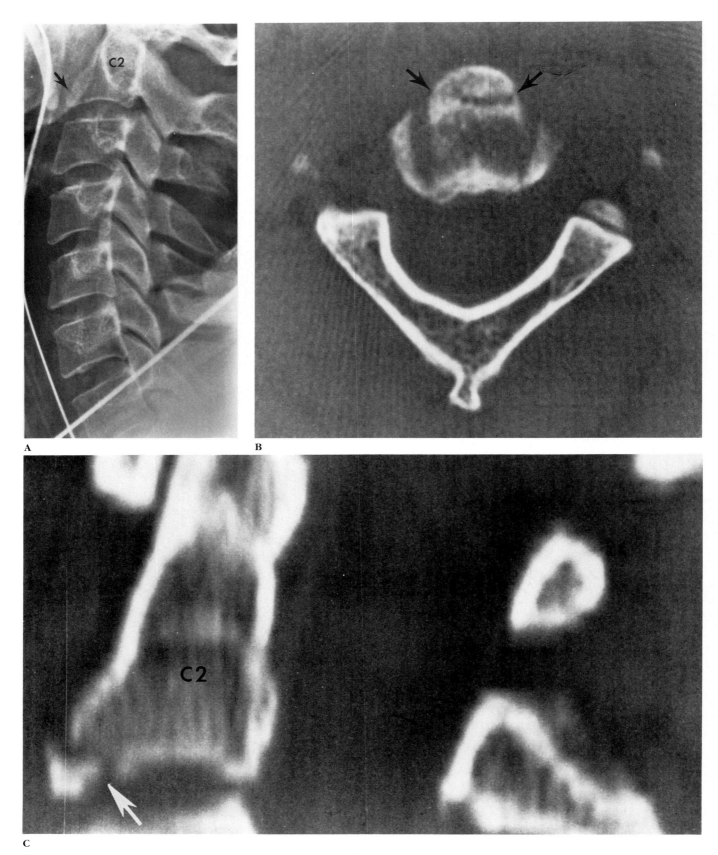

Figure 7-10   C2 Teardrop Fracture. **A.** *Teardrop fracture of C2 vertebral body is suggested from the plain film examination.* **B.** *CT is confirmatory.* **C.** *Sagittal reconstruction nicely demonstrates this fracture. Arrows = fracture line.*

Extension injuries (Fig. 7-11)

Extension injuries may go unrecognized because of the diversity and inconspicuousness of radiographic findings.[25,26] The following radiographic features have been stressed:[25–33]

1. Diffuse prevertebral soft tissue swelling with normally aligned cervical vertebrae (Fig. 7-11)
2. An avulsion fragment from the anterior aspect of the inferior end plate of the vertebra
3. Increased anterior height of the disk space, suggesting disruption of the anterior longitudinal ligament
4. Compressive fractures of the articular pillars, laminae, and spinous processes
5. Vacuum disk, or ''lucent cleft''
6. ''Hangman's'' fracture (traumatic spondylolisthesis of the axis)

A hyperextension type of injury should be considered likely if the patient demonstrates neurologic compromise with normal radiographic findings.

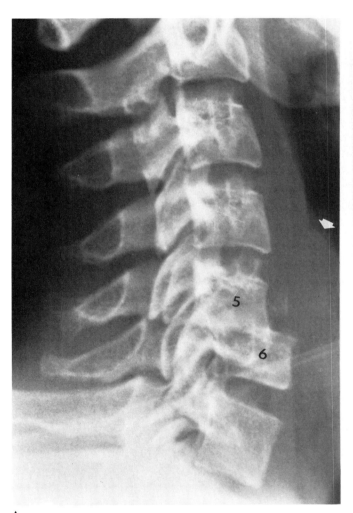

A

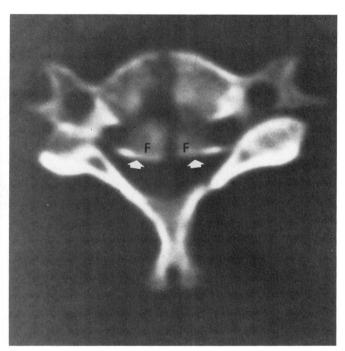

B

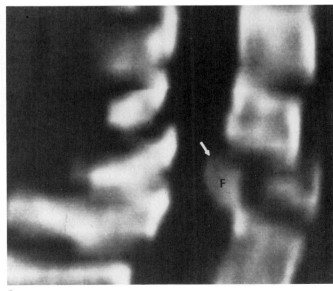

C

Figure 7-11   Hyperextension Comminuted Fracture. **A.** *Lateral radiograph following severe hyperextension injury shows diffuse prevertebral soft tissue swelling (arrow). There is posterior subluxation of C5 on C6 with a compression fracture of C6. The interspinous distances remain normal.* **B, C.** *Axial (B) and reformatted sagittal (C) CT images demonstrate a comminuted compression fracture of C6 with a retropulsed bony fragment (arrows) compromising 50 percent of the bony canal. F = retropulsed bony fragments.*

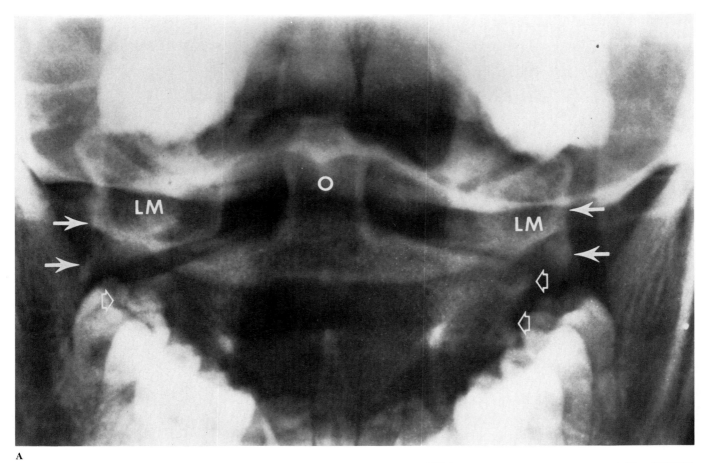

A

Compression injuries (Figs. 7-12 to 7-15)

This type of injury is usually caused by a vertical or axial loading force. This is typified by the following:[19,21–24,34,35]

1. Jefferson fracture (Fig. 7-12). This fracture is precipitated by a vertical force directed from the vertex of skull through the occipital condyles to the lateral masses of the atlas resulting in the following:
   (a) Lateral displacement of the articular masses of the atlas
   (b) Vertical fracture through one or both of the articular masses
   (c) Increased atlantoaxial interval of greater than 6 mm
   (d) Prevertebral soft tissue swelling
   (e) Fracture of the posterior arch of C1

2. Burst fracture (Figs. 7-13 to 7-15). This injury is caused by an axial loading force resulting in the following radiographic features.
   (a) Severe compression and communion of the vertebral body
   (b) Retropulsed bony fragments
   (c) Laminar fractures (unilateral or bilateral)
   (d) Disruption of the facet joints
   (e) Perivertebral hematoma

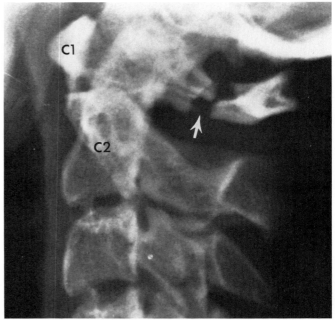

B

Figure 7-12 Jefferson Fracture. **A.** *Open-mouth view shows lateral displacement of the lateral masses of C1 (arrows) with respect to the C2 lateral masses (open arrows) and the odontoid process (O).* **B.** *Lateral radiograph shows fracture of the posterior arch of C1 (arrow). (Fig. 7-12C continues on the opposite page.)*

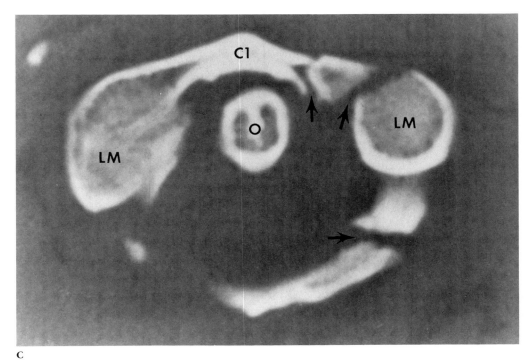

C

Figure 7-12 Jefferson Fracture (Continued). **C.** *Comminuted and displaced fracture (arrows) of the ring of C1 is clearly and best demonstrated with CT. LM = lateral mass of C1, O = odontoid process.*

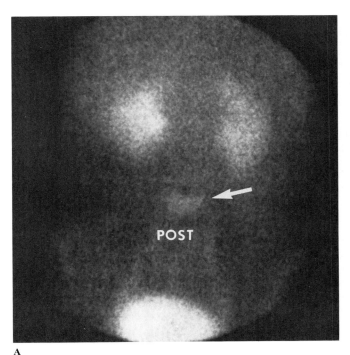

A

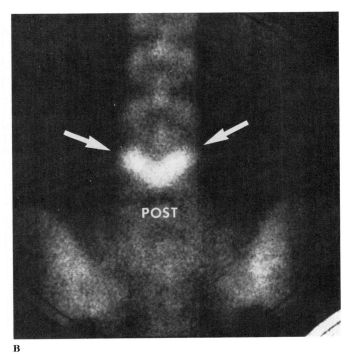

B

Figure 7-13 Acute Fracture of Vertebral Body (L4). **A.** *Initial blood pool image of TPBS. Faint nuclide activity is noted at L4. Posterior projection demonstrates excretion in the* kidneys, ureters, and bladder. Arrow = abnormal nuclide activity in the L4 vertebral body. **B.** *High-resolution delayed image, posterior projection. Butterfly, or V-shaped, nuclide activity is* noted in the L4 vertebral body. This pattern suggests a lumbar vertebral burst fracture. Arrows = area of increased nuclide activity. (Fig. 7-13C continues on next page.)

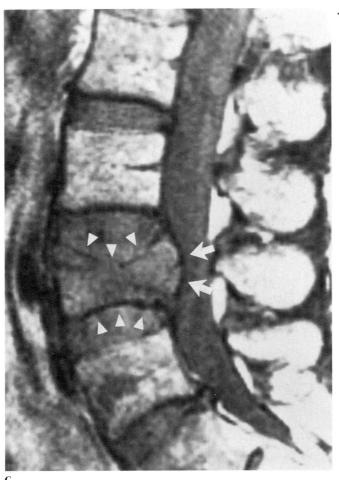

C

◀ **Figure 7-13** Acute Fracture of Vertebral Body (L4) (Continued). **C.** *MR scan of lower lumbar spine. Biconcave deformity of L4 vertebral body with posterior protrusion of the posterior bony cortex compressing the anterior aspect of the thecal sac. Arrowheads = concave appearing superior and inferior vertebral end plates; arrows = retropulsed posterior cortex of L4 indenting the anterior aspect of the thecal sac.*

Figure 7-14 Burst Fracture. **A.** *Lateral radiograph of the spine show a wedge fracture of the superior end plate of L1 (arrow) with minimal posterior displacement of bony fragments.* **B.** *CT clearly shows a 30 percent compromise of spinal canal by a posteriorly retropulsed fragment.* (Fig. 7-14C continues on the opposite page.)

▼

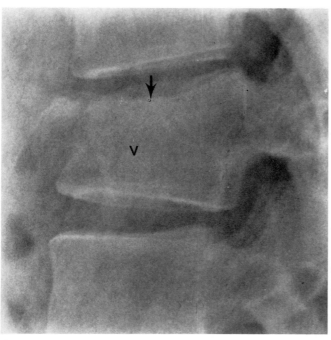

A

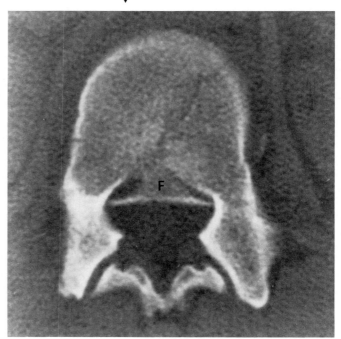

B

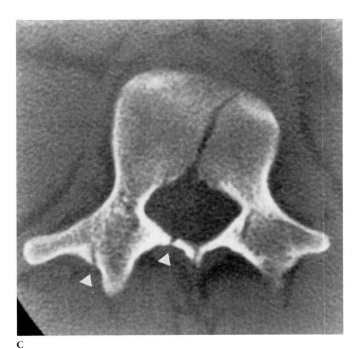

C

Figure 7-14   Burst Fracture (Continued). **C.** *Fractures of the right lamina and transverse process (arrowheads) are also present. F = retropulsed bony fragment; V = L1 vertebral body.*

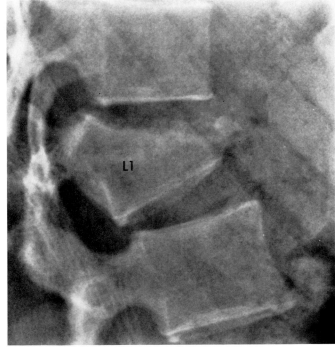

A

Figure 7-15   Burst Fracture L1. **A.** *Burst fracture with anterior compression of L1. There is posterior displacement of bony fragments.* **B.** *CT demonstrates burst fracture of L1 with 40 percent spinal canal compromise. Pedicle fractures are evident (arrows).* (Fig. 7-15C–E continues on following pages.)

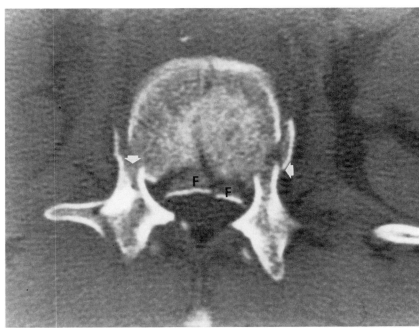

B

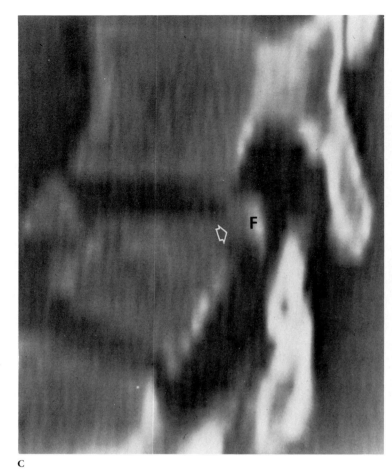

Figure 7-15   Burst Fracture L1 (Continued). **C.** *Retropulsed fragment (open arrow) causing canal compromise is well seen on this sagittal reconstruction.* **D.** *Coronal reconstruction shows longitudinal fractures of the right lamina (thick arrow) and right transverse process (thin arrow).* (Fig. 7–15E continues on the opposite page.)

C

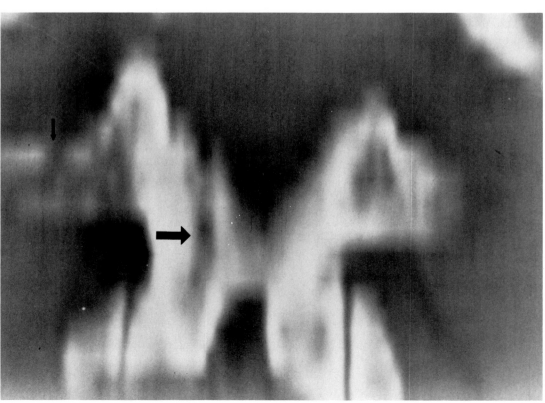

D

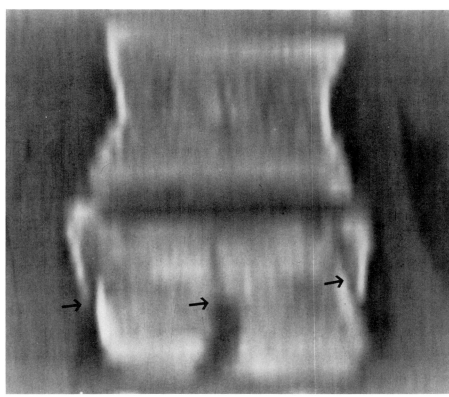

E

Figure 7-15 Burst Fracture L1 (Continued). **E.** *Multiple vertically oriented fractures (arrows) are shown on this coronal reconstruction. F = retropulsed fragment.*

Rotatory injuries (Figs. 7-16 to 7-21)

The combination of rotatory force with hyperflexion and hyperextension results in comminuted fractures of the articular masses, severe rotatory subluxation of the spine, and neurologic compromise. Asymmetric burst fractures, wedged vertebral body fractures, unilaterally locked facets, and asymmetric laminar fractures are frequently the result of this mechanism.[19,21–24]

Fractures (Figs. 7-4 and 7-5, 7-13 to 7-17, and 7-19 to 7-24)

Plain films are the initial diagnostic modality in the evaluation of fractures both in the acute and nonacute setting. Despite this, it is generally acknowledged that a significant number of fractures (greater than 25 percent) elude detection on plain films.[19,39] CT may visualize fractures not demonstrated by plain film radiographs (Figs. 7-16 and 7-17). However, MR is superior for the detection of associated soft tissue injury.[40–43]

Figure 7-16 Pedicle Fracture. **A.** *Lateral radiograph shows* ▶ *a fracture of the posterior elements of C5 as well as subluxation (arrow) of C5 on C6.* (Fig. 7-16B continues on next page.)

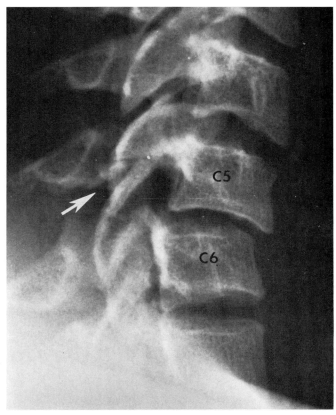

A

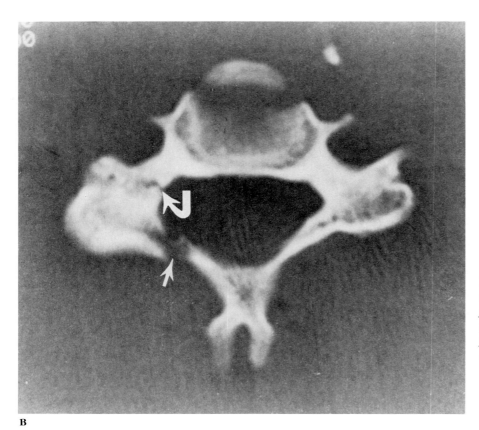

Figure 7-16 Pedicle Fracture (Continued). **B.** *CT demonstrates a fracture (curved arrow) of the right C5 pedicle, which was not seen on plain films, as well as a fracture of the right C5 lamina (arrow).*

B

Figure 7-17 Lateral Mass Fracture. *CT shows a vertical fracture through the right articular facet of C4 (arrow). This fracture could not be seen on the routine radiographs.*

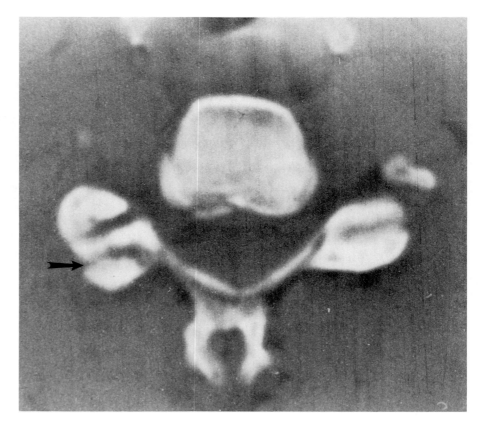

Acute fractures of the spine, even without distal cord symptoms, represent for the athlete a serious if not critical situation requiring, at the minimum, complete cessation of athletic activity. Several different scenarios can face the physician when vertebral body fracture is suspected. First, the radiograph may show abnormality in the area of pain, but uncertainty exists as to the chronicity of this finding. TPBS should be positive on all three phases for acute fracture (Figs. 7-4, 7-5, and 7-13).[11,20] The second diagnostic problem involves the athlete with a history of old or healing spinal fracture complicated by a new acute injury. Although TPBS shows increased nuclide activity for all phases of an acute fracture, a chronic or healing fracture is usually positive only on the delayed phase. Serial bone scans in aging fractures have shown that at 1 year almost 60 percent are normal on TPBS (approximately 40 percent will still be positive on scan) and at 2 years 90 percent show a normal scan appearance.[20]

MR imaging is required if spinal cord injury is a clinical consideration in the setting of spinal trauma.

Computed tomography is widely accepted for its accurate and definitive role in demonstrating and characterizing spine fractures.[44,45] It provides excellent depiction of the integrity of the vertebra and the patency of the spinal canal and intervertebral foramina. CT additionally allows the evaluation of adjacent organs that may be involved. It is unsurpassed in the demonstration of spinal instability that is primarily caused by fractures. These include

1. Vertebral body fracture close to the pedicles (Fig. 7-15)
2. Pedicle fracture (Fig. 7-16)
3. Facet and laminar fracture (Figs. 7-15, 7-17, and 7-19)
4. Retropulsed fragments (Figs. 7-14 and 7-15)
5. Pars interarticularis fracture (Fig. 7-22)

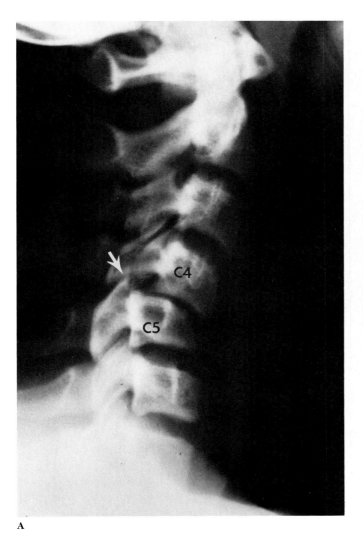
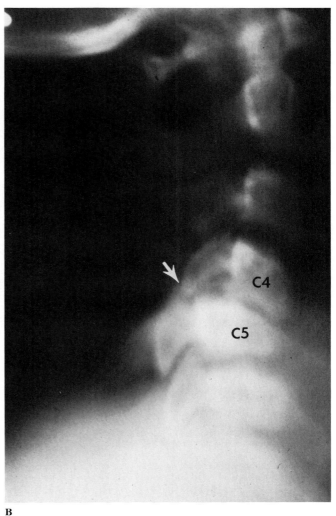

A

B

Figure 7-18   C4-C5 Subluxation with Perched Facet. **A.** *Lateral radiograph shows subluxation of C4 on C5 with perched facet (arrow).* **B.** *Perched facet (arrow) is better demonstrated on conventional tomogram.*

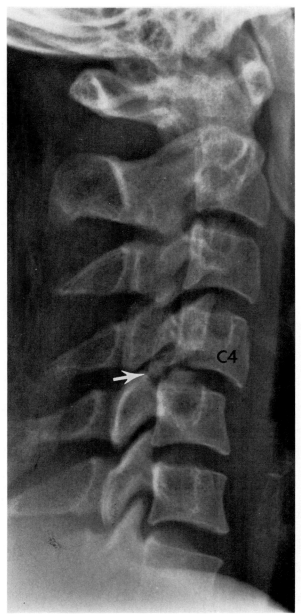

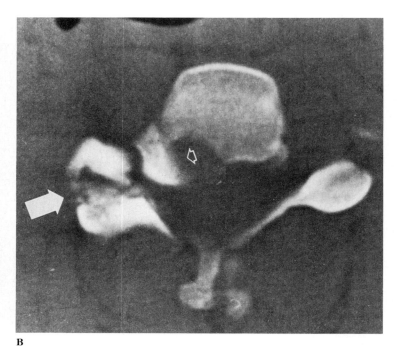

Figure 7-19   Rotatory Subluxation with Fractured Locked Facet. **A.** *Plain radiograph demonstrates rotation of C4 on C5 with unilaterally locked facet at that level (arrow).* **B.** *CT shows locked facet with fracture of right lateral mass (thick arrow) and bony fragment from superior end plate of C5 (open arrow).*

A

B

Acquisition of reformatted coronal and sagittal images from the axial study facilitates the detection and accurate analysis of the following:

1. Compression and comminuted vertebral fractures (Fig. 7-15)
2. Horizontally directed vertebral body fractures and articular pillar and pedicle fractures that could be missed on the axial study
3. Compromise of spinal canal by retropulsed fragments (Fig. 7-15)
4. Ligamentous injury suggested by widening of the interspinous distance and facet joints
5. Locked and/or perched facets (Figs. 7-20 and 7-21)

Reformatted CT images in the coronal and sagittal planes derived from the axial study (without added radiation) help in the thorough and complete evaluation of spinal fractures.

Pleuridirectional tomography has virtually been replaced by CT in the evaluation of fractures. Nevertheless, this modality can provide detailed images of fractures in the axial plane of some bony elements such as the articular pillars and the base of the odontoid process[46] (Figs. 7-23 and 7-24).

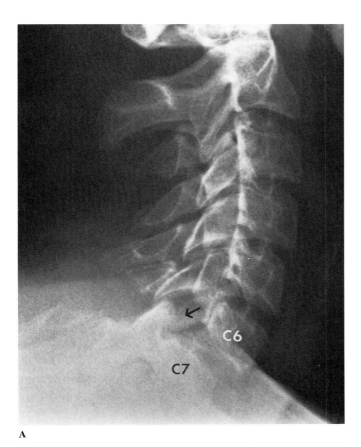

A

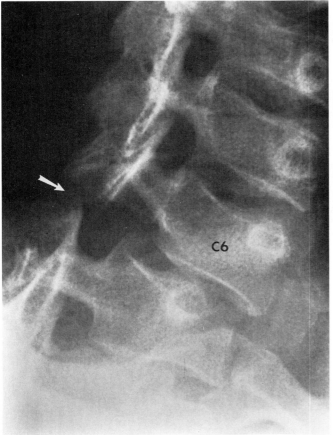

B

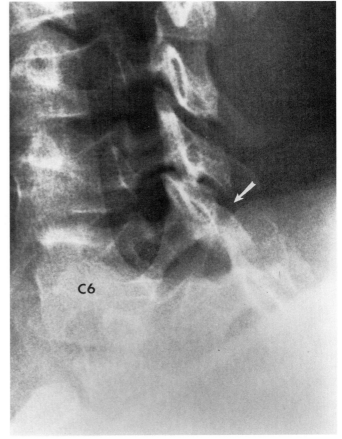

C

Figure 7-20 Bilateral Facet Dislocation. **A.** *Lateral radiograph shows subluxation of C6 on C7 with bilaterally disrupted facets (arrow).* **B, C.** *Oblique radiographs show perched facet of C6 (arrow) on right (B) and locked facet of C6 (arrow) on left (C).* (Fig. 7-20D–G continues on next page.)

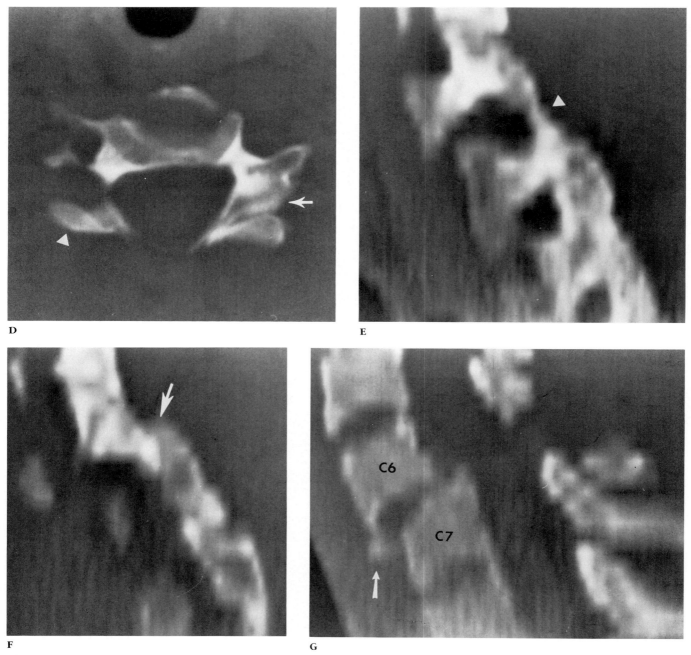

D

E

F

G

Figure 7-20 Bilateral Facet Dislocation (Continued). **D.** *Axial CT shows locked facet (arrow) and perched facet (arrowhead).* **E, F.** *Sagittal reconstructions show perched facet (E, arrowhead) and locked facet (F, arrow).* **G.** *Midline reconstruction shows anterior subluxation of C6 on C7. A teardrop fracture fragment (arrow) is now seen.*

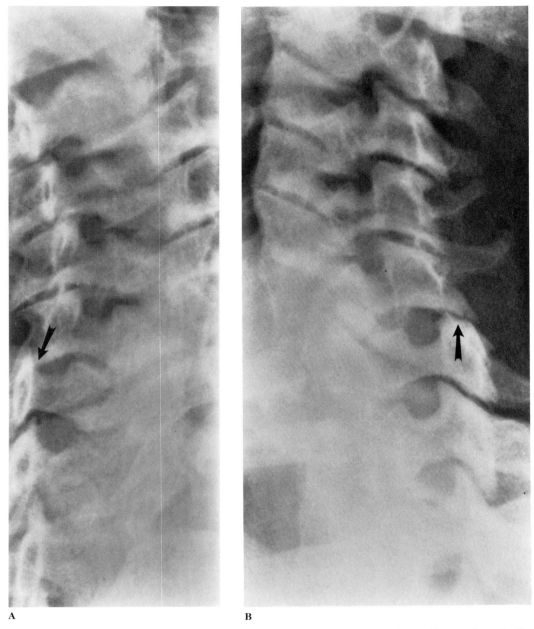

A

B

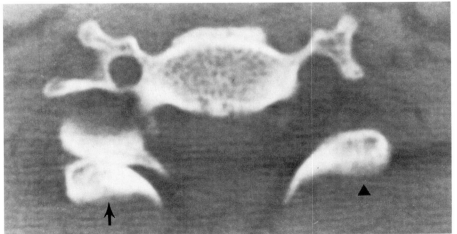

C

Figure 7-21 Facet Dislocation. **A, B.** *Oblique projections show locked facet (arrow) on right (A) and perched facet (arrow) on left (B).* **C.** *CT demonstrates locked facet (arrow) on right and perched facet (arrowhead) on left. (Fig. 7-21D and E continues on next page.)*

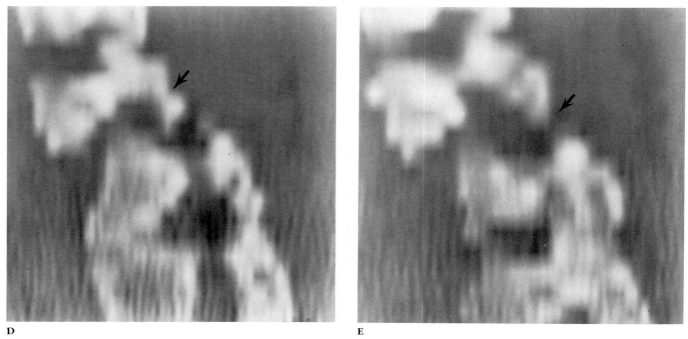

D   **E**

Figure 7-21 Facet Dislocation (Continued). **D, E.** *Sagittal reconstructions show locked right facet* (D) *and perched left facet* (E). *Arrows = abnormal facet.*

Figure 7-22 Bilateral Pars Interarticularis Defect (L5). **A.** *Right posterior oblique projection shows faint sclerotic abnormality (arrows) at the L5 pars.* (Fig. 7-22B and C continues on the opposite page.)

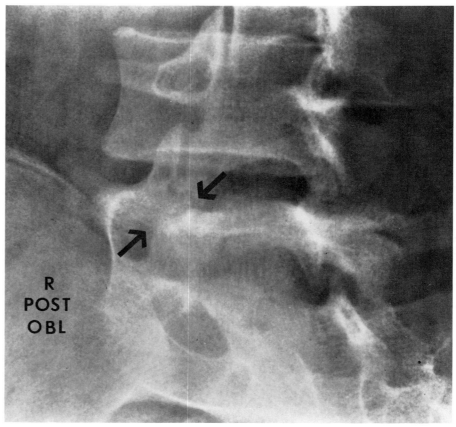

A

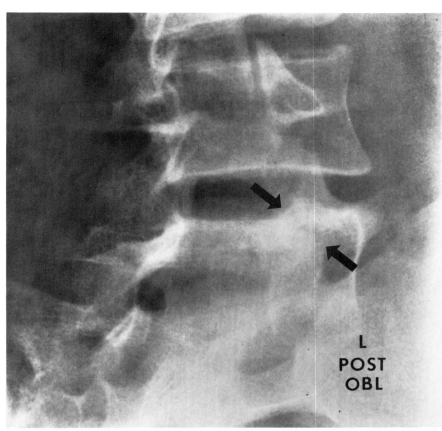

B

Figure 7-22   Bilateral Pars
Interarticularis Defect (L5)
(Continued). **B.** *Left posterior oblique
projection. Moderate sclerosis (arrows)
at left L5 pars with a faint, lucent line
through the pars.* **C.** *High-resolution
delayed posterior image from TPBS.
There is mildly increased activity at the
L5 pars on the left with minimally
increased activity on the right.* (Fig.
7-22D and E continues on next page.)

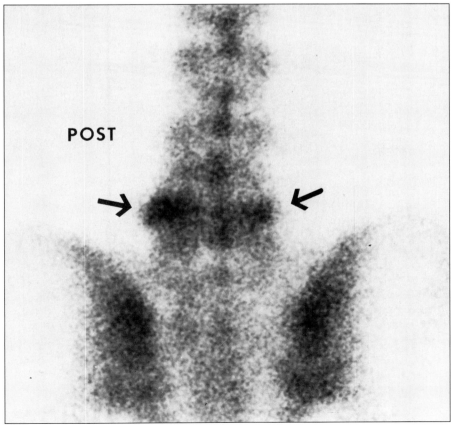

C

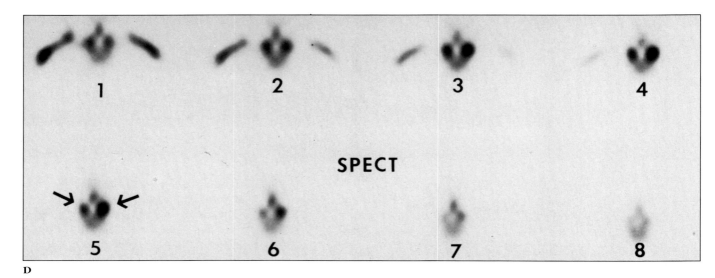

D

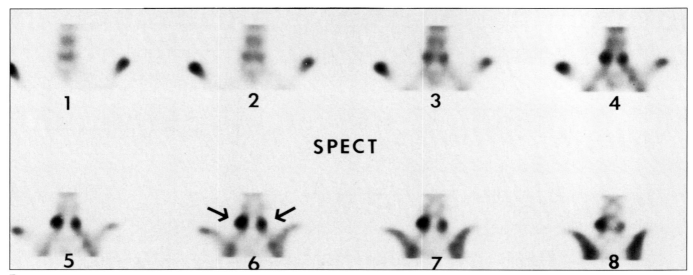

E

Figure 7-22 Bilateral Pars Interarticularis Defect (L5) (Continued). **D.** *SPECT scan in the transverse plane of TPBS, in the lower portion of the lumbar spine. Abnormal nuclide activity bilaterally (arrows) in the L5 pars which is more intense on the left side. Images are displayed sequentially from caudal to cranial, with #1 being most caudal and #8 most cranial.* **E.** *SPECT scan in the coronal plane. Abnormal nuclide activity bilaterally (arrows) in the L5 pars which is more intense on the left side. Images are displayed sequentially from anterior to posterior, with #1 being the most anterior and #8 the most posterior. Arrows = abnormal nuclide activity in the L5 pars bilaterally. SPECT imaging is a sensitive modality for detecting subtle or minimal abnormalities in the lumbar spine.*

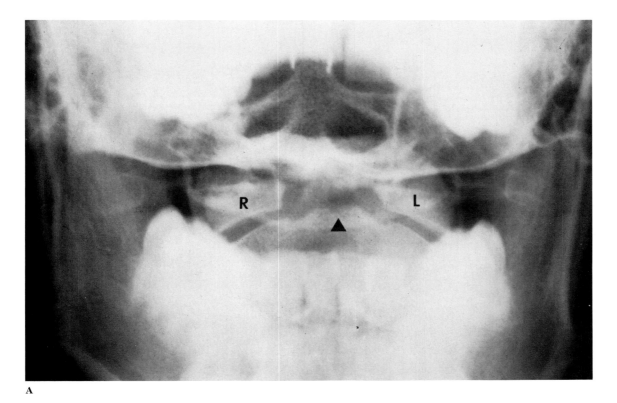

A

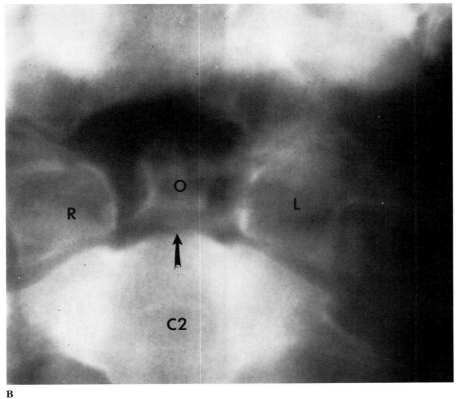

B

Figure 7-23 Odontoid Fracture (Type II). **A.** *Open-mouth radiograph reveals fracture (arrowhead) through the base of odontoid process, representing a type II fracture.* **B.** *Anteroposterior tomograph* *better demonstrates the fracture (arrow). Since the fracture line is parallel to the axial plane, routine multidirectional tomography more optimally demonstrates this abnormality than does axial CT. R* *= right lateral mass of C1; L = left lateral mass of C1; O = odontoid process, C2 = body of axis.*

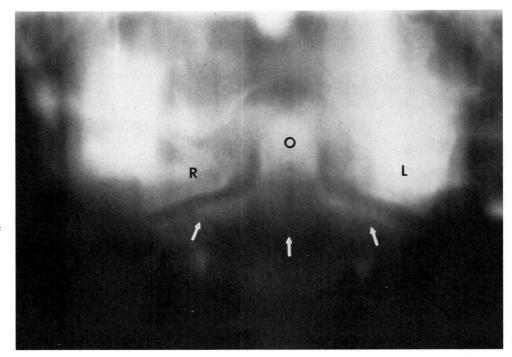

Figure 7-24 Odontoid Fracture (Type III). **A.** *Tomogram shows fracture (arrows) through the base of the C2 vertebral body, indicating type III fracture.* **B.** *Lateral radiograph confirms the fracture. R = right lateral mass of C1; L = left lateral mass of C1; O = odontoid process.*

A

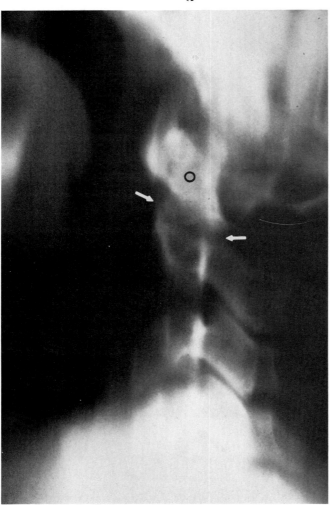

B

Spinal cord injury (Figs. 7-25 to 7-32)

A frequently unrecognized and underemphasized clinical condition that predisposes to severe traumatic spinal cord injury is *congenital stenosis* of the cervical portion of the spine[47] (Figs. 7-25 and 7-26). The existence of a narrow cervical spinal canal can be diagnosed when the posterior margins of the lateral elements overlap an imaginary line linking the spinolaminar junctions of the cervical vertebrae on a lateral plain film of the cervical spine (Fig. 7-26). The typical radiographic features of congenital spinal stenosis that are best shown by CT include the following:

1. Small sagittal and transverse diameters of the spinal canal (13 mm or smaller in the lumbar region and smaller than 10 mm in the cervical region)

2. Short and broad pedicles

3. Scanty epidural fat

4. Narrow lateral recesses

The currently favored diagnostic modality for the demonstration of bony compression of the spinal cord is MR imaging. MR noninvasively and accurately demonstrates spinal cord flattening and displacement by bony elements (Fig. 7-25).

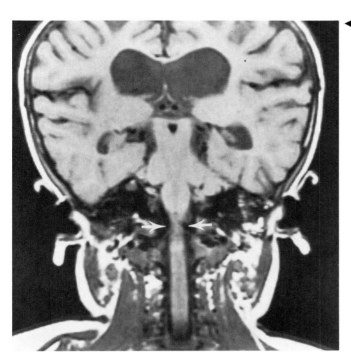

Figure 7-25 Congenital Spinal Stenosis. *Coronal T1-weighted image shows waistlike narrowing of upper cervical cord (arrows) at foramen magnum.*

Figure 7-26 Congenital Spinal Stenosis. **A.** *Lateral radiograph demonstrates features characteristic for congenital stenosis of the cervical spine. The posterior margins of the lateral masses (arrows) closely approximate an imaginary line through the spinolaminar junctions.* **B.** *Anteroposterior radiograph of the thoracolumbar spine of another patient shows large pedicles (P) and narrow interpedicular distances (arrows), indicating congenital spinal stenosis.*

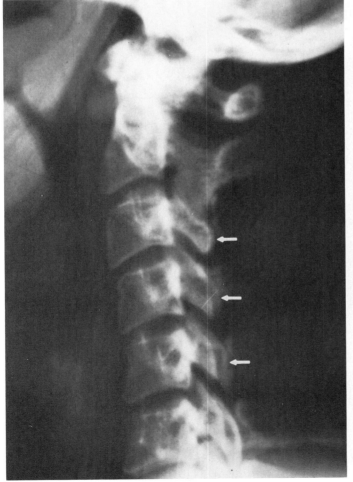

A

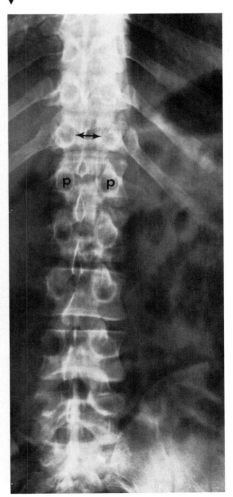

B

MR imaging has become the diagnostic modality of choice for the evaluation of posttraumatic spinal cord injury. Not only is it highly sensitive to the presence of acute and subacute contusion (Fig. 7-27), hematoma (Fig. 7-10), and edema (Fig. 7-28) but it is also useful in the assessment of chronic changes, which include posttraumatic cyst (Figs. 7-9, 7-29, and 7-30), myelomalacia, atrophy, and transection of the cord[40,48–50] (Fig. 7-31). The usual MR imaging sequences for the evaluation of spinal cord injury include the following:

1. T1-weighted axial and sagittal images (4 mm thick)

2. T2-weighted and proton density sagittal images (4 mm thick)

3. T2*-weighted gradient-recalled echo (GRE) sagittal and axial images (4 mm thick)

The diagnostic determination of parenchymal abnormality is based on characteristic features exhibited on the different imaging sequences (Table 7-1).

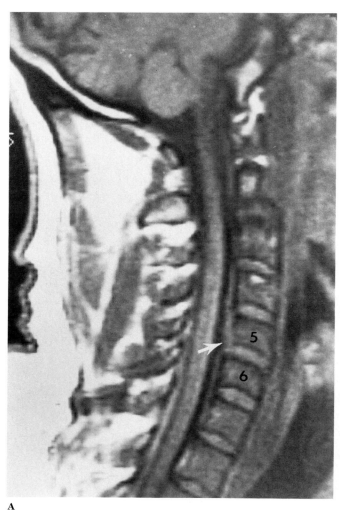

A

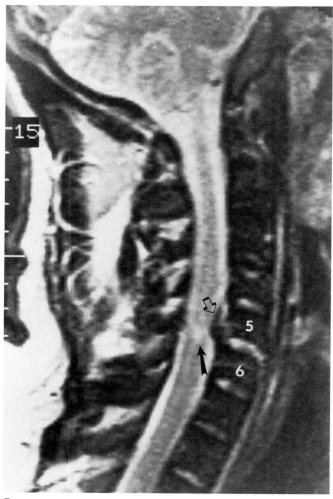

B

Figure 7-27   Herniated Nucleus Pulposus (HNP) C5-C6 with Cord Contusion. **A.** *T1-weighted MR image shows herniated C5-C6 disk with upward extension (arrow) posterior to C5.* **B.** *High-signal intensity focus (arrow) representing contusion of the spinal cord is evident on this T2-weighted image. Herniated disk (open arrow) is present.*

TABLE 7-1

MR imaging: traumatic spinal cord changes

Contusion hematoma	T1-weighted	T2-weighted
Acute (1–4 days) Deoxyhemoglobin	Hypointense to isointense	Hypointense to isointense

Subacute (5–10 days)
  Intracellular methemoglobin
  Extracellular methemoglobin
	Hyperintense	Hypointense to isointense
		Hyperintense

Chronic (weeks to months)	Foci of hyperintensity (methemoglobin) and hypointensity (hemosiderin)	Mixed hypo- and hyperintense
Edema	Isointense	Hyperintense
Myelomalacia	Iso- to hypointense	Hyperintense
Posttraumatic cyst and syringomyelia	Hypointense	Hyperintense

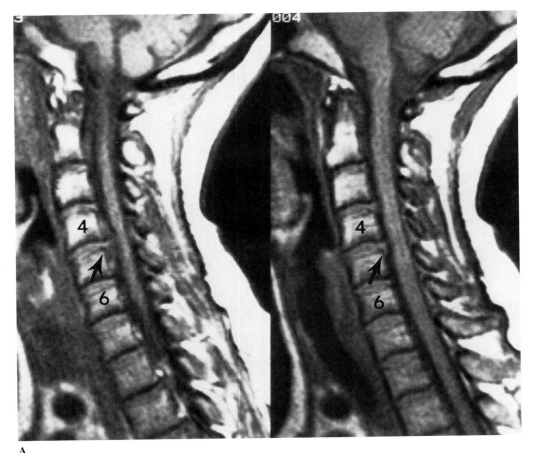

A

Figure 7-28 Cervical Disk Herniation. **A.** *Left parasagittal and midsagittal images demonstrate a left posterolateral herniation of the C4-C5 disk (arrow). Note the increased soft tissue behind the C4 and C5 vertebral bodies due to either epidural tissues or migrated/ extruded disk fragments. (Fig. 7-28B–D continues on following pages.)*

GRE imaging is extremely sensitive to the presence of *acute* hemorrhagic contusion within and outside the spinal cord and provides greater conspicuity of the lesion than do T1- and T2-weighted studies (Figs. 7-10 and 7-31). Spinal cord edema is best detected with combined T1- and T2-weighted imaging. GRE provides excellent contrast resolution, allowing distinction to be made between the subarachnoid space, spinal cord, dura, and bony margins. It is therefore an ideal sequence for the demonstration of spinal cord compression.

The availability of MR compatible life support equipment has facilitated the acceptance of this modality for the evaluation of the acutely injured spine. MR has essentially replaced both myelography and CT myelography for this purpose and has been shown to be the most accurate modality in evaluating traumatic spinal cord changes.[40,49–52] Recent studies have substantiated its capability to accurately detect spinal cord injury. Furthermore, MR imaging provides a method to separate hemorrhagic lesions (with serious prognostic implications) from edematous reaction (Fig. 7-32), thus allowing more accurate prediction of the clinical outcome of traumatic spinal cord injury.[40,48,51,53–55]

Herniated intervertebral disk (Figs. 7-27, 7-28, and 7-32 to 7-35)

Although data on the true incidence of herniated disk in the athletic population are lacking, disk herniation is not uncommonly related to trauma.[40,51] Generally, disk herniation is most commonly encountered at the L4-L5 and L5-S1 levels (90 to 95 percent of lumbar disk herniations)[56,57] and at C5-C6 and C6-C7 (90 percent of cervical disk herniation).[58,59] Symptomatic disk herniation in the thoracic region is rare.[60] In the lumbar region, disk herniation commonly presents with radiculopathy in addition to persistent and severe back pain. In the thoracic and cervical regions, myelopathy is usually seen in association with radiculopathy.[59,60] Myelopathy is the result of spinal cord compression with clinical manifestations of long tract signs of hyperreflexia, spasticity, and Babinski sign. Unilateral or bilateral extremity weakness, numbness and, when severe, loss of bowel and bladder control may also accompany the injury.[60,61]

Traumatic disk herniation can occur with either extension or flexion injuries but most commonly with a combined flexion-compression mechanism.[62] Disk herniation may ac-

Figure 7-28 Cervical Disk Herniation (Continued). **B.** *Gradient-recalled images corresponding to those in* A *clearly demonstrate the left posterolateral C4-C5 disk herniation (arrow) and the sharply defined displaced dura (arrowhead). Focal disk herniation has an intensity that is similar to the disk of origin. The soft tissues behind C4 and C5 shown in* A *represent prominent epidural tissues beneath the displaced dura; the herniated disk shows a slight caudal slope. (Fig. 7-28C continues on the opposite page.)*

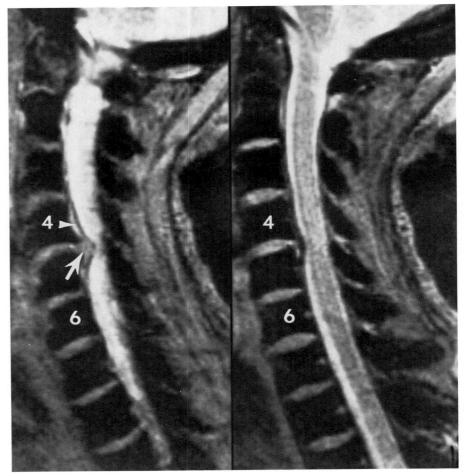

B

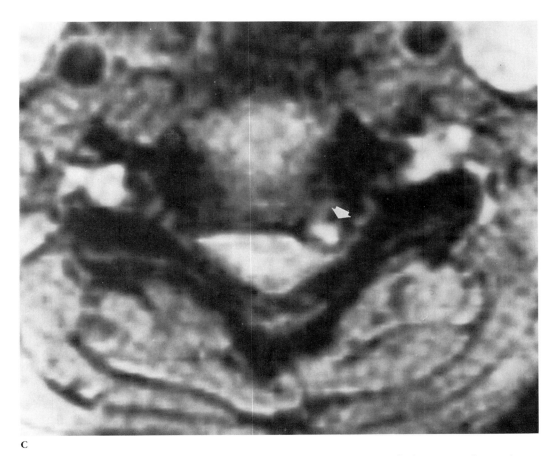

C

Figure 7-28   Cervical Disk Herniation (Continued). **C.** *Gradient-recalled image in the axial plane through the C4-C5 disk level clearly defines a left posterolateral disk herniation (arrow). A herniated disk usually displays high-signal intensity on gradient-echo imaging technique; hypertrophic spurs show hypointense signal intensity. (Fig. 7-28D continues on next page.)*

count for or contribute to spinal cord compression, contusion, and edema. In Flanders' series of 78 patients with acute traumatic cervical cord injury (including 19 percent diving-related and 9 percent recreational sports-related injuries), a 51 percent prevalence of herniated disk was reported. Forty-eight percent of patients with complete neurologic deficit (para/quadraplegic) had a radiologically demonstrated herniated disk.[51] Thus, detection of an associated disk herniation should constitute one of the major goals in the evaluation of spine trauma.

The current diagnostic modalities available for the evaluation of herniated disk are MR imaging, CT, and CTM. In comparative studies, the accuracy of MR imaging is equal to or greater than CT and CTM in the diagnosis of *lumbar disk* herniation.[63,64] The major advantages of MR imaging include its noninvasiveness, lack of ionizing radiation, multiplanar capability, and ability to simultaneously evaluate the conus medullaris. CT and CTM are highly accurate in the diagnosis of herniated lumbar disk, provide important detail regarding small traumatic bone fragments, and demonstrate

the contents of the subarachnoid space (conus medullaris, cauda equina, filum terminale) to great advantage.

In the screening and localization of traumatic thoracic and cervical disk herniation, MR imaging is the favored diagnostic tool.[40,51] Sagittal T1- and T2-weighted images provide an accurate survey of a long segment of the spine, a region where it is frequently difficult to accurately localize the exact level of radiculopathy and myelopathy. If a more detailed evaluation of a specific level is required, additional sequences such as axial GRE and T1-weighted images may be obtained to more completely evaluate a herniated disk. In the assessment of cervical radiculopathy, MR imaging correlates well with the surgical findings of disease.[65-67] CT and CTM, although highly accurate diagnostic modalities in their own right, maintain complementary roles in those instances where MR imaging fails to completely explain the clinical problem. CT remains most effective in the demonstration of cortical bony excrescences, calcifications, and bony fragments.

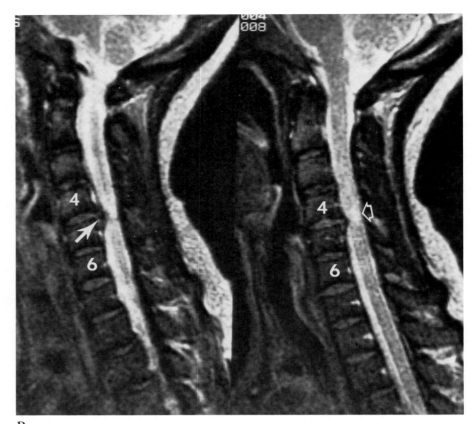

Figure 7-28 Cervical Disk Herniation (Continued). **D.** *T2-weighted sagittal images corresponding to* **A** *and* **B.** *The C4-C5 focal disk herniation (arrow) with slight downward protrusion is shown. In addition, an intramedullary edematous zone (open arrow), resulting from recent trauma, is also demonstrated. The T2-weighted imaging sequence is the most sensitive sequence for detection of spinal cord edema.*

D

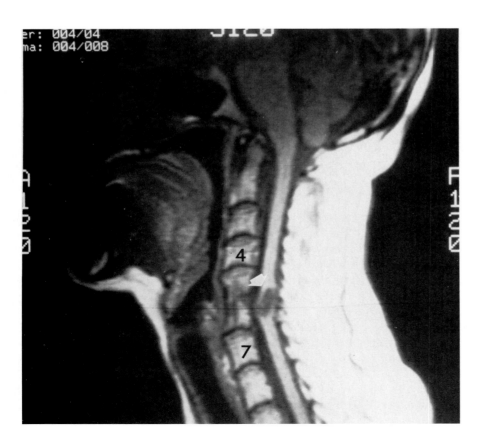

Figure 7-29 Posttraumatic Syrinx (Cervical Cord). *Hypointense syrinx (arrow) is shown on sagittal T1-weighted image. Note congenital anterior body fusion at the C5-C6 level.*

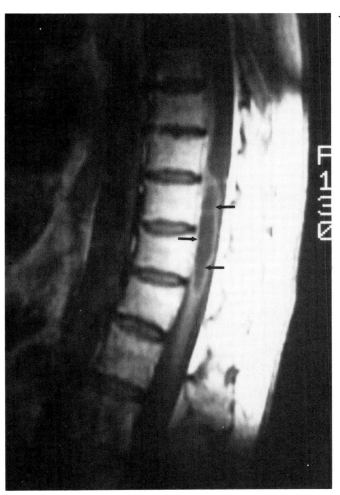

A

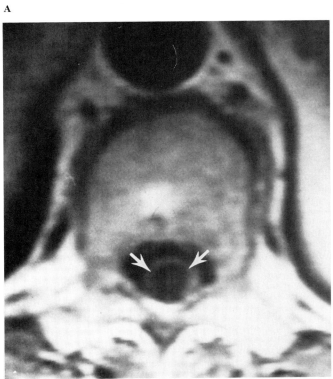

B

◀ **Figure 7-30** Posttraumatic Syrinx (Thoracic Cord). **A.** *Sagittal T1-weighted image demonstrates syrinx cavity (arrows) in the lower thoracic spinal cord.* **B.** *Axial T1-weighted images show syrinx cavity (arrows).*

▲
Figure 7-31 Cord Transsection. *Sagittal T1-weighted MR image shows interruption of the thoracic spinal cord from T9 to T12. Arrows point to the cord. Note compression fractures of T10 and T11.*

The diagnosis of *herniated disk* is made in the presence of a focal polypoid protrusion of disk material beyond the posterior margins of adjacent vertebral bodies (Figs. 7-27, 7-28, and 7-32 to 7-35). Disk herniations in the lumbar and cervical regions are frequently posterolateral; in the thoracic region disk herniations are usually posterocentral. Disk herniations are commonly associated with central or eccentric deformity of the subarachnoid space with displacement and flattening of the affected nerve root. In the cervical and thoracic regions, spinal cord flattening with rotation occurs.

Nerve root and spinal cord flattening and displacement are best appreciated in the *axial plane*.

Lateral disk herniation is an extruded disk into the intervertebral foramen that may or may not affect the dorsal root ganglion and exiting motor nerve root (Fig. 7-28). Axial images confirm this most accurately.[68] Diagnosis of lateral disk herniation by MR imaging requires the additional observation of obliteration of the intraforaminal fat on parasagittal images.

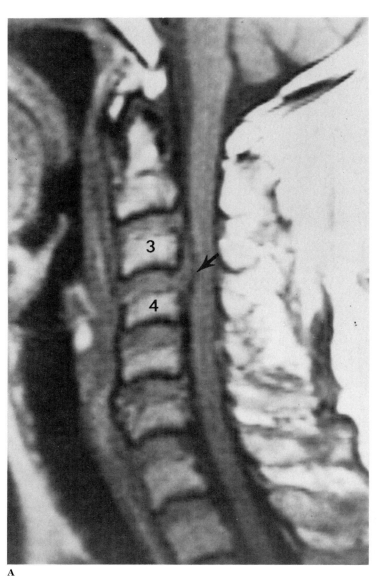

A

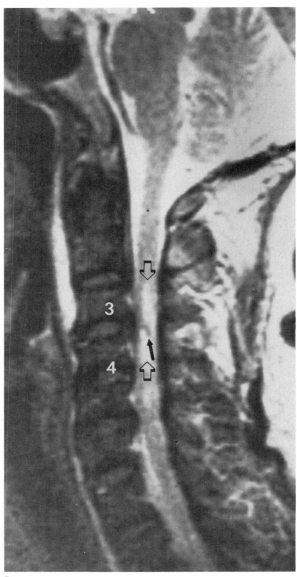

B

Figure 7-32   HNP C3-C4 with Cord Contusion. **A.** *T1-weighted sagittal image shows herniated C3-C4 disk (arrow) extending superiorly and posteriorly to the C3 vertebral body causing mild spinal cord compression.* **B.** *T2-weighted MR image demonstrates cord contusion (open arrows) and hemorrhage (thin arrow) not seen on T1-weighted image. (Fig. 7-32C and D continues on the opposite page.)*

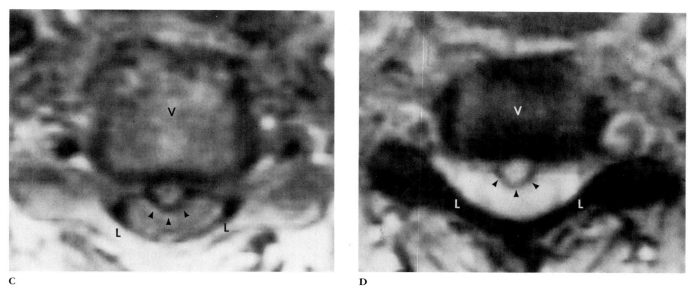

C   D

Figure 7-32 HNP C3-C4 with Cord Contusion (Continued). **C.** *Axial T1-weighted image shows disk herniation (arrowheads) and spinal cord compression.* **D.** *Gradient echo image confirms this finding (arrowheads). V = vertebral body; L = lamina.*

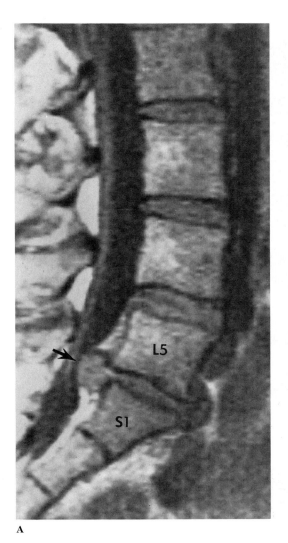

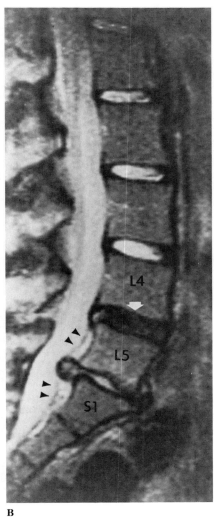

Figure 7-33 Herniated Lumbar Disk. **A.** *T1-weighted midsagittal MR image demonstrates a polypoid protrusion of the L5-S1 disk (arrow) well beyond the posterior margins of the vertebral bodies. Note the similarity in intensity between the herniated disk and the disk of origin. The subarachnoid space is deformed by the herniated disk.* **B.** *On this T2-weighted study the deflected dura can be delineated (arrowheads). The T2-weighted MR sequence is sensitive to the presence of degenerative disk disease, which is commonly hypointense because of dessication. This is seen at L4-L5 (arrow). Note the normal hyperintense disks at the levels above.*

A   B

An *extruded* and *migrated disk fragment* is characteristically separate from the disk of origin and may have migrated from the disk space above or below (Fig. 7-34).

Disk herniation at any level of the spine should be carefully distinguished from a diffuse disk bulge, a smooth, usually degenerative disk protrusion which is not commonly associated with radiculopathy or myelopathy. When disk herniation is suspected, consecutive 3-mm (lumbar) or 1.5-mm (thoracic and cervical) axial CT images should be obtained through the region of clinical interest. Acquisition of angled axial images coplanar to the disk space completes the examination. Intravenous injection of iodinated contrast medium enhances the accuracy of CT in the diagnosis of herniated cervical disk. Such examination provides excellent delineation of the nonenhancing herniated disk and nerve roots from the enhancing epidural tissues.[69]

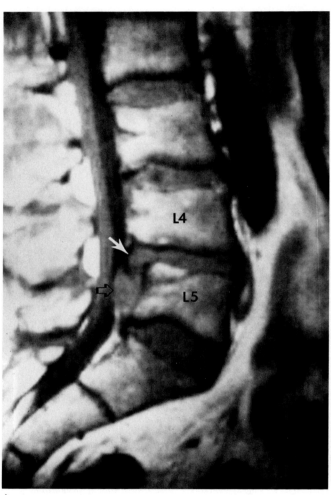

A

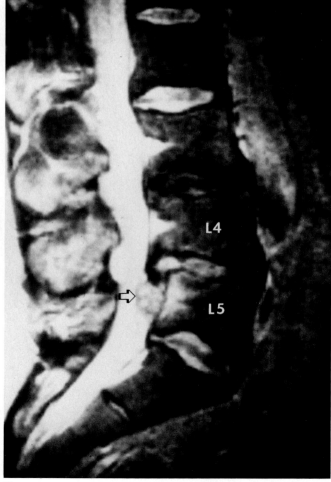

B

Figure 7-34 Herniated and Migrated (Extruded) Disk. **A.** *Sagittal T1-weighted MR image shows a focal herniated disk (arrow) at L4-L5 with an intensity similar to the disk of origin. In addition, a larger polypoid migrated disk can be delineated behind the L5 vertebral body (open arrow).* **B.** *Sagittal T2-weighted image shows the disk to appear hyperintense, typical of a migrated or extruded disk (open arrow). The hypointense cortical margins of the vertebral bodies are in sharp contrast to the hyperintense subarachnoid space.*

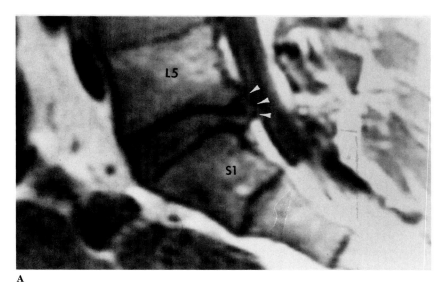

A

Figure 7-35   HNP L5-S1. **A.** *Sagittal T1-weighted image shows disk herniation with superior tonguelike protrusion (arrowheads).* **B.** *Axial T1-weighted image shows disk herniation (arrows) with impingement on the right S1 nerve root (open arrow).* **C.** *High-signal intensity disk herniation (arrows) is evident on this gradient echo image.*

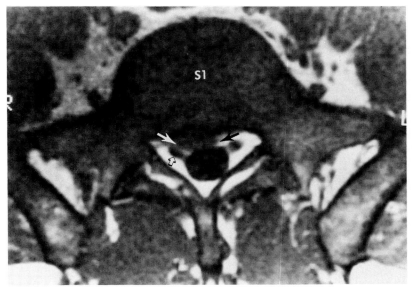

B

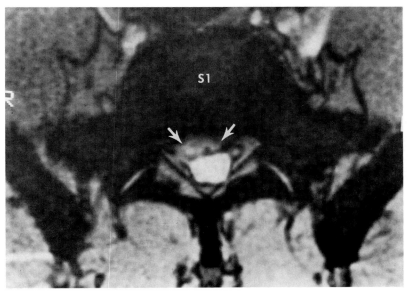

C

The diagnosis of a herniated disk by MR imaging requires careful examination of the focality of disk protrusion and its signal intensity. The spatial resolution is improved by the use of appropriate surface coils and motion suppression techniques. Routinely, 4-mm-thick spin-echo T1- and T2-weighted sagittal images are obtained to visualize disk herniations. Focal disk herniations characteristically have a signal intensity isointense to the disk of origin on both T1- and T2-weighted images. Extruded disk fragments show a soft tissue signal on T1-weighted images and a hyperintense signal on T2-weighted studies.[70] GRE imaging sequences offer the advantage of faster image acquisition and better separation between bone, dura, and cerebrospinal fluid. These sequences increase our ability to distinguish herniated disk from hypertrophic spurs and calcifications. Herniated disks show a relatively high-signal intensity, while degenerative hypertrophic spurs are usually markedly hypointense.[67,71] The use of GRE imaging sequences has been particularly effective in examination of the cervical and thoracic regions.

CHRONIC PROBLEMS

Posttraumatic morbidity and disability can be due to a variety of spine injuries, a majority of which relate to at least one of the following:

1. Undetected or inadequately treated ligamentous injuries
2. Undetected or incompletely healed fractures
3. Spinal instability (related to items 1 and 2)
4. Reparative and proliferative bony and soft tissue changes
5. Disk herniations
6. Intrinsic spinal cord posttraumatic changes

The majority of chronic abnormalities (items 1 to 4) of the *bony* spine can be accurately evaluated by plain films and computed tomography. Instability is best detected by lateral radiographs done with flexion and extension of the spine. Occasionally oblique weight-bearing films may prove diagnostic. CT provides accurate demonstration of bony and soft tissue overgrowths leading to foraminal narrowing with nerve root compression.

MR imaging is most effective in the evaluation of spinal cord compression and in the detection of cord changes from myelomalacia, fissures, and cysts.[49,50,52] The exact mechanism and time of evolution of posttraumatic cyst or syrinx remain incompletely understood. The combined result of posttraumatic contusion/hematoma, edema, and eventual necrosis is considered to antedate the development of a glial-lined cavity, which enlarges secondary to surrounding adhesions. Progressive central cavitation of the spinal cord, believed to be related to scar and venous pressure elevation, could be the cause of ascending myelopathy. MR imaging

accurately defines an expansile cyst that characteristically exhibits a low-signal intensity (cerebrospinal fluidlike content) or a high-signal intensity (highly proteinaceous fluid content) on T1- and T2-weighted sequences. Recognition of such entities as bony spurs or an expansile syrinx producing myelopathy is necessary in order to plan effective surgical decompression.[50,52]

With an active older population participating in all types of recreational and competitive sports, it is not unusual for patients in their 50s, 60s, and 70s to present to a sports medicine clinic complaining of low back pain. Many of these patients will have a preexisting, unrelated radiographic abnormality. TPBS affords the opportunity to distinguish those abnormalities which are "active" metabolically and possibly responsible for symptoms from those which are inactive. In the older age group, degenerative disk disease is frequent, and it becomes important to separate that underlying abnormality from other causes of low back pain (Fig. 7-2).[18]

Spondylolysis (Figs. 7-22, 7-36, and 7-37)

The most common spine-related complaint is that of "low back pain." This descriptive phrase has become a nonspecific "symptom complex." In the young athlete, overuse injuries causing low back pain are thought to be due to one of four conditions: (1) spondylolysis (stress fracture of the pars interarticularis), (2) mechanical low back pain (musculotendinous, facet disease, etc.), (3) disk herniation, and (4) vertebral apophysitis (Scheuermann's disease).[17] Radionuclide bone imaging in the evaluation of spondylolysis and low back pain in both children and adolescent athletes is well accepted[6,11,17,72–75] (Figs. 7-22, 7-36, and 7-37). Numerous studies attest to its clinical usefulness, accuracy, and safety. The development of single photon emission computed tomography (SPECT) imaging of the lumbar spine, which has occurred in the last decade, has greatly increased accuracy and specificity in identifying pathologic areas[76] (Fig. 7-3).

Numerous studies discuss the etiology of stress injuries of the pars interarticularis.[77–81] Most agree that repetitive flexion and extension cause a concentration of stress in the pars, especially at the L5 level. A pars defect is, therefore, most likely secondary to chronic overuse and represents a stress fracture. It is not surprising that this entity is seen in a higher percentage of the athletic population than in the general population.[4,12,15,20,73,75,79] Additionally, with a stress fracture of one pars, there is often an associated increased stress on the contralateral side leading to secondary reactive sclerosis (and increased nuclide activity) of that pars.[82]

Radionuclide bone scanning in suspected pars stress injuries is useful in two different clinical settings. First, if there is low back pain and radiographs (including oblique views) are normal, then TPBS and SPECT scans should be performed to evaluate a possible occult stress fracture of the pars (Figs. 7-36 and 7-22). If, on the other hand, the radiographic study is abnormal, showing a lucent or sclerotic

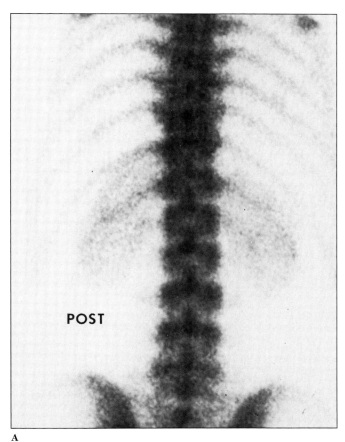

A

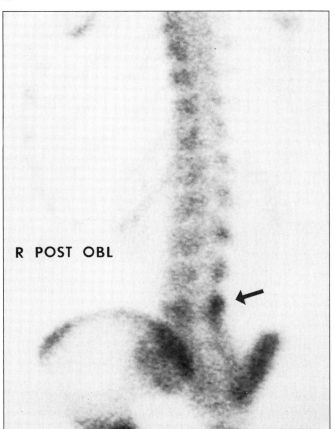

B

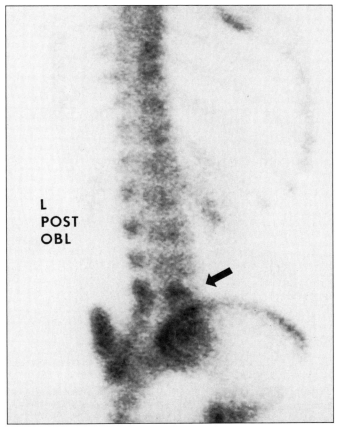

C

Figure 7-36   Unilateral Pars Defect (L5). **A.** *High-resolution delayed posterior projection from TPBS of the thoracolumbar region, shows no abnormality.* **B.** *High-resolution delayed image of TPBS in right posterior oblique projection shows focally increased activity within the left L5 pars. Arrow = abnormal activity.* **C.** *High-resolution delayed image in left posterior oblique projection shows abnormal nuclide activity within the left L5 pars. Arrow = abnormal activity.* (Fig. 7-36D continues on next page.)

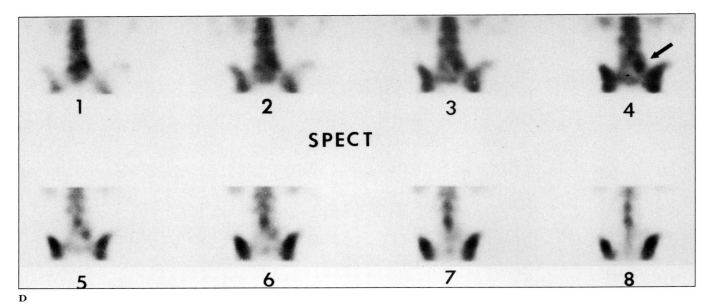

D

Figure 7-36 Unilateral Pars Defect (L5) (Continued). **D.** *Coronal SPECT images show a focal abnormality in the left L5 pars. This was not visible on the planar posterior projection and* *could be seen only vaguely on the posterior oblique projections. SPECT enhances both the sensitivity and the anatomic detail in this region. Images are displayed sequentially from* *anterior to posterior, with #1 being the most anterior and #8 the most posterior. Arrow = increased nuclide activity of L5 pars representing stress injury.*

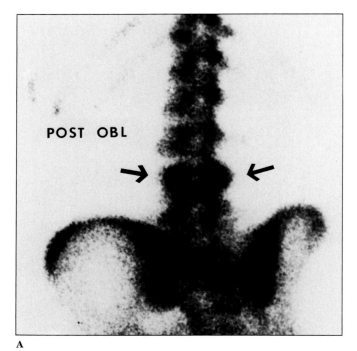

A

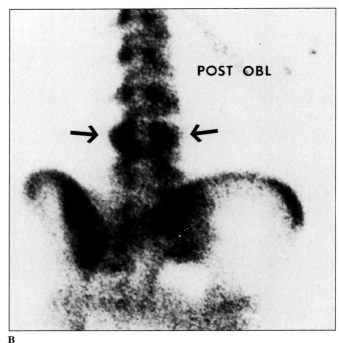

B

Figure 7-37 Bilateral Pars Interarticularis Defect. **A.** *High-resolution delayed image in the right posterior oblique projection from* *TPBS.* **B.** *High-resolution delayed image in the left posterior oblique projection. There is abnormal nuclide activity bilaterally involving L4 pars consistent* *with bilateral pars stress injury. The posterior oblique projection optimally displays the pars abnormality. Arrows = increased uptake in L4 pars bilaterally.*

defect in the pars, then a radionuclide bone scan will likely be helpful in determining the presence or absence of "metabolically active" disease as would be expected if the pars defect were the cause of low back pain. Often the pars defect is obvious on planar imaging, and SPECT scanning is not needed. If the combination of plain radiographs and planar nuclear scanning is indeterminate for a confident diagnosis, then SPECT imaging should be performed.[11] It is important to realize that most athletes with low back pain do not have a pars injury but rather have either musculotendinous or ligamentous injury. One study showed that of 27 athletes with low back pain only 6 proved to have pars stress injury. The diagnosis of a soft tissue (nonosseous) cause for low back pain can be made with a higher degree of certainty once a negative bone scan has been obtained.[6]

DIAGNOSTIC PROBLEMS

Back pain in athletes may be due to a nonathletic cause, creating "pitfalls" that could preclude prompt and accurate diagnosis.[83]

Diskitis (Figs. 7-38 and 7-39)

Diskitis is an inflammatory process that commonly affects the disk space with progression to involve the vertebral end plates. It is a serious medical problem in which diagnosis is often delayed because of the nonspecific findings often associated with this condition. In general, a radionuclide bone scan is ordered to evaluate possible occult fracture or pars injury, and diskitis is noted incidentally.[11,84] TPBS is highly sensitive to the presence of diskitis (Fig. 7-38). On MR imaging, diskitis typically shows increased intensity of the narrowed disk space on a T2-weighted study (Fig. 7-39). *Osteomyelitis* is the term applied to an infectious process that primarily affects the vertebral body and appendages. Osteomyelitis exhibits increased vertebral hyperintensity on T2-weighted imaging sequences because of increased water accumulation and hyperemia. In this era of widespread use of antibiotic therapy and steroids, it is not uncommon to discover etiologic organisms other than staphylococci and streptococci. Tuberculosis may present as destructive osteomyelitis. Radionuclide bone scanning is effective in detecting early diskitis and osteomyelitis.

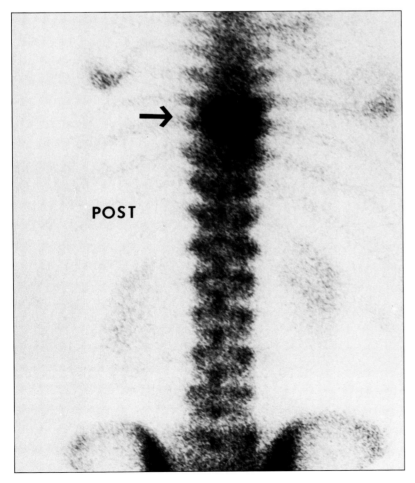

POST

Figure 7-38 Diskitis. *High-resolution posterior delayed images from TPBS. Abnormal nuclide activity seen at the T7-T8 disk level representing disk infection. Once identified on the bone scan, a ^{67}Ga scan, ^{111}In white cell scan, or MRI is confirmatory. Arrow demonstrates level of disk space infection.*

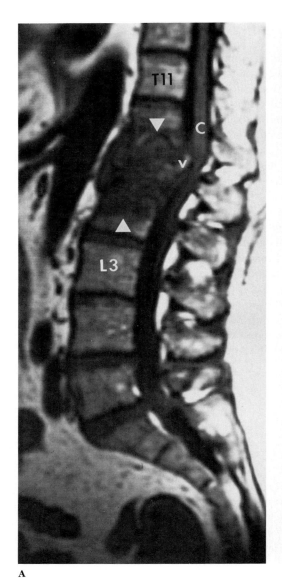

A

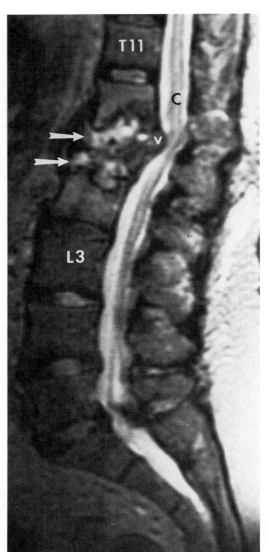

B

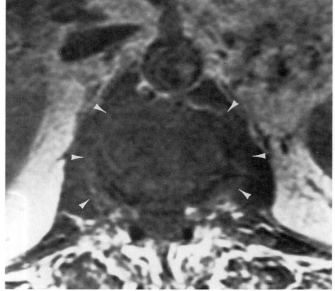

C

Figure 7-39 Diskitis. **A.** *Sagittal T1-weighted image demonstrates decreased signal intensity in the T12, L1, and L2 vertebral bodies (arrowheads). There is loss of height with diminished signal intensity of the T12-L1 and L1-L2 intervertebral disks. Almost complete destruction of the L1 vertebral body has occurred. Note compression of conus medullaris (C) by a retropulsed remnant of the L1 vertebral body (V). **B.** Increased signal intensity (arrows) is seen in the involved vertebral bodies and disks on this T2-weighted sagittal image. **C.** Axial T1-weighted image reveals paravertebral extension of inflammatory process (arrowheads).*

Genitourinary lesions (Fig. 7-40)

Occasionally an athlete with low back pain may be found to have hydronephrosis as the cause of symptoms. This serendipitous finding is often incidentally detected on bone scan, since the kidneys are the major route of excretion of isotope.[85,86] Congenital ureteropelvic junction obstruction is an uncommon but not a rare cause of abdominal and/or flank pain (Fig. 7-40).[87] Once found, sonography, intravenous pyelography, and retrograde pyelography as well as renal radionuclide studies are useful in further evaluation.

Neoplasms (Figs. 7-41 to 7-44)

Tumors of the spine, whether primary or secondary, benign or malignant, must be considered as possible causes of back pain.

Skeletal *hemangioma* commonly involves the spine (particularly the thoracic portion) and is often seen in middle-aged females. Hemangiomas are usually discovered inciden-tally. However, trauma could initiate hemorrhage and fracture within these vascular tumors.[88,89] Typically, on plain films and CT, vertebral hemangiomas show pronounced vertical trabeculations. On radioisotope studies, they exhibit marked radionuclide uptake. On MR imaging, high-intensity signal on both T1- and T2-weighted images is commonly observed. MR imaging enhances the recognition of a hemorrhagic event by demonstrating different adjacent intensity regions which are related to hemorrhagic components.

Osteoblastoma (ages 10 to 30 years), *giant cell tumors* (ages 20 to 40 years), and *osteoid osteoma* (ages 10 to 30 years) may involve the spine.[90,91] Osteoid osteoma of the spine involves the posterior elements and may not be visualized with routine radiographs (Figs. 7-41 and 7-42). It often presents with nocturnal pain that responds to salicylates. The exuberant perilesional sclerosis facilitates its detection by CT but is not always present. Osteoblastoma is an expansile lesion without any perifocal bone formation.[43,91] If it involves the neural arch, it may result in cord and nerve root compression. Nuclear scans characteristically show increased activity and are useful in assessing the pre- and postoperative patient for both osteoid osteoma and osteoblastoma.[92–97]

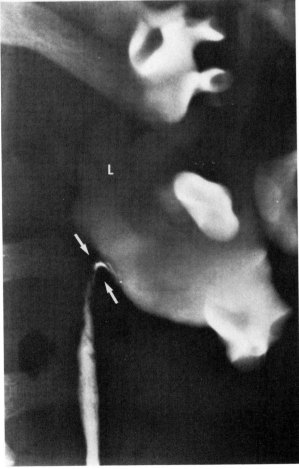

A

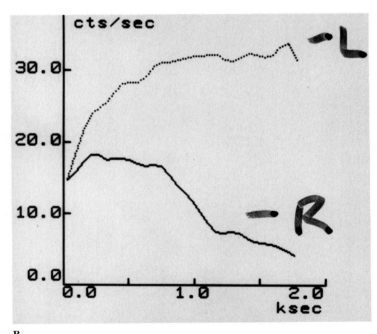

B

Figure 7-40 Left Hydronephrosis Secondary to Congenital Ureteropelvic Junction (UPJ) Obstruction. *This 16-year-old football player presented with the gradual onset of left flank pain 48 h after a game.* **A.** *Left-sided retrograde pyelogram demonstrates marked narrowing (arrows) at left UPJ with proximal hydronephrosis.* **B.** *Renogram curve from iodine hippuran 131 renal scan. Normal excretion curve on right and abnormal curve on left consistent with obstructive uropathy.*

Figure 7-41 Osteoid Osteoma. **A.** *Axial T1-weighted image demonstrates decreased signal intensity (arrowheads) in the right pedicle and neural arch of L4.* **B.** *Increased signal intensity (arrowheads) is present on this sagittal T2-weighted image.* **C.** *CT scan reveals the nidus (arrow), characteristic for this neoplasm, in the right pedicle of L4.*

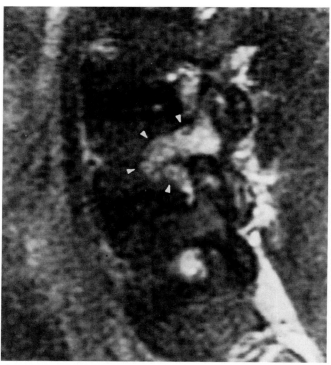

A

B

C

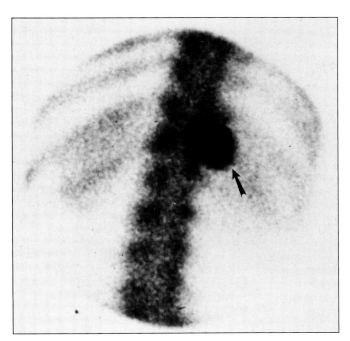

Figure 7-42 Osteoid Osteoma, T11 Vertebral Body. *College athlete presents with severe back pain without any history of trauma. High-resolution posterior projection of the thoracolumbar spine shows intense nuclide activity on the right side of T11. Biopsy demonstrated osteoid osteoma. Arrow = abnormal nuclide activity in the T11 vertebral body.*

Giant cell tumors are locally aggressive lesions of the mature skeleton and only rarely affect the spine. The lesions are well vascularized and cause ill-defined lytic destruction, usually of the vertebral bodies in the sacral or thoracic region.[43,98] Aneurysmal bone cyst can simulate any of these lesions both radiographically and clinically (Fig. 7-43).

Neurofibroma (neurilemmona, schwannoma) and *meningioma* are the most common intradural benign soft tissue neoplasms seen in young adults. Neurofibroma frequently involves the nerve root and presents as an eccentric soft tissue mass causing foraminal enlargement and erosion (Fig. 7-44). Meningiomas most commonly affect young women and tend to be located in the thoracic portion of the spine. Meningiomas are more frequently calcified than are neurilemmomas. On MR imaging, both these tumors are seen as soft tissue masses that significantly enhance following the intravenous injection of paramagnetic contrast agents.

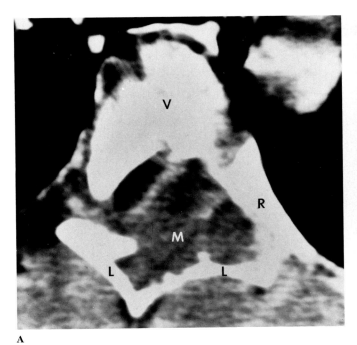

A

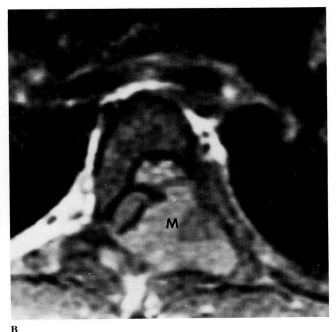

B

Figure 7-43 Aneurysmal Bone Cyst. **A, B.** *CT* (A) *and axial T1-weighted MR images* (B) *show an expansile mass (M) of the posterior elements extending into the left pedicle, eroding the proximal portion of the left rib, and compressing the spinal cord.* (Fig. 7-43C and D continues on next page.)

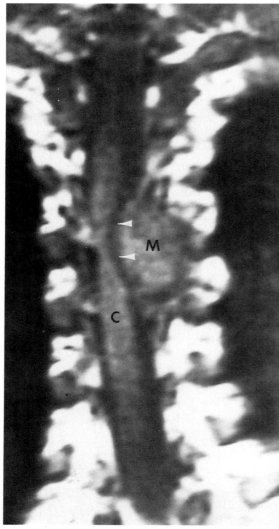

C

Figure 7-43 Aneurysmal Bone Cyst (Continued). **C.** *Coronal T1-weighted image demonstrates indentation of spinal cord (arrowheads).* **D.** *Sagittal T1-weighted image following intravenous enhancement with gadolinium-DTPA shows enhancing tumor (M) extending into the pedicle and vertebral body. V = vertebral body; L = lamina; R = rib; C = spinal cord.*

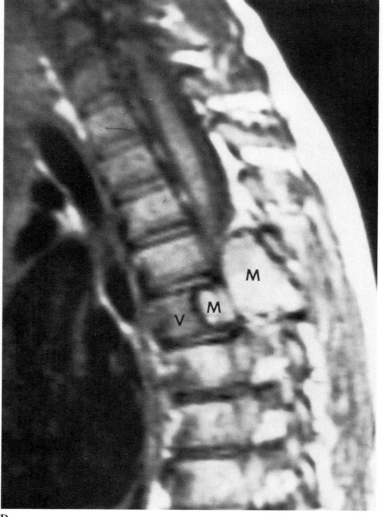

D

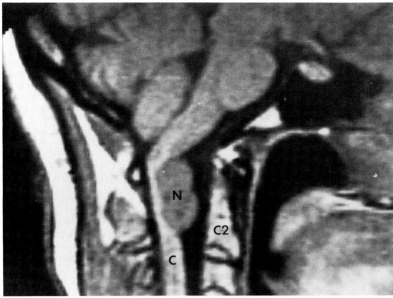

A

Figure 7-44 Neurofibroma. **A.** *Sagittal T1-weighted image shows a mass (N) demonstrating decreased signal intensity relative to the spinal cord (C) at the level of C1 and C2.* **B.** *Axial T1-weighted image shows bilobed neurofibroma (N) compressing and displacing the spinal cord (C) to right.*

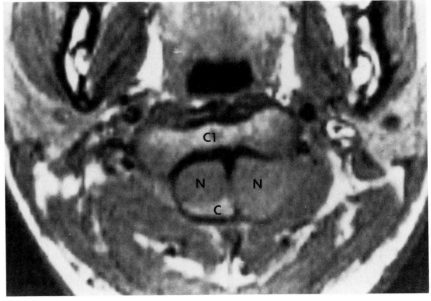

B

REFERENCES

1. Basford JR: Weightlifting, weight training and injuries. Orthopedics 8:1051–1056, 1985.
2. Ferguson RJ, McMaster JH, Stanitski CL: Low back pain in college football linemen. J Sports Med 2:63–80, 1974.
3. Holder LE, Matthews LS: The nuclear physician and sports medicine, in Freeman L, Weissman H (eds): *Nuclear Medicine Annual 1984.* Raven, New York, 1984, pp 88–140.
4. Jackson DW, Wiltse LL, Cirincione RJ: Spondylolysis in the female gymnast. Clin Orthop 117:68–73, 1976.
5. Maroon JC: Catastrophic neck injuries from football in Western Pennsylvania. Phys Sports Med 9:83–86, 1981.
6. Rupani HD, Holder LE, Espinola DA, et al.: Three phase radionuclide bone imaging in sports medicine. Radiology 156:187–196, 1985.
7. Tator CH, Edmonds VE, New ML: Diving: frequent and potentially preventable cause of spinal cord injury. Can Med Assoc J 124:1323–1324, 1981.
8. Garrick JG, Webb DR: *Sports Injuries: Diagnosis and Management.* Saunders, Philadelphia, 1990.
9. Vinger PF (ed): *Sports Injuries: the Unthwarted Epidemic,* 2d ed. PSG Publishing, Littleton, Mass., 1986.
10. Abel MS: Jogger's fracture and other stress fractures of the lumbosacral spine. Skeletal Radiol 13:221–227, 1985.

11. Martire JR: The role of nuclear medicine scans in evaluating pain in athletic injuries. Clin Sports Med 6:713–737, 1987.

12. Tehranzadeh J, Serafini AN, Pais MJ: *Avulsion and Stress Injuries of the Musculoskeletal System.* Karger, Basel, 1989.

13. Clancy EG, Micheli LJ, Jackson DW, et al.: Low back pain in athletes. Am J Sports Med 7:361–369, 1979.

14. Clark A, Stanish WD: An unusual cause of back pain in a young athlete: A case report. Am J Sports Med 13:51–54, 1985.

15. Jackson DW: Low back pain in young athletes: Evaluation of stress reaction and discogenic problems. Am J Sports Med 7:364–366, 1979.

16. Micheli LJ: Low back pain in the adolescent: Differential diagnosis. Am J Sports Med 7:362–364, 1979.

17. O'Neill BD, Michelli LJ: Overuse injuries in the young athlete. Clin Sports Med 3:591–610, 1988.

18. Stanish W: Low back pain in middle-aged athletes. Am J Sports Med 7:367–369, 1979.

19. Gehweiler JA, Osborne RL, Becker RF: *The Radiology of Vertebral Trauma.* Saunders, Philadelphia, 1980.

20. Matin PM: Appearance of bone scans following fractures including immediate and long term studies. J Nucl Med 20:1227–1231, 1979.

21. Goldberg AL, Daffner RH, Schapiro RL: Imaging of acute spinal trauma: An evolving multi-modality approach. Clin Imaging 14:11–16, 1990.

22. Whitley JF, Forsythe HF: Classification of cervical spine injuries. Am J Roentgenol 83:633–644, 1960.

23. Roaf R: International classification of spine injuries. Paraplegia 10:78–84, 1972.

24. Holdsworth F: Fractures, dislocations and fracture-dislocations of the spine. J Bone Joint Surg 52(A):1534–1551, 1970.

25. Edeiken-Monroe B, Wagner LK, Harris JH Jr.: Hyperextension dislocation of the cervical spine. AJNR 7:135–140, 1986.

26. Taylor AR, Blackwood W: Paraplegia in hyperextension cervical injuries with normal radiographic appearances. J Bone Joint Surg 30(B):245–248, 1948.

27. Forsyth HR: Extension injuries of the cervical spine. J Bone Joint Surg 46(A):1792–1797, 1964.

28. Marar BC: Hyperextension injuries of the cervical spine. J Bone Joint Surg 56(A):1655–1662, 1974.

29. Clark WH, Gehweiler JA, Laib R: Twelve significant signs of cervical spine trauma. Skeletal Radiol 3:201–205, 1979.

30. Penning L: Prevertebral hematoma in cervical spine injury: Incidence and etiologic significance. AJNR 1:557–565, 1980.

31. Reymond RD, Wheeler RS, Parovic M, et al.: The lucent cleft, a new radiologic sign of cervical disc injury or disease. Clin Radiol 23:188–192, 1972.

32. Grogono BJS: Injuries of the atlas and axis. J Bone Joint Surg 36(B): 397–410, 1954.

33. Schneider RC, Livingston KE, Cave AJE, Hamilton G: ''Hangman's fracture'' of the cervical spine. J Neurosurg 22:141–154, 1965.

34. Nykamp PW, Levy JM, Christensen F, et al.: Computed tomography for a bursting fracture of the lumbar spine. J Bone Joint Surg 60(A):1108–1109, 1978.

35. Jefferson G: Fracture of the atlas vertebra. Report of four cases and a review of those previously recorded. Br J Surg 7:407–422, 1920.

36. Webb JK, Broughton RBK, McSweeney T, et al.: Hidden flexion injury of the cervical spine. J Bone Joint Surg 58(B):322–327, 1976.

37. Green JD, Harle TS, Harris JH Jr.: Anterior subluxation of the cervical spine: Hyperflexion sprain. AJNR 2:243–250, 1981.

38. Scher AT: Anterior cervical subluxation: An unstable position. AJR 133:275–280, 1979.

39. Bohlman HH: Acute fractures and dislocations of the cervical spine: An analysis of three hundred hospitalized patients and review of the literature. J Bone Joint Surg 61(A):1119–1142, 1979.

40. Mirvis SE, Geisler FH, Jelinek JJ, et al.: Acute cervical spine trauma: Evaluation with 1.5T MR imaging. Radiology 166:807–816, 1988.

41. Beale SM, Pathria MN, Masaryk TJ: Magnetic resonance imaging of spinal trauma. Top Magn Reson Imaging 1:53–62, 1988.

42. McArdle CB, Crofford MJ, Mirfakhraee M, et al.: Surface coil MR of spinal trauma: Preliminary experience. AJNR 7:885–893, 1986.

43. Huvos AG: *Bone Tumors. Diagnosis, Treatment and Prognosis,* 2d ed. Saunders, Philadelphia, 1991.

44. Handel SF, Lee YY: Computed tomography of spinal fractures. Radiol Clin North Am 19:69–83, 1981.

45. Post MJD, Green BA, Quencer RM, et al.: The value of computed tomography in spine trauma. Spine 7:417–431, 1982.

46. Yetkin Z, Osborn AG, Giles DS, Haughton VM: Uncovertebral and facet joint dislocations in cervical articular pillar fractures: CT evaluation. AJNR 6:633–637, 1985.

47. Pavlov H, Torg JS, Robie B, Jahre C: Cervical spinal stenosis: Determination with vertebral body ratio method. Radiology 164:771–775, 1987.

48. Hackney DB, Asato R, Joseph PM, et al.: Hemorrhage and edema in acute spinal cord compression: Demonstration by MR imaging. Radiology 161:387–390, 1986.

49. Post MJD, Quencer RM, Green BA, et al.: Radiologic evaluation of spinal cord fissures. AJNR 7:329–335, 1986.

50. Quencer RM, Sheldon JJ, Post MJD, et al.: Magnetic resonance imaging of the chronically injured cervical spinal cord. AJNR 7:457–464, 1986.

51. Flanders AE, Schaefer DM, Doan HT, et al.: Acute cervical spine trauma: Correlation of MR imaging findings with degree of neurologic deficit. Radiology 177:25–33, 1990.

52. Takahashi M, Yamashinta Y, Sakamoto Y, et al.: Chronic cervical cord compression: Clinical significance of increased signal intensity on MR images. Radiology 173:219–224, 1989.

53. Allen WE, D'Angelo CM, Kier EL: Correlation of microangiographic and electrophysiologic changes in experimental spinal cord trauma. Radiology 111:107–115, 1974.

54. Wagner FC Jr, Dohrman GJ, Bucy PC: Histopathology of transitory traumatic paraplegia in the monkey. J Neurosurg 35:272–276, 1971.

55. Sasaki S: Vascular changes in the spinal cord after impact injury in the rat. Neurosurgery 10:360–363, 1982.

56. Peterson HO, Kieffer SA: Radiology of intervertebral disk disease. Semin Roentgenol 7:260–276, 1972.

57. Hudgins WR: The predictive value of myelography in the diagnosis of ruptured lumbar discs. J Neurosurg 32:152–162, 1970.

58. Shapiro R: *Myelography,* 4th ed. Year Book Medical Publishers, Chicago, 1984.

59. Spurling RG: *Lesions of the Cervical Intervertebral Disc.* Springfield, IL, Charles C Thomas, 1956.

60. Baker HL Jr, Love JG, Uihlein A: Roentgenologic features of protruded thoracic intervertebral disks. Radiology 84:1059–1065, 1965.

61. DePalma AF, Rothman RH: *The Intervertebral Disc.* Saunders, Philadelpha, 1970.

62. Pratt ES, Green DA, Spengler DM: Herniated intervertebral disc associated with unstable spinal injuries. Spine 7:662–666, 1990.

63. Modic MT, Masaryk TJ, Boumphrey F, et al.: Lumbar herniated disk disease and canal stenosis: Prospective evaluation by surface coil MR, CT and myelography. AJNR 7:709–717, 1986.

64. Edelman RR, Shoukimas GM, Stark DD, et al.: High-resolution surface-coil imaging of lumbar disk disease. AJNR 6:479–485, 1985.

65. Brown BM, Schwartz RH, Frank E, et al.: Preoperative evaluation of cervical radiculopathy by surface-coil MR imaging. AJNR 9:859–866, 1988.

66. Modic MT, Masaryk TJ, Mulopoulos GP, et al.: Cervical radiculopathy: Prospective evaluation with surface coil MR imaging, CT with metrizamide, and metrizamide myelography. Radiology 161:753–759, 1986.

67. Tsuruda JS, Norman D, Dillon W, et al.: Three-dimensional gradient-recalled MR imaging as a screening tool for the diagnosis of cervical radiculopathy. AJNR 10:1263–1271, 1989.

68. Williams AL, Haughton VM, Daniels DL, et al.: CT recognition of lateral disk herniation. AJNR 3:211–213, 1982.

69. Russell EJ, D'Angelo CM, Zimmerman RD, et al.: Cervical disk herniation: CT demonstration after contrast enhancement. Radiology 152:703–712, 1984.

70. Masaryk TJ, Ross JS, Modic MT, et al.: High-resolution MR imaging of sequestered lumbar intervertebral disks. AJNR 9:351–358, 1988.

71. Hedberg MC, Drayer BP, Flom RA, et al.: Gradient echo (GRASS) MR imaging in cervical radiculopathy. AJNR 9:145–151, 1988.

72. Gelfand MJ, Strife JL, Kereiakes JG: Radionuclide bone imaging in spondylolysis of the lumbar spine in children. Radiology 140:191–195, 1981.

73. Jackson DW, Wiltse LL, Dingeman RD, et al.: Stress reactions involving the pars interarticularis in young athletes. Am J Sports Med 9:304–312, 1981.

74. Papanicolaou N, Wilkinson RH, Emans JB, et al.: Bone scintigraphy and radiology in young athletes with low back pain. AJR 145:1039–1044, 1985.

75. Pennel RG, Maurer AH, Bonakdarpour A: Stress injuries of the pars interarticularis: Radiologic classification and indications for scintigraphy. AJR 145:763–766, 1985.

76. Collier BD, Johnson RP, Carrera GF, et al.: Painful spondylosis or spondylolisthesis studied by radiography and single-photon emission computed tomography. Radiology 154:207–211, 1985.

77. Farfan HF, Osteria V, Lamy C: The mechanical etiology of spondylosis and spondylolisthesis. Clin Orthop 117:40–67, 1976.

78. Hoshina H: Spondylolysis in athletes. Phys Sports Med 9:75–79, 1980.

79. Letts M, Smallman T, Afanasiev R, et al.: Fracture of the pars interarticularis in adolescent athletes: A clinical-biomechanical analysis. J Pediatr Orthop 6:40–46, 1986.

80. Rossi F: Spondylolysis, spondylolisthesis and sports. J Sports Med 18:317–340, 1978.

81. Wiltse LL, Widell EH Jr, Jackson DW: Fatigue fracture: The basic lesion in isthmic spondylolisthesis. J. Bone Joint Surg 57(A):17–22, 1975.

82. Sherman FC, Wilkinson RH, Hall JE: Reactive sclerosis of a pedicle and spondylosis in the lumbar spine. J Bone Joint Surg 59(A):49–54, 1977.

83. Baker BE, Levinsohn EM, Coren AB: Pitfalls to avoid in diagnosing pain in the athlete. Clin Sports Med 6:921–934, 1987.

84. Gates GF: Scintigraphy of discitis. Clin Nucl Med 2:20–25, 1980.

85. Biello DR, Coleman RE, Stanley RJ: Correlation of renal images on bone scan and intravenous pyelogram. AJR 127:633–636, 1976.

86. Haden HT, Katz PG, Kondering KF: Detection of obstructive uropathy by bone scintigraphy. J Nucl Med 29:1781–1785, 1988.

87. Leslie SW, Tudor RB: Congenital ureteropelvic junction obstruction: Abdominal pain in runners. Phys Sports Med 13:105–109, 1985.

88. Kagan EM: The problem of hemangiomas of the bone skeleton. Vestn Rentgenol Radiol 3:17–24, 1960.

89. Robbins LR, Fountain EN: Hemangioma of cervical vertebrae with spinal cord compression. N Engl J Med 258:685–687, 1958.

90. Dahlin DC: Giant-cell tumor of vertebrae above the sacrum—A review of 31 cases. Cancer 39:1350–1356, 1977.

91. Jackson RP, Reckling RW, Mantz FA: Osteoid osteoma and osteoblastoma: Similar histologic lesions with different natural histories. Clin Orthop 128:303–313, 1977.

92. Ghelman B, Vigorita VJ: Postoperative radionuclide evaluation of osteoid osteomas. Radiology 146:509–512, 1983.

93. Gore DR, Mueller HA: Osteoid osteoma of the spine with localization aided by ^{99m}Tc-polyphosphate bone scan: Case report. Clin Orthop 113:132–134, 1975.

94. Sim FH, Dahlin DC, Beabout JW: Osteoid osteoma: Diagnostic problems. J Bone Joint Surg 57(A):154–159, 1975.

95. Smith FW, Gilday DL: Scintigraphic appearance of osteoid osteoma. Radiology 137:191–195, 1980.

96. Swee RG, McLeod RA, Beabout JW: Osteoid osteoma: Detection, diagnosis and localization. Radiology 130:117–123, 1979.

97. Winter PF, Johnson PM, Hilal SK, et al.: Scintigraphic detection of osteoid osteoma. Radiology 122:177–178, 1977.

98. Smith J, Wixon D, Watson RC: Giant-cell tumor of the sacrum—Clinical and radiologic features in 13 patients. J Can Assoc Radiol 30:34–39, 1979.

INDEX

Page numbers followed by *f* indicate figures; page numbers followed by *t* indicate tables.